LP 026872901 3

AF598348

WITHDRAWN

Advances in ___________________

Pharmacology

Volume 21

Advisory Board

Advances in 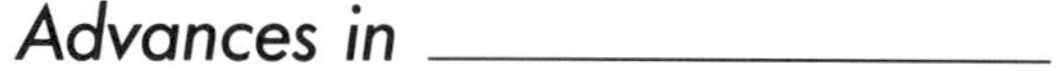

Pharmacology

Volume 21

Edited by

Tom August
Department of Pharmacology
Johns Hopkins University
Baltimore, Maryland

M. W. Anders
Department of Pharmacology
University of Rochester
Rochester, New York

Ferid Murad
Pharmaceutical Products Division
Abbott Laboratories
Abbott Park, Illinois

Alan Nies
Clinical Pharmacology
University of Colorado Health Sciences Center
Denver, Colorado

Academic Press, Inc.
Harcourt Brace Jovanovich, Publishers
San Diego New York Boston
London Sydney Tokyo Toronto

This book is printed on acid-free paper. ∞

ACADEMIC PRESS, INC.
San Diego, California 92101

United Kingdom Edition published by
ACADEMIC PRESS LIMITED
24-28 Oval Road, London NW1 7DX

LIBRARY OF CONGRESS CATALOG CARD NUMBER: 61-18298

ISBN 0-12-032921-2 (alk. paper)

PRINTED IN THE UNITED STATES OF AMERICA
90 91 92 93 9 8 7 6 5 4 3 2 1

Contents

Erythropoietin: Regulation of Erythropoiesis and Clinical Use
Emmanuel N. Dessypris and Sanford B. Krantz

DNA Topoisomerases as Anticancer Drug Targets
Erasmus Schneider, Yaw-Huei Hsiang, and Leroy F. Liu

Multidrug Resistance and Chemosensitization: Therapeutic Implications for Cancer Chemotherapy
Elias Georges, Frances J. Sharom, and Victor Ling

Peptides: Chemistry, Biology, and Pharmacology
Amrit K. Judd and Gary K. Schoolnik

Contributors

Numbers in parentheses indicate the pages on which the authors' contributions begin.

A. Claudio Cuello (1), Department of Pharmacology and Therapeutics, McGill University, Montreal, Quebec H3G 1YG, Canada

Emmanuel N. Dessypris (127), Department of Medicine, Division of Hematology, Vanderbilt University and VA Medical Center, Nashville, Tennessee 37232

Charles Flexner (51), Departments of Medicine, and Pharmacology and Molecular Sciences, Division of Clinical Pharmacology, The Johns Hopkins University School of Medicine, Baltimore, Maryland 21205

Elias Georges (185), The Ontario Cancer Institute, and the Department of Medical Biophysics, University of Toronto, Toronto, Ontario M5S 1A1, Canada

Yaw-Huei Hsiang (149), Department of Biological Chemistry, The Johns Hopkins University School of Medicine, Baltimore, Maryland 21205

Amrit K. Judd (221), SRI International, Menlo Park, California 94025

Sanford B. Krantz (127), Department of Medicine, Division of Hematology, Vanderbilt University and VA Medical Center, Nashville, Tennessee 37232

Victor Ling (185), The Ontario Cancer Institute, and the Department of Medical Biophysics, University of Toronto, Toronto, Ontario M5S 1A1, Canada

Leroy F. Liu (149), Department of Biological Chemistry, The Johns Hopkins University School of Medicine, Baltimore, Maryland 21205

Richard J. Miller (101), Department of Pharmacological and Physiological Sciences, University of Chicago, Chicago, Illinois 60637

Ian J. Reynolds (101), Department of Pharmacology, University of Pittsburgh, Pittsburgh, Pennsylvania 15261

Erasmus Schneider (149), Department of Biological Chemistry, The Johns Hopkins University School of Medicine, Baltimore, Maryland 21205

Gary K. Schoolnik (221), Howard Hughes Medical Institute/Stanford University, Stanford, California 94305

Frances J. Sharom (185), Department of Chemistry and Biochemistry, Guelph-Waterloo Centre for Graduate Work in Chemistry, University of Guelph, Guelph, Ontario N1G 2W1, Canada

Preface

Pharmacology is a field of extraordinarily rapid growth. One driving force is the great advances in biological and chemical sciences, another is the growing recognition of the possibilities for applying these advances to the benefit of mankind in the prevention and treatment of disease. The vastly increased understanding of cell and tissue function that come from all branches of biological science provide an ever expanding base on which to construct models and experiments of pharmacologic relevance. An understanding of the interplay between the molecular mechanisms of cell function and of drug action provides an intellectual basis both for the experimental approach to the design and application of new medicines and for the appropriate usage of modern medicines. Knowledge of these advances and their relationship to pharmacology is critical to individuals whose activities range from clinical sciences to basic research.

Advances in Pharmacology will seek to incorporate these discoveries as they apply to pharmacology, drawing openly from all branches of biology, chemistry, and medicine. The emphasis will be on the new and on the molecular basis of drug action, whether applied or experimental. This approach is deliberately diverse, in the expectation of providing a reference source for developments that encompass all specialized fields of investigation that are relevant to pharmacology. In the broadest sense it will serve to draw the reader's attention to new developments that impact on pharmacology and may provide stimulus for new investigation or understanding; in the immediate focus, it will provide detailed information on topics of specialized interest. It is hoped that the readers will include all those whose research, teaching, or clinical activities involve the study of drug development, function, and application from either an experimental or clinical perspective.

The volumes will include both a serial volume, published yearly, and thematic volumes on specialized topics. The topics and their authors are drawn from the experience of the Editors and the suggestions of our Editorial Board of distinguished and active scientists whose research and training encompass a wide range of pharmacologic applications. As the new editors of *Advances in Pharmacology*, we hope you will find this and subsequent volumes interesting and enlightening.

Tom August
M. W. Anders
Ferid Murad

Glycosphingolipids That Can Regulate Nerve Growth and Repair

A. Claudio Cuello

Department of Pharmacology and Therapeutics
McGill University
Montreal, Quebec
H3G 1Y6, Canada

I. Introduction

The concept that the mammalian central nervous system is unable to repair itself has been imprinted in the minds of many generations of biologists and medical doctors. The roots of this idea can probably be traced to the insightful work of Ramón y Cajal (1928), who brilliantly described the degeneration and regeneration of neurons in the peripheral nervous system.

His remarkably accurate drawings of the repair of peripheral axons remain of contemporary value. When he pointed out the notable capacity of peripheral neurons to regenerate and establish new contacts, he also stated that in the central nervous system (CNS) "the paths are incapable of regeneration, for the majority of the regenerative acts described in man and laboratory animals are temporary reactions, aborted restorative processes, incapable of bringing about a complete and definitive repair of the interrupted paths . . ." (Ramón y Cajal, 1928).

Advances in Pharmacology, Volume 21

Nevertheless, he indicated the possibility that future scientific endeavors might change this rigid rule and "[they] must work to impede or moderate the gradual decay of the neurons, to overcome the almost invincible rigidity of their connections, and to re-establish normal nerve paths, when disease has severed centers that were intimately associated."

Recent developments in the neurosciences have given credence to this assertion. These include the successful grafting of nervous tissue within the CNS (Björklund *et al.*, 1988) and the evidence that centrally located neurons can regenerate and establish new contacts if adequate conditions are provided (Aguayo, 1985). In addition to the above dramatic experimental data showing regeneration of CNS neurons, there is the equally startling evidence that a plethora of endogenous factors can modulate trophic functions in the CNS. The concept that trophic molecules can regulate the number and organization of cells of peripheral neuronal populations emerged with the discovery of the nerve growth factor (NGF) (for review, see Levi-Montalcini and Calissano, 1986). Only much later were its effects recognized on neurons of the CNS as well (Levi-Montalcini and Aloe, 1985; Thoenen *et al.*, 1987). At present, many peptides with trophic properties in the developing and adult brain have been described (Varon *et al.*, 1988; Hefti, 1989). Some of these peptides, notably NGF, can attenuate and prevent degeneration or promote regeneration after injury of centrally located neurons. In addition to peptides, other molecules are able to elicit some of these responses in experimental circumstances. Of these, the glycosphingolipids are a particularly interesting group. The fact that some endogenous peptides such as NGF, and naturally occurring molecules such as gangliosides, can be employed experimentally to prevent damage or induce repair of CNS neurons opens up the attractive possibility of pharmacological intervention to enhance regeneration of the nervous system. Although this recent offshoot of neuropharmacology is still in its infancy, the pace of current research promises the development of more effective drugs which will correct or counterbalance the mechanisms leading to neuronal degeneration or death.

This review covers aspects of the biology and experimental uses of glycosphingolipids in general, and sialogangliosides in particular, which can be included as potential tools in the neuropharmacology of neural repair. As it is impractical to cover all of the abundant literature on the subject, reference is made only to select contributions in the hope that this will provide an overall impression of the field.

II. Characteristics of Glycosphingolipids

Glycosphingolipids were identified in the brain as early as 1874 by the father of modern neurochemistry Joham L. W. Thudichum (Drabkin, 1958). They share a common structure consisting of a hydrophobic portion (the ceramide) and a hydrophilic portion (the oligosaccharide). Hydrolysis of the ceramide yields a fatty acid tail and sphingosine, a long-chain unsaturated amino alcohol. According to Hakomori (1986), there are about 130 known forms of glycosphingolipids. They vary both in their sugar and ceramide composition, and are classified into major groups (ganglio-, globo-, galacto- series) according to the sequence and nature of chemical bonds between the sugars and the presence of sialic acid (see Table I). Figure 1 illustrates the general pattern of glycosphingolipids in the ganglioside series. Much of the chemistry of this group has been elucidated by Svennerholm (1980), to whom we are indebted for establishing the most widely used classification of gangliosides (see Table II).

Glycosphingolipids are widely distributed in the body but are particularly concentrated in the brain. The majority of glycosphingolipids are normal constituents of cell membranes and significantly contribute to their asymmetry. The hydrophobic ceramide portion is inserted in the outer leaflet of the lipid bilayer while the sugar moiety extends toward the extracellular space (see Fig. 1). They are therefore located in a rather privileged position where they may interact with other membranous constituents of the same or a neighboring cell and with other molecules which come in contact with the cell surface such as hormones, toxins, or various factors (trophic?) of diverse nature. The ganglioside series accounts for a large portion of the naturally occurring glycosphingolipids.

In the brain, the gangliosides are known to be distributed in a differential pattern across species, brain regions, and cell types. In addition, there is ample evidence that the ganglioside population in nervous tissue changes during ontogeny in a temporospatial manner. The expression of these diverse membrane-bound gangliosides is largely dependent on the equilibrium established between

Table I

Schematic Structure of Selected Neural Glycosphingolipids

	Trivial designation	Schematic structure[a]
Glucosylceramide		Glcβ 1′Cer
Lactosylceramide	AGM3, GA3 CDH	Galβ1 4Glcβ 1′Cer
Tetrahexosylceramide	AGM1, GA1	Galβ1 3GalNAcβ1 4Galβ1 4Glcβ1 1′Cer
Globoside		GalNAcβ1 3Galα1 4Galβ1 4Glcβ1 1′Cer

[a] Glc, Glucose; Cer, ceramide; Gal, galactose; GalNAc, *N*-acetylgalactosamine.

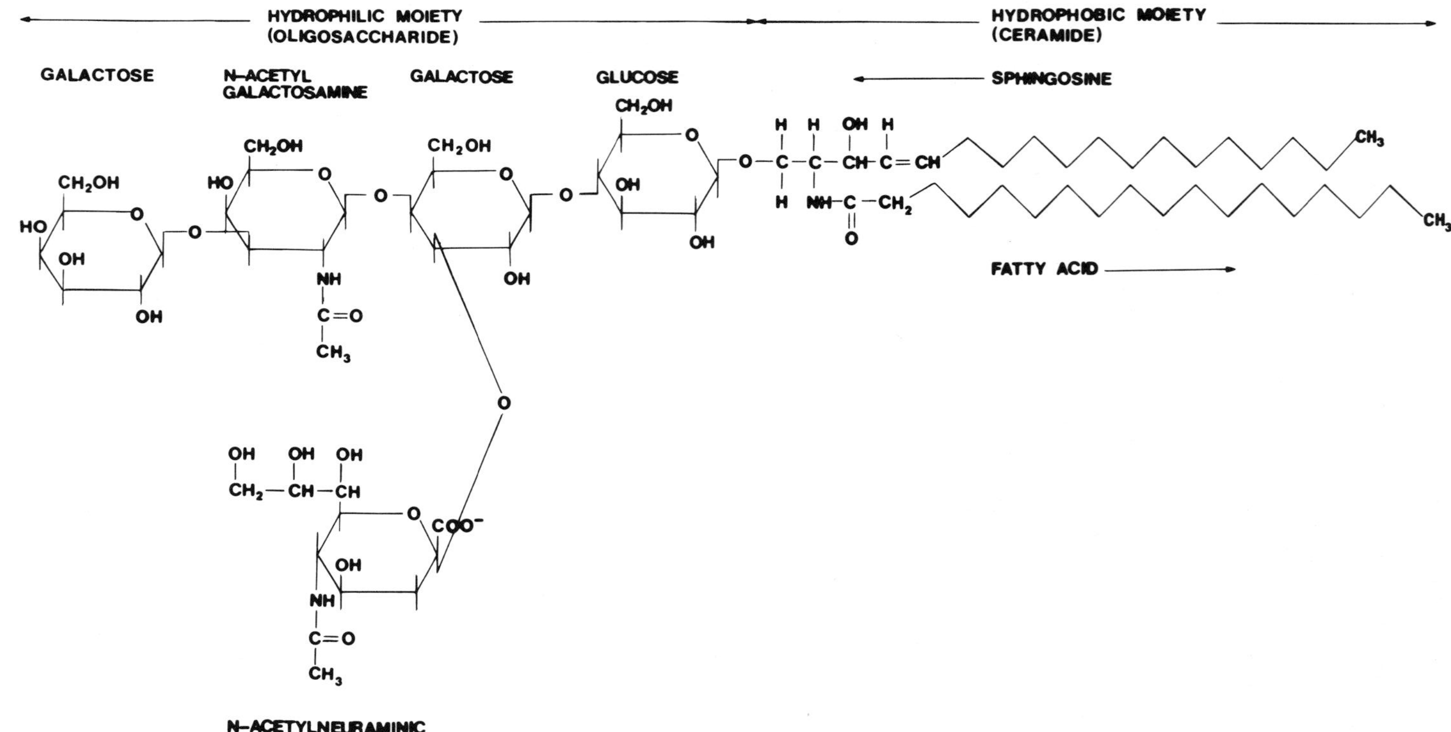

Fig. 1 General pattern gangliosides. (GM1, as an example.)

Table II
Schematic Structure of Selected Gangliosides

Svennerholm's classification (1980)	Schematic structure[a]
GM4	NeuAcα2 3Galβ1 1'Cer
GM3	NeuAcα2 3Galβ1 4Glcβ1 1'Cer
GM2	GalNAcβ1 4(NeuAcα2 3)Galβ1 4Glcβ 1'Cer
GM1, GM1a	Galβ1 3GalNAcβ1 4(NeuAcα2 3)Galβ1 4Glcβ1 1'Cer
GD3	NeuAcα2 8NeuAcα2 3Galβ1 4Galβ1 1'Cer
GD2	GalNAcβ1 4(NeuAcα2 8NeuAcα2 3)Galβ1 4Glcβ1 1'Cer
GD1a	NeuAcα2 3Galβ1 3GalNAcβ1 4(NeuAcα2 3)Galβ1 4Glcβ1 1'Cer
GD1b	Galβ1 3GalNAcβ1 4(NeuAcα2 8NeuAcα2 3)Galβ1 4Glcβ1 1'Cer
GT3	NeuAcα2 8NeuAcα2 8NeuAcα2 3Galβ1 4Glcβ1 1'Cer
GT1b	NeuAcα2 3Galβ1 3GalNAcβ1 4(NeuAcα2 8NeuAcα2 3)Galβ1 4Glcβ1 1'Cer
GQ1b	NeuAcα2 8NeuAcα2 3Galβ1 3GalNAcβ1 4(NeuAcα2 8NeuAcα2 3)Galβ1 4Glcβ1 1'Cer
GQ1c	NeuAcα2 3Galβ1 3GalNAcβ1 4(NeuAcα2 8NeuAcα2 8NeuAcα2 3)Galβ1 4Glcβ1 1'Cer

[a] Glc, Glucose; Gal, galactose; GalNAc, *N*-acetylgalactosamine; GlcNAc, *N*-acetylglucosamine; Man, mannose; Cer, ceramide; NeuA, *N*-acetylneuraminic acid.

biosynthetic glycosyltransferases and lysosomal degradative enzymes. Figure 2 depicts the possible biosynthetic pathway for the most conspicuous gangliosides via a multiglycosyltransferase system as proposed by Roseman and collaborators (Roseman, 1970; Basu *et al.*, 1973) and Caputto and collaborators (1976). According to this scheme, gangliosides are synthesized through the stepwise addition of activated sugar residues to the ceramide or the ceramide–sugar acceptor. These sugar-activated residues are then bound to nucleotide carriers. The biosynthesis of gangliosides apparently occurs in the Golgi apparatus since glycosyltransferases are associated with these subcellular organelles (Yusuf *et al.*, 1983). The Golgi membrane-bound lipid acceptors do not freely exchange with exogenously supplied lipids (Arce *et al.*, 1971). It is thought that newly synthesized gangliosides are transported from the Golgi apparatus to the plasma membrane via vesicular flow and then incorporated into its external leaflet. These glycosphingolipid-enriched vesicles are also the presumptive carriers for the bidirectional axonal transport of the glycolipids (Aquino *et al.*, 1987). Although the exact regulation of ganglioside synthesis remains an open question, feedback mechanisms on ganglioside synthetases are thought to be involved. The differential expression of sphingolipids also depends on the genetics of the glycosyltransferases and their subcellular assembly. Degradation of gangliosides is mediated

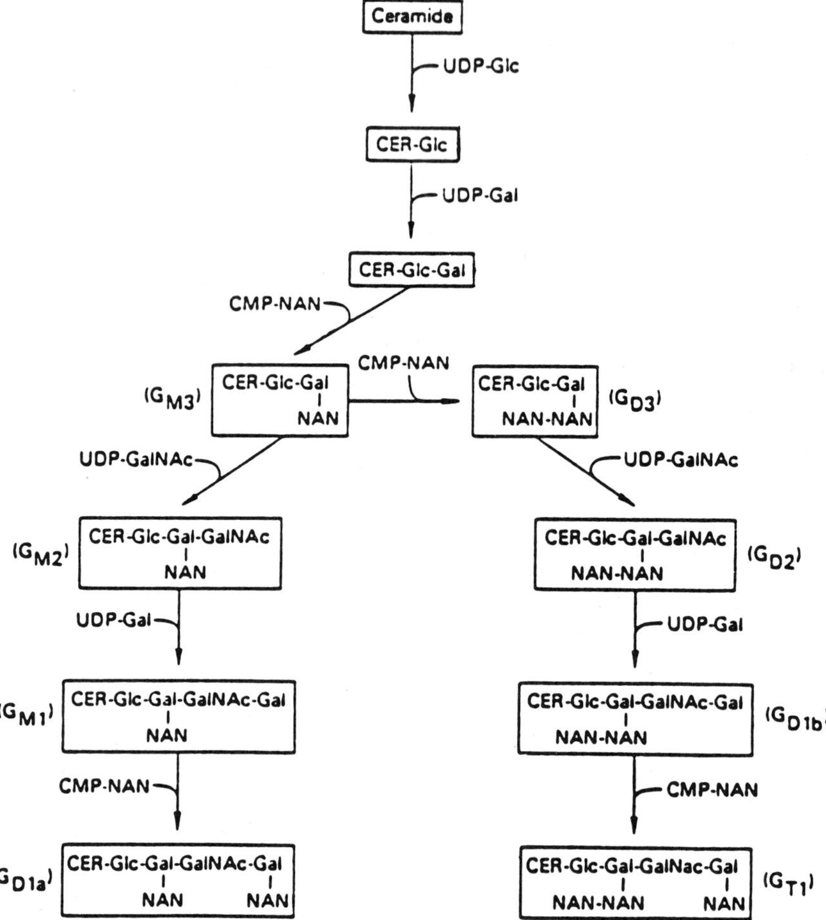

Fig. 2 Possible pathway for the biosynthesis of gangliosides. Each reaction is catalyzed in a stepwise fashion by a specific glycosyltransferase. CER, Ceramide; Gal, galactose; GalNAc, *N*-acetylgalactosamine; Glc, glucose; NAN, *N*-acetylneuraminic acid (sialic acid); UDP, uridine diphosphate; CMP, cytidine monophosphate (Fishman and Brady, 1976).

by neuraminidases or glycosidases, which sequentially hydrolyze the neuraminic acid (sialic acid) and sugar residues, respectively. Neuraminidase activity has been detected at the plasma membrane level (Scheel *et al.*, 1985), although most of the ganglioside degradation is believed to occur at the lysosomal level following endocytosis of plasma membrane. There is evidence that the lipid products of this hydrolysis can be recycled and reused in the biosynthesis of glycosphingolipids and phosphoglycerolipids. The cellular fate of glycosphingolipid molecules is schematically represented in Fig. 3.

Distribution of Exogenous Gangliosides

The intramuscular administration to rats of radiolabeled gangliosides (which have tritium incorporated into their sphingosine component) revealed that exogenous gangliosides distribute widely within the body. The major accumulation occurred in the liver while the lowest accumulation was found in the brain (Lang, 1981). Approximately 90% of the incorporated gangliosides remained unchanged during the first 24 hours, decreasing to about 50% after 8 days. In mice, administered radiolabeled gangliosides bind in micellar form to serum albumin and are incorporated into the brain later than into the liver, muscle, or kidney. Most of the radioactive material could be recovered both in particulate (membrane-bound) and soluble (presumably internalized) forms (Orlando *et al.*, 1979; Tettamanti *et al.*, 1981). Based on studies by Orlando and collaborators (1979) and Tettamanti and collaborators (1981), differences in peak concentrations of radioactive

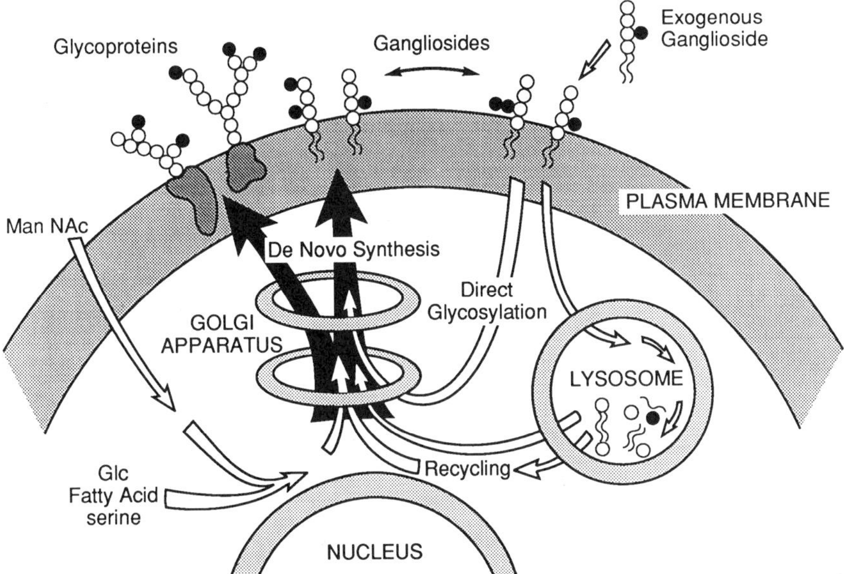

Fig. 3 The different routes of ganglioside metabolism. The processes of *de novo* biosynthesis, direct glycosylation of internalized gangliosides, lysosomal degradation, and biosynthetic recycling of catabolic byproducts are shown (Tettamanti, 1988).

gangliosides between brain and liver suggest that approximately 1 to 2% of this compound can cross the blood–brain barrier.

Toffano and co-workers (1980) have demonstrated that exogenously administered GM1 ganglioside can be incorporated into membranes of nervous tissue. Insertion of exogenous glycosphingolipids into the cell membranes results in complex localized biophysical changes, some of which restrict lateral mobility of the lipid bilayer (Goins *et al.*, 1986). These alterations depend, of course, on other membrane components (proteins and lipids) and on the nature of the glycosphingolipids. A number of possible models for interaction can be envisaged. Figure 4 represents a simplified scenario of possible localized membrane changes resulting from the insertion of gangliosides into the outer leaflet of cell membranes as conceptualized by Maggio and collaborators (1988).

III. Gangliosides in Human Pathology

The notion that gangliosides could somehow induce aberrant or regenerative processes came from observations of pathological material from human and animal gangliosidoses. Gangliosidoses are rare diseases caused by inborn defi-

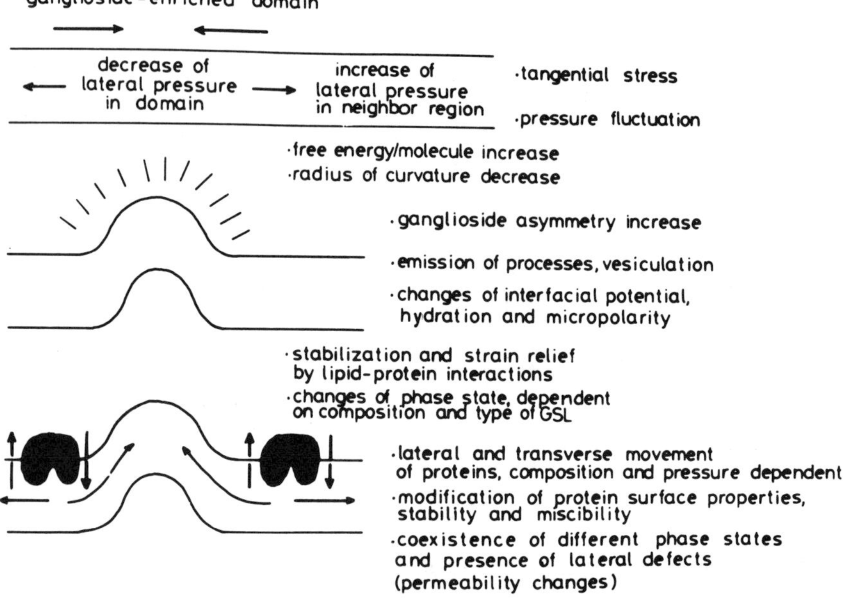

Fig. 4 Postulated effects of gangliosides on the interfacial properties, organization, and morphology of membranes (Maggio *et al.*, 1988).

ciencies of lysosomal enzymes responsible for hydrolysis of the sugar moiety of glycosphingolipids (Crome and Stern, 1981; Brady and Barranger, 1981). An excessive accumulation of glycosphingolipids results, with gangliosidosis being the most common outcome. For example, deficiency of β-galactosidase produces generalized GM1 gangliosidosis, whereas deficiencies of hexosaminidases (A and B), which are required for the hydrolytic cleavage of the terminal *N*-acetyl-galactosamine from GM2, result in accumulation of GM2. There are two forms of this latter pathology, the deficit in hexosaminase A producing the variant known as Tay-Sachs disease. This gangliosidosis is generalized but particularly marked in the CNS, where gangliosides can be concentrated up to 100 times their normal content. The neuropathological observation of Tay-Sachs material reveals enlarged neurons with occasionally swollen dendrites. At the electron microscopic level, the affected neurons display numerous concentrically laminated structures which are referred to as membranous cytoplasmatic bodies (MCBs) (Terry and Weiss, 1963). Of great interest in the context of this review is the finding that ganglioside storage diseases are associated with growth of aberrant neuritic processes. This was observed for the first time in biopsy material from a 14-month-old child with suspected gangliosidosis who experienced seizures, motor retardation, and anomalous responses to sound (de Baecque *et al.*, 1975). Diagnosis was made of a rapidly progressing AB variant of GM2 gangliosidosis. This material was also examined microscopically by Purpura and Suzuki (1976), who, with application of the Golgi method, found that small- and medium-sized pyramidal neurons possessed enlargements interposed between the cell body and the initial axonal portion. These axonal expansions were named "meganeurites." The meganeurites, in turn, revealed spinelike protuberances which were suggestive of new growth processes and had characteristics of ectopic dendrites (see Fig. 5). Some of these newly formed spines displayed actual synaptic contacts. The child died 2 years later, and the postmortem examination revealed even more bizarre meganeurites with more extended dendritic outgrowths bearing multiple synaptic spines (Purpura, 1978).

Access to feline animal models of gangliosidosis (Baker *et al.*, 1971, 1976) allowed Purpura and co-workers (Purpura and Baker, 1977, 1978; Purpura *et al.*, 1978) to undertake more stringent morphological studies of the pathological nervous tissue. These studies confirmed the development of meganeurites and other anomalies in feline gangliosidosis. Furthermore, electron microscopic observations confirmed the existence of synapses in the aberrant dendrites (Purpura *et al.*, 1978; Walkley *et al.*, 1981). In a recent Golgi study of feline GM1 gangliosidosis, Walkley (1987) revealed neuronal and regional differences in expression of meganeurites. He proposed that meganeurites are the result of constraints on somatic expansion resulting from ganglioside accumulation, while secondary neurites and spines are due to genuine neuritogenesis and synaptogenesis. It now appears that, besides gangliosidosis, other metabolic disturbances

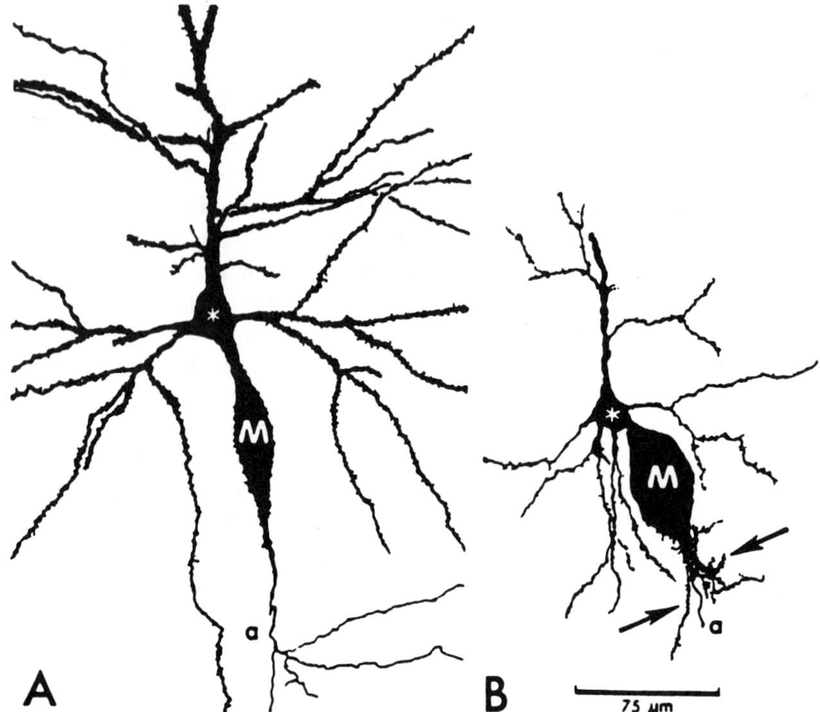

Fig. 5 Camera lucida drawings of Golgi rapid preparations of layer III pyramidal neurons from a child with GM2-gangliosidosis, AB variant. (A) Characteristics of well-developed neuron with prominent early meganeurite (M) at the time of diagnostic cortical biopsy, 14 months of age (the photomicrograph of this neuron is shown in Fig. 1A). (B) Progressive growth and elaboration of the meganeurite, secondary dendrites, and dendritic spines (arrows) in a neuron from postmortem brain tissue 2.5 years after the diagnostic biopsy. Note the marked atrophy of the apical and basilar dendrites in the face of continuing differentiation of secondary dendrites arising from the meganeurite. a, Axon. Magnification bar applies to A and B (Purpura, 1978).

such as sphingomyelin lipodosis and α-mannosidosis also lead to the formation of meganeurites and aberrant processes (Walkley and Baker, 1984; Walkley and Siegel, 1985).

Changes in the distribution pattern of gangliosides in postmortem brain of Alzheimer's and other diseases have been described. However, these studies have failed to provide a consistent picture. Recent interesting data have appeared, linking the presence of antibodies against glycosphingolipids or glycoconjugates with neurological disorders. For example, a number of IgM monoclonal antibodies produced in paraproteinemic neuropathies showed reactivities to glycoproteins associated with myelin and glycosphingolipids (Ilyas *et al.*, 1985a).

Furthermore, cases of such conditions were identified in which the antibody activity was directed against endogenous gangliosides (Ilyas *et al.*, 1985b; Quarles *et al.*, 1986). Latov and co-workers (1988) have found human monoclonal IgMs in two patients with gammopathy associated with motor neuron disease which reacted to GM1, GD1b, and glycoconjugates frequently present in gangliosides. In this study, antibodies from the patients bound to neurons in the spinal cord and to motor end plates. Also, Ilyas and collaborators (1988) have found high titers of antibodies to gangliosides in 5 out of 26 patients suffering from Guillain-Barré syndrome, a demyelinating polyneuropathy of unknown etiology. A closer correlation (57 out 73 patients) between antibodies against the gangliosides GM1 and GD1a was found in victims of amyotrophic lateral sclerosis (ALS) (Pestronk *et al.*, 1989).

All these observations are of relevance in the understanding of sphingolipid involvement in human disease. In simple terms, there is an indication that gangliosidosis leads to the formation of excessive, aberrant neurites while antibodies to gangliosides are often associated with demyelination or dysfunction of peripheral nerves. The latter observation relates well to the proposition that immunization against gangliosides may be a model for experimental allergic neuropathy (Nagai *et al.*, 1976). In this context, it is worth commenting that sugar sequences characteristic of sphingolipids have been used for the immunological recognition of primary sensory neuron subsets (Dodd and Jessell, 1985), and that gangliosides themselves might be transmitter- (Ferretti and Borroni, 1986) or territory specific-markers.

IV. Effects of Gangliosides on Neural Cells *in Vitro*

The interest in the actions of gangliosides and other sphingolipids on *in vitro* neuronal systems sprang from a variety of earlier observations and findings, including a pathological neuritogenic capacity (see Section III), peripheral reinnervation (Ceccarelli *et al.*, 1976) (see section V,A), and receptor activity (see Section VI,A).

On the basis of the historical background indicated, studies on the effects of exogenously applied gangliosides to neural cells *in vitro* have been directed at exploring whether these molecules are able to modulate differentiation, survival rate, or synaptogenesis. Thus, Obata and collaborators (1977) observed stimulation of synapse formation in spinal cord–skeletal muscle cocultures in the presence of low concentrations of the ganglioside GM1, and the opposite effect at high concentrations. Morgan and Seifert (1979) applied gangliosides to "serum-starved" cultures of transformed neuronal cells (clone B 104). This clonal line, derived from chemically induced rat brain tumors, survived and even divided in the presence of ganglioside. At 14 to 30 days the cells acquired a multipolar morphology with numerous radiating neurites. Neurite extension was stimulated by the application of gangliosides to hippocampal primary cultures but not to PC12 cells (Seifert, 1981). Seifert (1981) characterized these effects as those of a "differentiating factor," analogous to those of NGF on PC12 cells. In the neuroblastoma cell line Neuro-2a, Dimpfel and collaborators (1981) noted that the ganglioside-induced neurite formation occurs rapidly and that there is an initial correlation with cAMP content in the cultures. Roisen and co-workers (1981a) found that a bovine ganglioside mixture increased the length and number of processes in the small cell line and the rate of elongation of neurites in primary cultures of sensory neurons. In addition, the content of ornithine decarboxylase, a biochemical indicator of cell growth, was elevated 2-fold by the ganglioside mixture. Similar effects were obtained by Leon and colleagues (1982), who showed a concomitant increase in cAMP levels. Whether the neuritogenic effects of gangliosides could be ascribed to the mixture, contaminants, or a particular ganglioside was investigated by Byrne and co-workers (1983). These authors found that the application of highly purified GM1 preparations produced similar neuritogenic effects on neuroblastoma cells as did a mixture of gangliosides. In another study, Facci and co-workers (1984) showed that stimulation of Neuro-2a cell differentiation by GM1 correlated with the incorporation of the ganglioside into these cells.

Roisen and collaborators (1981b, 1984; Spero and Roisen, 1984) have produced detailed and convincing microscopic evidence for the formation of processes by neuroblastoma cells in response to gangliosides (see Fig. 6). Changes include the formation of microvilli and ruffled membranes, as well as redistribution of intermediate filaments into bundles forming the core of microvilli.

Ganglioside Interactions with Trophic Factors *in Vitro*

Explant cultures of different ganglia have been instrumental in demonstrating that environmental conditions such as a balance between inhibiting and promoting influences (factors?) are crucial for the ganglioside induction of neurite extension (Skaper and Varon, 1985; Skaper *et al.*, 1985). For example, the presence of NGF or ciliary neuronotrophic factor (CNTF) is required for the chick sympathetic and ciliary ganglia to respond to exogenous gangliosides. Whether these constraints are primarily due to the presence of specific trophic factors is an aspect of theoretical and practical relevance. In this regard, antibodies against GM1 have been reported to inhibit the regenerative responses in goldfish retinal explants (Spirman *et al.*, 1982), and, more specifically, to inhibit the NGF-induced sprouting in dissociated cell cultures of chick dorsal root ganglia (Schwartz and Spirman, 1982). Antibodies against GM2 only moderately inhibited such responses. However, in a similar tissue culture preparation, well-

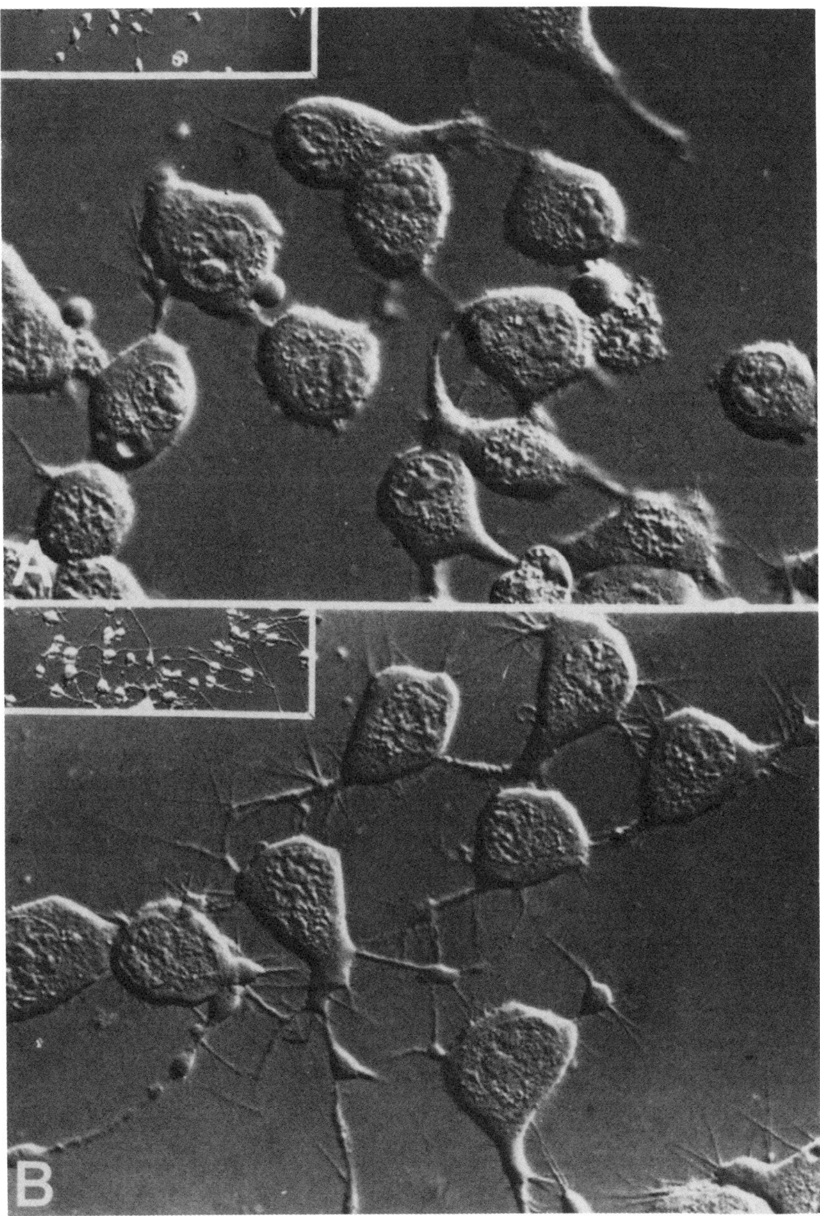

Fig. 6 Representative Nomarski photomicrographs illustrating the effect of gangliosides on Neuro-2a morphology after 44 hours *in vitro* on a glass surface. Magnification: 600×; inserts 30×: (1) Control medium. (B) Control medium supplemented with 250 μg/ml bovine brain gangliosides. More numerous and longer processes than in the control can be seen (Roisen *et al.*, 1981a).

characterized affinity-purified polyclonal antibodies against GM1 failed to modify fiber outgrowth or neuronal survival dependent on the presence of NGF (Doherty and Walsh, 1987). In an earlier report, Doherty and co-workers (1985) found that the ganglioside GM1 was able to enhance the NGF-induced neurite regeneration in dorsal root neurons. This phenomenon was accompanied by an increment in the expression of neurofilament proteins. Gangliosides are also known to promote the neurite outgrowth from PC12 cells primed with NGF (Ferrari *et al.*, 1983; Katoh-Semba *et al.*, 1984; Varon *et al.*, 1986). In chick explants of ciliary ganglia and spinal cord grown in conditioned medium (muscle and Schwannoma cells), Spoerri and Roisen (1988) found that GM1 or a bovine ganglioside mixture potentiated the neuritogenic effects of unknown (non-NGF) growth-promoting substances present in the cultures.

To what extent cells of the CNS can respond directly or indirectly to gangliosides is yet to be determined. It is possible that CNS neurons and glial cells would respond quite differently to exogenously applied gangliosides depending on their developmental state, as well as to the chemical environment in which they are grown. In support of this, Hefti *et al.* (1985a) demonstrated that the addition of gangliosides did not modify the survival or neuritic pattern of cultured dissociated cells from embryonic rat septal nucleus but reduced the number of astroglial elements. In those experiments, a mixture of gangliosides modified the morphology of astroglial cells and elicited a significant increase in the enzymatic activity of the biosynthetic enzyme for acetylcholine, choline acetyltransferase (ChAT) (see Fig. 7), but did not alter the NGF-induced increase in ChAT activity. We have adopted this tissue culture model to investigate the trophic effects of two substances, NGF and GM1 (Cuello *et al.*, 1989). In our experiments, the dissociated septal cells (a mixed neuronal–glial population) were maintained in monolayer culture in the presence of serum-supplemented medium. The presence of ChAT-immunoreactive neurons and astroglia in the culture system was confirmed with anti-ChAT monoclonal (Eckenstein and Thoenen, 1982) and anti-GFAP (glial fibrillary acidic protein) (Bignami *et al.*, 1972) antibodies, respectively. In agreement with Hefti and co-workers (1985a) and Hatanaka and Tsukui (1986), ChAT activity in these septal cells was found to be modulated by either NGF or GM1. A dramatic increase in ChAT activity was noted after a 7-day exposure to exogenous NGF. This increase was dose-dependent, detectable at concentrations as low as 10^{-13} *M*, and maximal in the nanomolar range, as previously observed by Hefti and co-workers (1985a). In our mixed glial–neuronal, serum-supplemented culture, GM1 produced a moderate (15–30% over control) increase in ChAT activity which was detected only when cells were exposed to 10^{-6} to 10^{-5} *M* GM1 (Cuello *et al.*, 1989). Higher concentrations tended to diminish ChAT activity (D. Maysinger *et al.*, unpublished results), while lower concentrations of GM1 (e.g., 10^{-7} *M*) were ineffective. In these culture conditions, we

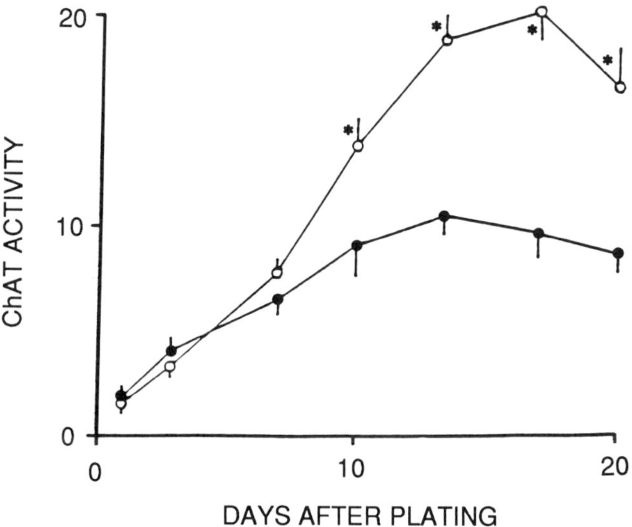

Fig. 7 Effect of gangliosides on ChAT activity in cultures of dissociated septal cells. The cells were grown in the absence (○) or presence (●) of a ganglioside mixture (0.5 mg/ml, present during the entire culture time). Bars represent SEM; *, significantly different from corresponding control levels; $p < 0.01$; $n = 4$ to 12 (Hefti *et al.*, 1985b).

have found that gangliosides can enhance NGF responses within a narrow range of concentrations.

When effective concentrations of GM1 (10^{-5} *M*) were added in combination with NGF, a potentiation of the effects of the latter factor was observed (Fig. 8A). In combination with 10^{-5} *M* GM1, submaximal (10^{-13} *M*) and maximal (10^{-9} *M*) concentrations of NGF produced an increase in ChAT activity which was significantly greater than that obtained with NGF alone. This potentiating effect of GM1 was most evident when applied in combination with submaximal concentrations of NGF. The idea of cooperativity between these factors was further supported by the finding that ineffective GM1 concentrations (10^{-7} *M*) potentiated the NGF-induced increase in ChAT activity (Fig. 8B). How much of the ganglioside effects in the *in vivo* situation is dependent on the presence of glial cells or other cellular elements has yet to be established. The culture of neurons in chemically defined media can help to elucidate some of the direct actions of gangliosides.

In tissue culture conditions, the sialic acid residues seem crucial for the stimulation of neuritogenesis in a neuroblastoma cell line (Neuro-2a) (Tsuji *et al.*, 1988), although these effects are independent of the nature of the hydrophobic

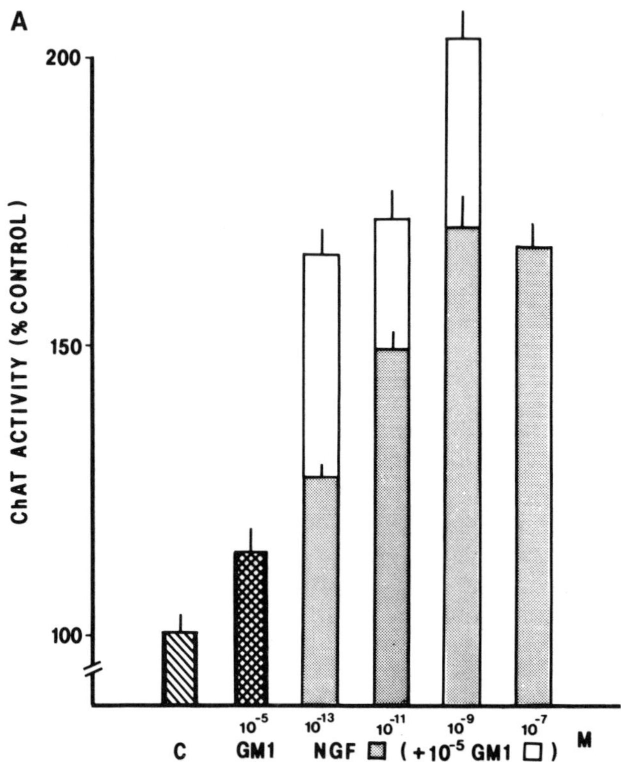

Fig. 8 (A) Effect of 10 μ*M* GM1, alone or in combination with various concentrations of β-NGF, on ChAT activity in cultures of dissociated septal cells. Septal cells were grown for 7 days in the absence of GM1 and β-NGF [control (C), hatched bar], in the presence of 10 μ*M* GM1 (cross-hatched bar), or in the presence of 0.1 p*M*, 10 p*M*, 1 n*M*, or 0.1 μ*M* β-NGF alone (stippled bars), or in combination with 10 μ*M* GM1 (open bars). Bars represent the means ± SEM from quadruplicate culture wells from sister culture preparations. Control absolute value was 4.5 nmol of acetylcholine per milligram of protein per hour (Cuello *et al.*, 1989). (B) Effect of a subthreshold concentration (0.1 μ*M*) of GM1, alone or in combination with

molecule (cholesterol, ceramide, or alkyl glycerol ether) to which they are coupled.

V. Effects of Gangliosides in Damaged Nervous Tissue

A. Peripheral Nervous System

1. Motor, Sensory and Autonomic Neurons

Early experiments of Ceccarelli and collaborators (1976) stimulated a great deal of interest in the potential uses of sphingolipids in neural repair. Furthermore,

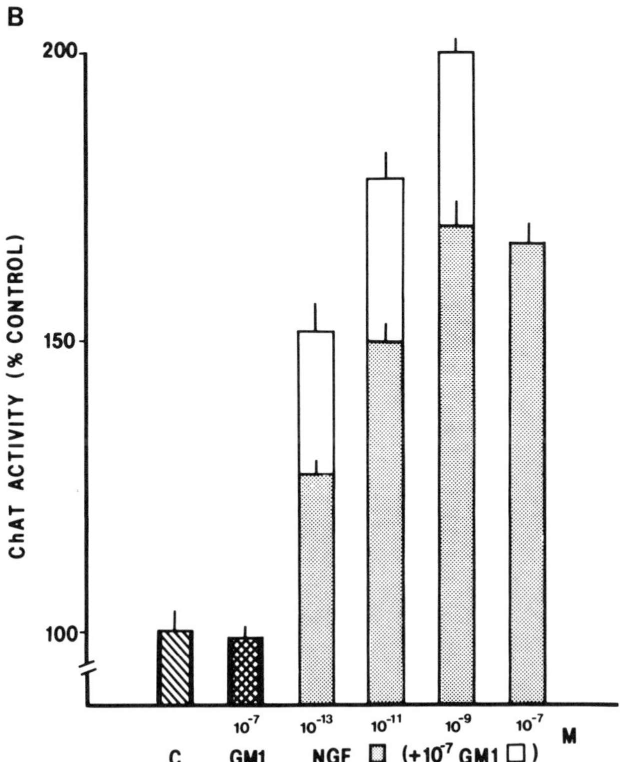

Fig. 8 (*Continued*)
various concentrations of β-NGF, on ChAT activity in cultures of dissociated septal cells. Septal cells were grown for 7 days in the absence of GM1 and β-NGF [control (C), hatched bar], in the presence of 10 μ*M* GM1 (cross-hatched bar), or in the presence of 0.1 p*M*, 10 p*M*, 1 n*M*, or 0.1 μ*M* β-NGF alone (stippled bars), or in combination with 10 μ*M* GM1 (open bars). Bars represent the means ± SEM from quadruplicate culture wells from sister culture preparations. Control absolute value was 4.5 nmol of acetylcholine per milligram of protein per hour (Cuello *et al.*, 1989).

they addressed contemporary questions related to the effects of theses glycolipids, namely, their site of action and transmitter specificity. These investigators noted a marked improvement in the rate of recovery of the contractile responses of sympathetically denervated (pre- and postganglionic) nictitating membrane in ganglioside-treated animals (Ceccarelli *et al.*, 1976). An improvement in denervated skeletal muscle was subsequently reported by Caccia and co-workers (1979). These early observations were followed by an extensive series of investigations by Gorio and colleagues (Gorio *et al.*, 1980, 1983a; Carmignoto *et al.*, 1983), who observed that the administration of a ganglioside mixture can accelerate the process of reinnervation of skeletal muscle in the extensor digitorum following sciatic nerve crush. They observed that maximal reinnervation, as determined electrophysiologically (percentage of double innervated muscle fibers), occurred at day 25 postcrush, while in the ganglioside-treated group, this was observed a week earlier. Morphological evidence for fiber sprouting and formation of new motor end plates was also obtained at light and electron microscopic levels (Gorio *et al.*, 1983a). Further experiments were undertaken to examine the sprouting capacity of intact motor neurons in rats in which the soleus muscle was partially denervated by the removal of the L_5 component of the sciatic nerve (Gorio *et al.*, 1983b). Thirty days following surgery, the morphology of silver-stained axons and the muscle isometric tension measurements after stimulation were used to monitor the degree of reinnervation. The authors established an index for motor sprouting based on the ratios of isometric responses obtained after surgery and of responses obtained in normal muscle. Such ratios showed an improvement of 50% in the "index of sprouting" in ganglioside-treated rats compared with untreated rats (Gorio *et al.*, 1983b).

Other investigators have also reported reparative effects of gangliosides in skeletal muscle reinnervation. Robb and Keynes (1984) communicated that gangliosides induce a very fast (days) production of nerve terminal sprouting and functional recovery following partial denervation of the gluteus maximus in the mouse, while Kleinebeckel (1982) found electromyographical evidence for ganglioside-induced muscle reinnervation. Reports by Mengs and collaborators (1984) determined an improvement in peripheral nerve conduction following the application of large doses of a ganglioside mixture, "Cronassial" (GM1 21%, GD1a 40%, GD1 16%, GT1b 19%). The same group also provided morphological evidence showing an increase in the diameter and number of remaining axons following nerve crush in ganglioside-treated rats (Mengs *et al.*, 1986; Mengs and Stotzen, 1987). In nonmammalian species, Maier and Singer (1984) reported a rapid increase of regenerating axons (up to 45%) in the limb buds of newts which were either injected with or immersed in ganglioside solutions. The goldfish optic nerve, in contrast to that of mammals, has a capacity to regenerate in an analogous fashion to that observed in mammalian peripheral nerves. In this classical model for neuronal regeneration, Sparrow and collaborators (1984) found evidence of a possible role for endogenous gangliosides in regeneration because antibodies against these molecules disrupted the regenerative process.

The peripheral neurotoxic effects of the false transmitter 6-hydroxy-dopamine (6-OH-DA), capsaicin, and blockers of axonal transport can be arrested (at least partially) by the timely administration of gangliosides. One such example has been provided by Jonsson and co-workers (1984), who showed that gangliosides can increase the recovery rate of noradrenaline-containing fibers following 6-OH-DA administration in neonatal and adult animals. These authors postulated a possible participation of NGF in the recovery of these neurons. Such a contention received further indirect support from the finding that GM1 can partially diminish the depletion of substance P-immunoreactive material in the superficial layers of the spinal cord caused by capsaicin (Gorio *et al.*, 1986), an agent which preferentially affects small-caliber-peptide-containing primary sensory neurons (Jancso *et al.*, 1977; Jessell *et al.*, 1978). These two systems, sympathetic and sensory, are known to be NGF dependent (Levi-Montalcini and Calissano, 1986). Furthermore, Otten and collaborators (1983) have shown that devastating neurotoxic damage on substance P-containing primary sensory neurons, induced by neonatally administered capsaicin, can clearly be counterbalanced by early treatment with NGF. More compelling evidence for a ganglioside–growth factor interaction in the peripheral nervous system was provided by Vantini and colleagues (1988). These authors confirmed that the long-lasting damage on peripheral noradrenergic neurons (spleen and heart) induced by vinblastine, a blocker of axonal transport (Menessini Chen *et al.*, 1977; Zieher and Jaim-Etcheverry, 1983), can be ameliorated by the administration of NGF. Furthermore, Vantini and collaborators (1988) provided clear evidence for a cooperative interest between GM1 and NGF on reestablishing the levels of noradrenaline in the heart (see Fig. 9).

2. Diabetic Neuropathy

The efficacy of gangliosides in diabetic neuropathy is a subject of great interest because treatment of this disease offers an indication of the therapeutic value of gangliosides (Cronassial) in a number of European countries. Horowitz (1986), in a controlled, double blind study, examined a group of 28 patients with moderate diabetic neuropathy and found that 14 patients who received Cronassial showed a significant improvement in clinical and electrophysiological scores over the placebo group. Comprehensive reports on the toxicology and efficacy of gangliosides in the clinic are awaited.

In experimental animals, Gorio and colleagues (Vitadello *et al.*, 1983) determined that the mutant mouse C57BL/Ks (db/db) develops a peripheral neuropathy in which the axonal atrophy and diminution of conduction velocity are accompanied by a decreased transport of the enzyme acetylcholinesterase (AChE). In these animals, gangliosides improved peripheral nerve function only if applied in a later (insulin-insensitive) phase of the neuropathy (Norido *et al.*, 1984). Furthermore, in a separate study, the impaired axonal flow of AChE observed in rats with alloxan-induced experimental diabetes was also shown to be antagonized by gangliosides (Marini *et al.*, 1986).

B. Central Nervous System

1. Effects of Gangliosides on Diverse CNS Lesions and Behavioral Correlates

Unilateral or bilateral lesions of the entorhinal cortex in rats produce a rapid (24–48 hours) and marked loss of learned alternation behavior and induce signs of

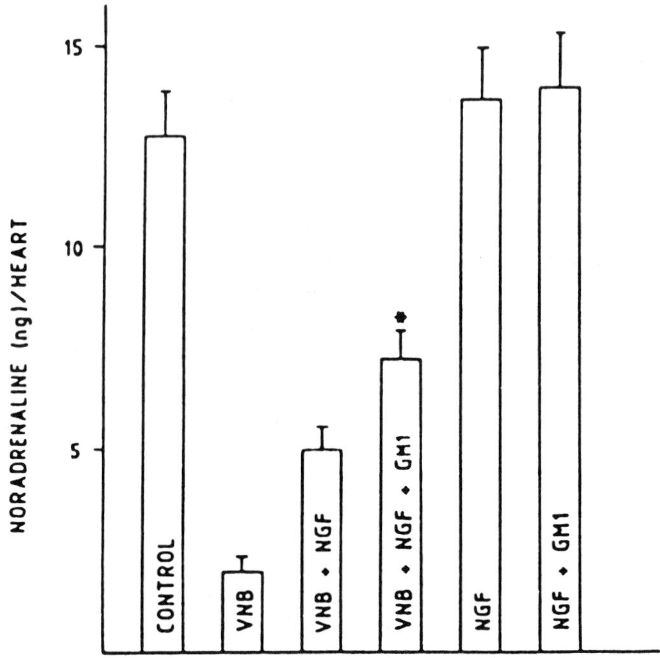

Fig. 9 Effect of vinblastine (VNB) and/or NGF ± GM1 treatments on the noradrenaline (NA) content in heart of 6-day-old rats. Single injections of VNB (0.15 mg/kg) were given on postnatal day 3 (P3). GM1 (30 mg/kg) was administered daily on P3, P4, and P5. In VNB-treated animals NGF was given 30 minutes after VNB administration. On P3, GM1 was administered 1.5 hours following NGF injection. Animals were killed 20 hours after the last GM1 injection. Each value represents the mean ± SEM of 10–12 animals. *, Significant difference ($p < 0.05$) from the VNB + NGF-treated group (Vantini *et al.*, 1988).

locomotor hyperactivity. The systemic administration of gangliosides has been shown to attenuate these behavioral deficits and, furthermore, to reduce the high level of mortality following these lesioning procedures (Karpiak, 1983; Fass and Ramirez, 1984; Ramirez *et al.*, 1987).

Sabel *et al.* (1984) applied GM1 ganglioside (30 mg/kg/day) to rats receiving large, bilateral, electrolytic lesions of the caudate putamen. In these experiments, brain sections obtained from ganglioside-treated animals did not show any obvious histological differences (Nissl staining) from those of the nontreated group, although a significant improvement in their behavior in an active avoidance paradigm was noted. This research group (Sabel *et al.*, 1985) also found a behavioral improvement in apomorphine-induced rotational asymmetries in ganglioside-treated rats with brain hemitransections (see Section V,B,2). This was accompanied by relatively greater success in the retrograde labeling of substantia nigra neurons with horseradish peroxidase (HRP) implanted in the caudate putamen.

2. Ganglioside Effects on Transmitter-Specific Systems

a. Dopaminergic Neurons In 1983, two studies demonstrated the capability of gangliosides to protect partially dopaminergic nigral neurons in the rat from anterograde and retrograde degeneration following brain hemitransections (Toffano *et al.*, 1983; Agnati *et al.*, 1983b). This was shown by examining tyrosine hydroxylase (T-OH) activity in the caudate putamen and T-OH immunoreactivity in the substantia nigra (Toffano *et al.*, 1983) (see Fig. 10). Chronic administration of the ganglioside GM1 (10 mg/kg/i.p./day) for 56 days resulted

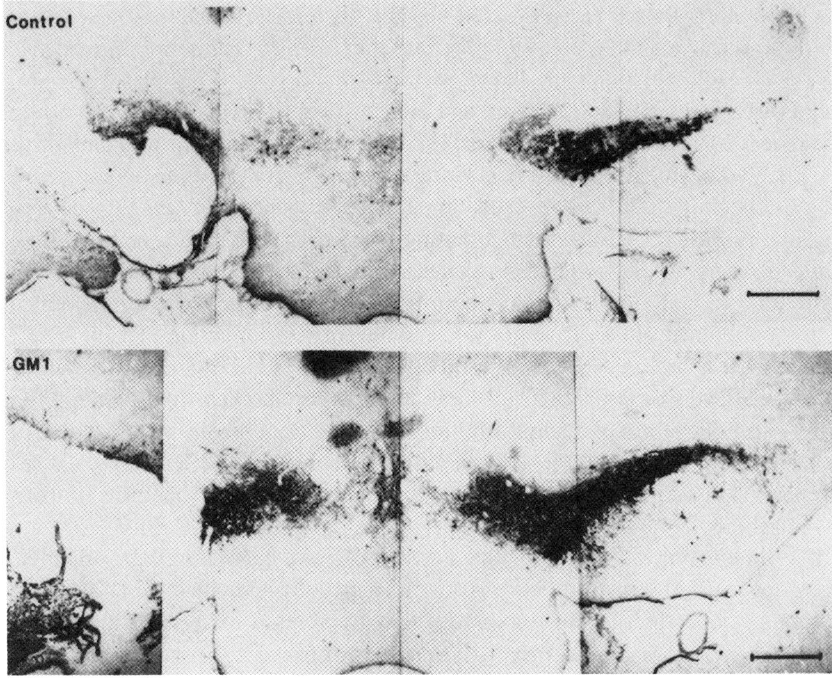

Fig. 10 Transverse sections of rat brain at rostral level of substantia nigra, stained by peroxidase–antiperoxidase immunocytochemistry, utilizing antibodies against tyrosine hydroxylase (T-OH). The rats were hemitransected and started on saline or GM1 treatment (30 mg/kg i.p.) 48 hours after surgery. Rats were sacrificed 28 days following the lesion. Note that GM1 treatment induces an increased survival of TOH immunopositive cell bodies which were not primarily affected by the lesion (left side) (Consolazione *et al.*, 1988).

in a remarkable protection of the morphology, biochemical indicators, and behavioral parameters of the dopaminergic nigrostriatal system following these extensive lesions (Agnati *et al.*, 1983a). In this fairly comprehensive study, the preservation of immunoreactivity, both at the cell body (substantia nigra) and terminal network (caudate putamen) sites, was demonstrated by applying a rigorous image analysis approach. In both these communications, evidence was presented for an increased dendritic length in dopaminergic nigral neurons. These observations support the idea that protection induced by gangliosides facilitates the salvage of neurons following injury by promoting new dendrodendritic interactions and thus reestablishing trophic support for the cells (Agnati *et al.*, 1983b). This is a plausible situation because dendrodendritic interactions (Groves *et al.*, 1975) and dendritic release of transmitters have been documented both *in vitro* (Geffen *et al.*, 1976; Cuello and Iversen, 1978) and *in vivo* (Korf *et al.*, 1976; Nieoullon *et al.*, 1977; Cheramy *et al.*, 1981). However, the possibility that gangliosides may interact with an endogenous "dopaminergic trophic factor" should be considered because such a substance has been postulated (Tomozawa and Appel, 1986; Ferrari *et al.*, 1988). Furthermore, evidence for spontaneous repair of the damaged nigrostriatal system has also been provided (Reis *et al.*, 1978; Björklund and Stenevi, 1979; Gilad and Reis, 1979). In this model, Agnati and collaborators (1983b) provided biochemical (quantitative receptor radioautography) and behavioral (locomotor responses to apomorphine with unilaterally denervated caudate putamen) evidence of ganglioside (10 mg/kg/i.p./day, for 45 days) ameliorating the denervation supersensitivity. In a consecutive study, Toffano and co-workers (1984) found that mechanical but not neurotoxic (6-OH-DA) lesions of the nigrostriatal pathway could be prevented with the administration of gangliosides. A recent reexamination (Tilson *et al.*, 1988) of the neurotoxic effects of 6-OH-DA in this system showed a normalization in the levels of dopamine (DA) and its main metabolites with the daily (25 and 50 kg) intraventricular administration of a mixture of bovine gangliosides. In the same report, the subcutaneous (s.c.) administration of GM1 (20 mg/kg/day) to Fischer 344 rats significantly reduced the haloperiodol-induced supersensitivity to apomorphine.

It is interesting to note that the internal ester of GM1 (AGF2), which is converted to GM1 in the bloodstream, is more effective than GM1 itself in protecting dopaminergic neurons in the hemitransection model (Aldino *et al.*, 1984). These authors found that AGF2 preserved striatal T-OH activity at lower doses than GM1, while agents used for reduction of cerebral edema, such as dexamethasone or mannitol, were ineffective. Ganglioside-induced recovery of uptake was also noted by Raiteri and collaborators (1985). However, there was no improvement in the success rate of substantia nigra grafts after GM1 administration (Freed, 1985).

Recently, a great deal of attention has been paid to the use of 1-methyl-4-

phenyl-1,2,3,6-tetrahydropyridine (MPTP) in mouse and primate for the development of animal models for Parkinsons's disease (Burns *et al.*, 1983; Langston *et al.*, 1984; Heikkila *et al.*, 1984). This compound produces neurotoxic effects in human which are identical to the neurological and neuropathological changes seen in Parkinsonism (Langston *et al.*, 1983; Ballard *et al.*, 1985). Using the mouse MPTP model, Hadjiconstantinou and colleagues (1986) have demonstrated that the chronic administration of GM1 restores DA content in the striatum. In a more extensive study, Hadjiconstantinou and Neff (1988) indicated that the degree of restoration of the DA content and its metabolite dihydroxyphenylacetic acid (DOPAC) correlated with the duration of GM1 treatment (see Table III). Moreover, delaying the onset of GM1 treatment for several days proved ineffective (see Fig. 11). This situation is analogous to that observed with central cholinergic neurons of the NBM (Stephens *et al.*, 1987). Hadjiconstantinou and Neff (1988) also found that AGF2, the internal ester of GM1, was at least as effective as GM1 in protecting dopaminergic neurons from the neurotoxic effects of MPTP. An unresolved aspect of this study was that neither GM1 nor

Table III

Evaluation of Various GM1 Treatment Schedules on the Catechol Content of MPTP-Treated Mice[a]

	Protein (pmol/mg)	
Treatment	DA	DOPAC
Saline[b]	664 ± 21	164 ± 8
MPTP 7	282 ± 12[c]	88 ± 7[c]
MPTP 30[b]	335 ± 21[c]	144 ± 11[c]
GM1	657 ± 30	182 ± 14
Cotreatment		
GM1 + MPTP 7	245 ± 28[c]	90 ± 10[c]
GM1 + MPTP 30	530 ± 26[d]	127 ± 12[c]
Pretreatment		
GM1 + MPTP 7	269 ± 14[c]	86 ± 9[c]
GM1 + MPTP 30	566 ± 26[d]	162 ± 7[d]
Posttreatment		
MPTP 30 + GM1[b]	570 ± 24[d]	158 ± 13[d]

[a] From Hadjiconstantinou and Neff (1988).

[b] Data from Hadjiconstantinou *et al.* (1986).

[c] $p < 0.05$ when compared with saline or GM1 treatment.

[d] $p < 0.05$ when compared with the corresponding MPTP alone treatment.

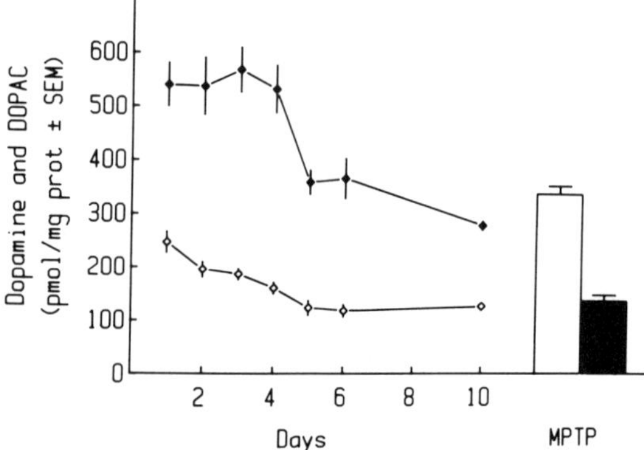

Fig. 11 The consequence of delayed treatment with GM1 ganglioside on the dopamine (DA) and 3,4-dihydroxyphenylacetic acid (DOPAC) content of MPTP-treated mice. Mice were treated with 1-methyl-4-phenyl-1,2,3,6-tetrahydropyridine (MPTP), 30 mg/kg i.p., for 7 days. Treatment with GM1 was started after ≥24 hours, as indicated. Once initiated, treatment was continued for 23 days. The open column represents the striatal DA content, and the solid column represents the DOPAC content for MPTP treatment alone. Data are mean ± SEM (bars) values for 12–15 mice (Hadjiconstantinou and Neff, 1988).

AGF2 corrected the MPTP-induced deficits of DA uptake into striatal synaptosomes (see Table IV).

b. Cholinergic Neurons The interest in studying potential reparative effects of gangliosides in cholinergic neurons is highlighted by their apparent responsiveness to NGF (Kromer, 1987; Levi-Montalcini and Calissano, 1986) and the marked involvement of this transmitter system in Alzheimer's disease (Davies and Maloney, 1976; Bowen *et al.*, 1976). The possibility that this condition is a result of defective or diminished trophic factor function has been proposed (Appel, 1981; Hefti, 1983). In experimental animals, basal forebrain cholinergic neurons display NGF binding sites and NGF receptor immunoreactivity (for review, see Whittemore and Seiger, 1987). There is a good correlation between the density of cholinergic innervation in the CNS and the expression of NGF mRNA or the peptide (Korsching *et al.*, 1985). The functional merit of such an association is strengthened by the finding that NGF is retrogradely transported to cell bodies of cholinergic but not dopaminergic neurons (Schwab *et al.*, 1979). More importantly, in the adult, these cholinergic neurons respond to exogenous NGF following partial or total damage of the septohippocampal pathway (Hefti, 1986; Kromer, 1987; Williams *et al.*, 1986).

Prior to the dramatic observations showing a reparative role of NGF on injured cholinergic neurons, Wojcik and co-workers (1982) demonstrated that ganglio-

Table IV

GM1 or AGF2 Do Not Correct the Loss of DA Uptake into Striatal Synaptosomes Induced by Treatment with MPTP[a]

Treatment	DA uptake (pmol/mg of protein/6 min)	Percentage change
Saline	232 ± 13	
GM1	193 ± 13	
AGF2	217 ± 11	
MPTP 7	167 ± 15[b]	−32
MPTP 30	130 ± 6[c]	−47
MPTP 30 ± GM1	109 ± 7[c]	−52
MPTP 30 ± AGF2	117 ± 8[c]	−50

[a] From Hadjiconstantinou and Neff (1988).
[b] $p < 0.05$ compared with saline-treated mice.
[c] $p < 0.05$ compared with the MPTP 7 group.

side mixtures promoted the anterograde regeneration of cholinergic fibers in the hippocampus of rats with septal nucleus lesions. A similar effect was observed by the same group after partial deafferentation of the septohippocampal pathway (Oderfeld-Nowak *et al.*, 1984). Consequently, Oderfeld-Nowak and colleagues (Gradkowska *et al.*, 1986; Skup *et al.*, 1987) demonstrated that pure GM1 preparations produced similar effects and that the degree of recovery obtained in hippocampal markers was dependent on the extent of the lesion (i.e., the number of fibers affected). Thus, a more pronounced recovery of the cholinergic deficit was observed in animals bearing unilateral knife lesions of the lateral fimbria rather than in those with fimbria–fornix lesions (see Fig. 12).

The nucleus basalis magnocellularis (NBM) is a major basal forebrain cholinergic ascending projection (Johnston *et al.*, 1981; Lehman *et al.*, 1982; Mesulam *et al.*, 1986). In man, this nucleus, as well as its cortical fiber network, is highly involved in the pathology of Alzheimer's disease (Davies and Maloney, 1976; Bowen *et al.*, 1976; Whitehouse *et al.*, 1982). Cytotoxic stereotaxic lesions of the NBM lead to the anterograde degeneration of cortically projecting fibers with a concomitant loss of cholinergic markers and behavioral deficits (Dunnett *et al.*, 1985; Fine *et al.*, 1985; Wenk *et al.*, 1980; Flicker *et al.*, 1983). Pedata and collaborators (1984) have demonstrated that long-term administration of GM1 (30 mg/kg/i.p./day) in NBM-lesioned animals can prevent this anterograde degeneration, as judged by high-affinity choline uptake (HACU) in the cerebral cortex of NBM-lesioned animals. In addition, treatment improved the

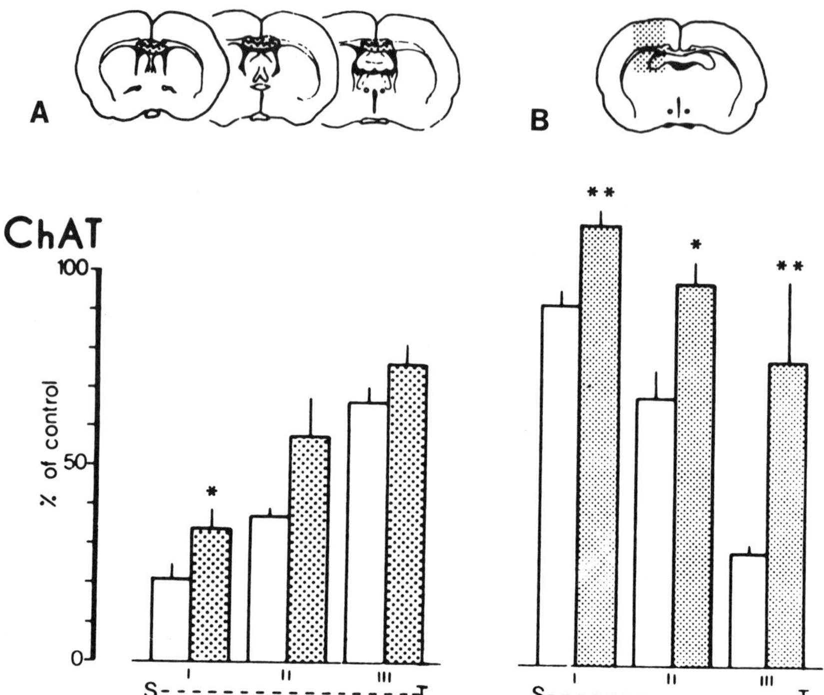

Fig. 12 Effect of GM1 treatment on ChAT activity in the hippocampus 6 days after partial lesions of the dorsal hippocampal afferents: (A) after bilateral electrolytic lesion in the supracallosal area encroaching upon fornix superior (upper scheme) (Skup *et al.*, 1987) and (B) after unilateral knife lesion of lateral fimbria (upper scheme) (Skup *et al.*, unpublished). I–III, Hippocampal parts from septal (S) to temporal (T) end. Open bars represent data from buffer-treated rats; dotted bars, data from GM1-treated rats. Number of rats in experimental groups equals to 4–7. Differences between values from operated GM1-treated and operated buffer-treated rats were significant at * $p < 0.05$ and ** $p < 0.01$ (Student's t-test). Average control values (in μmol ACh/100 mg protein/hr) are equal to I, 5.47 ± 0.48; II, 6.61 ± 0.30; III, 7.42 ± 0.26 (Oderfeld-Nowak *et al.*, 1984).

rate of recovery of the ChAT enzymatic activity and behavioral performance (Casamenti *et al.*, 1985).

The involvement of the cholinergic neurons in the NBM in Alzheimer's disease could be either a primary factor in the pathology or, alternatively, secondary to a primary cortical lesion. With this in mind, we have developed an animal model to study the retrograde degenerative involvement of immunocytochemically identifiable cholinergic neurons in the NBM. Thus, it has been demonstrated that extensive devascularizing neocortical lesions lead to retrograde damage of cholinergic cells in this nucleus (Sofroniew *et al.*, 1983). This retrograde involvement is expressed by loss of neurites and shrinkage in the ChAT-immunoreactive neurons. The lesioning also leads to a concomitant depletion of ChAT enzymatic activity in microdissected samples of the NBM, but not in other areas (Stephens *et al.*, 1985). The administration of large doses of GM1 (30 mg/kg/i.p./day) from the time of onset of the lesion for 30 days resulted in total protection of the neurons from retrograde shrinkage, as determined by the cross-sectional area of immunostained neurons and ChAT enzymatic activity (Cuello *et al.*, 1986) (see Table V). Using this model, Elliott and co-workers (1989) noted a significant improvement in the behavioral performance of GM1-treated rats, as assessed by the Morris water maze and passive avoidance tests, which correlated with the improvement in biochemical cholinergic parameters.

In order to achieve more effective drug delivery to the CNS, we have explored the use of microencapsulated gangliosides in the NBM–cortex cholinergic lesion model (Maysinger *et al.*, 1989). The animals were immediately treated with either microencapsulated GM1 or human serum albumin (HSA) microcapsules containing no drug. Treatment with GM1 in this manner prevented the decrease in ChAT activity and cell shrinkage. These observations are of potential value in considering long-term treatment strategies.

The retrograde responses of the medial septum to hippocampal ablation or fornix–fimbria transections include the apparent loss of the immunostained medial septum neurons (see Fig. 13). Whether the failure in immunocytochemically detecting cholinergic neurons after axotomy or removal of target sites is a

Table V

Effects of GM1 on Cross-Sectional Areas of ChAT Immunoreactive Neurons in the Nucleus Basalis of Control and Operated Animals[a,b]

Experimental conditions	Number of cases	Mean cross-sectional area (μm^2)	SEM
Control	6	319	26.1
Control + GM1	3	328	35.8
Operated	10	234*	18.0
Operated + GM1	3	323	43.9

[a] From Cuello *et al.* (1986).
[b] Values represent the mean and standard error of the mean (SEM) of 50 randomly selected ChAT immunoreactive neurons, per case.
*$p < 0.001$.

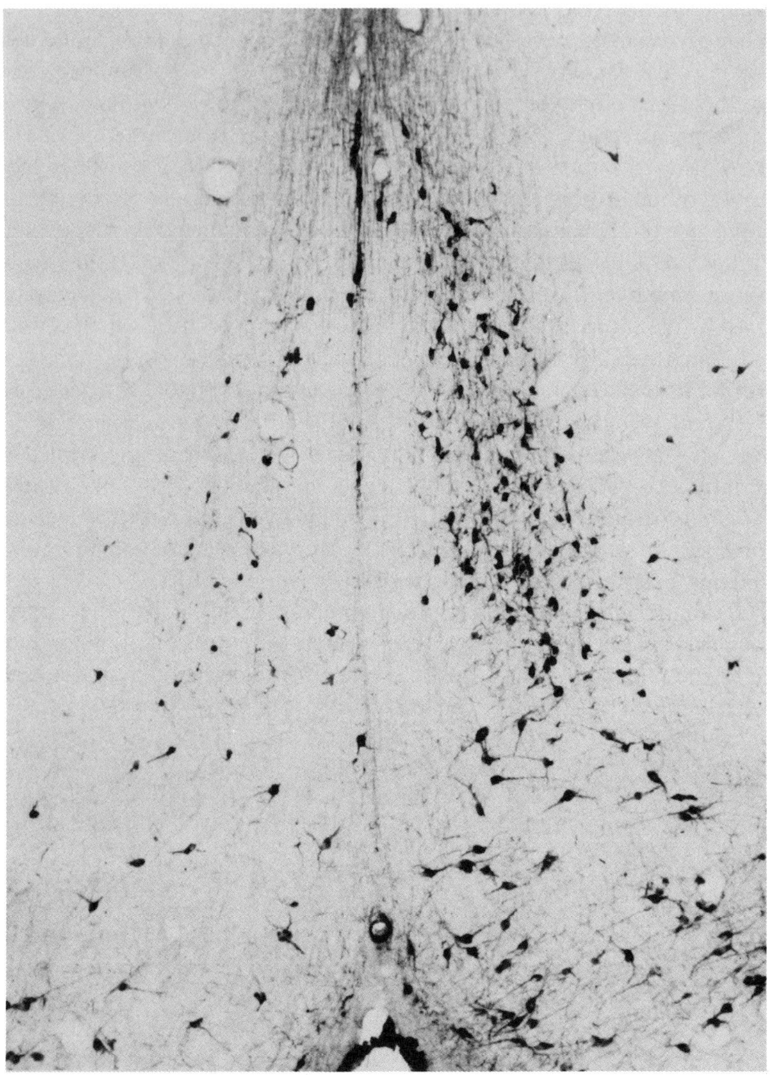

Fig. 13 The unilateral (left side) cell loss of cholinergic neurons in the rat medial septum which follows removal of the hippocampus is illustrated. Chronic application of exogenous gangliosides secured the survival of most cells (Table VI). Cholinergic neurons were defined by immunoreactivity toward a rat monoclonal antibody against ChAT (Eckenstein and Thoenen, 1982).

reflection of actual cell death or extreme cell shrinkage with diminished expression of antigenic sites remains to be resolved. In a unilateral hippocampal ablation model, the continuous administration of GM1 rendered a substantial protection in the numbers of identifiable cholinergic neurons of the medial septum (Sofroniew *et al.*, 1986) (see Table VI). This result is comparable to that ensuing from the intra-cerebroventricular (i.c.v.) administration of NGF in analogous situations (Hefti *et al.*, 1984; Williams *et al.*, 1986; Kromer, 1987). However, when lesions were more extensive, i.e., involving the fornix bilaterally, NGF but not GM1 protected the numbers of cholinergic neurons (Kromer, 1989). This could be explained by the concept that gangliosides require "permissive conditions" to exert reparative effects (see Section V,B,5). The severity of the lesion in the latter model may result in maximal retrograde damage because it occurs close to the cell body (for example, see Liu, 1955). The correlation between proximity of lesion to cell body location and retrograde cell damage has been confirmed specifically for the cholinergic septohippocampal projection (Sofroniew and Isacson, 1988).

In the NBM–cortex model, we also found that gangliosides were unable to prevent retrograde cholinergic damage if treatment were delayed for 10 days (a 2-day delay still allowed full protection) (Stephens *et al.*, 1987). In the same study using a treatment protocol which was effective for young or mature rats, we were unable to prevent NBM degeneration in lesioned aged rats (Stephens *et al.*, 1987).

Another example in which ganglioside treatment proved ineffective was after application of neurotoxins such as ethyl choline mustards and kainic acid. Of these toxins, ethyl choline mustard aziridinium ion (AF64-A) has been proposed

Table VI

Effects of Unilateral (Left) Hippocampal Removal and Ganglioside Administration, in Rats, on ChAT Immunoreactive Cell Numbers in the Medial Septum[a]

	ChAT immunoreactive cell number (mean ± SEM)		
Treatment	Ipsilateral	Contralateral	Difference (%)
Unoperated + vehicle	682.3 ± 41.3	687.3 ± 22.7	−0.7
Unoperated + GM1	647.7 ± 23.6	645.5 ± 36.6	+0.4
Lesioned + vehicle	170.0 ± 25.8	637.3 ± 45.8	−73.3*
Lesioned + GM1	639.0 ± 30.3	752.5 ± 20.6	−14.7

[a] From Sofroniew *et al.* (1986).
* $p < 0.001$.

as a selective cholinergic toxin (Fisher and Hanin, 1980), although in practice its specificity is very limited. In the hippocampal system, Johnson and collaborators (1988) were unable with GM1 to counteract the fall in ChAT activity and high affinity choline uptake subsequent to the i.c.v. administration of AF64-A. In our hands, chronic application of gangliosides i.p. did not prevent cholinergic damage resulting from the injection of kainic acid into the cerebral cortex (Stephens *et al.*, 1988). These findings are somewhat in contrast to the positive effects obtained with gangliosides following the use of neurotoxic agents which affect aminergic neurons, (see Sections V,A,1 and V,B,2,a). The contradictory results suggest that subsets of CNS neurons may possess markedly different regenerative capacities and thereby influence the "permissive conditions" for ganglioside protection. In favor of such a view, Johnson and colleagues (1988) found that even NGF was unable to protect cholinergic neurons after the application of neurotoxins, although vitamin E partially attenuated the deficits.

c. Neurotransmitter Release While most studies *in vivo* have concentrated on vital morphological and/or biochemical parameters in the systems analyzed, few studies have examined functional correlates. The ability of lesioned neurons to synthesize and release their transmitter(s) is of paramount importance. Addressing this issue, Florian and associates (1987) used the classical cortical cup technique to demonstrate that chronic administration of gangliosides to animals with unilateral electrolytic lesions of the NBM prevented the otherwise diminished ipsilateral output of ACh. Compensatory enhancement in ACh was also detected in the contralateral cortex. More recently, Maysinger and collaborators (1988) used microdialysis to record the output of ACh from contralateral and ipsilateral remaining neocortices in rats which had undergone extensive devascularizing lesions (see Section V,B,2,b) and were treated with either saline or GM1 (5 mg/kg/i.c.v.). In these studies, measurements of ACh levels in the cortical interstitial space during basal and high K^+ molarity conditions revealed that the evoked-to-basal ratio of transmitter release was enhanced in GM1-treated animals.

3. Nerve Growth Factor and Gangliosides in the CNS

More recently, our laboratory has initiated studies to compare the actions of NGF and gangliosides in the NBM–cortex model of cholinergic injury in order to examine whether these factors might act in a cooperative manner (Cuello *et al.*, 1987). In contrast to the *in vitro* studies (see Section IV), there was no direct evidence for interaction between these two factors *in vivo*. We have observed that the i.c.v. administration of NGF in doses of 12 μg/day for 7 days, commencing at the time of cortical lesioning, prevented the decrease of ChAT activity in the microdissected NBM after partial cortical infarction (Cuello *et al.*, 1987, 1989). In this model, the NGF protective effect was comparable to that obtained with the i.c.v. administration of GM1 alone (5 mg/kg/day) (Table VII). The combined administration of NGF and GM1 to the decorticated animals slightly increased ChAT activity above control levels in the ipsilateral NBM (Table VII). Immunocytochemical analysis revealed not only full protection of the cholinergic neurons from retrograde cell shrinkage and loss of neuritic extensions, but also an apparent increase in the number of ChAT-immunoreactive processes in the neuropil (see Fig. 14). In the aforementioned experiments, ChAT activity in the remaining ipsilateral cortex of lesioned untreated animals did not differ significantly from that of the unlesioned contralateral side. Treatment with either NGF or GM1 increased ChAT activity over control levels in the remainder of the ipsilateral cortex. Interestingly, their combined administration resulted in ChAT activity of the remaining ipsilateral neocortex increasing to over 200% of control values (Table VII). The notion that cooperative interactions may occur between NGF and sialogangliosides in this specific *in vivo* model was reinforced by observations noted in cortically lesioned animals which were treated with ineffective doses of GM1. Doses of GM1 (0.5 mg/kg/day/i.c.v./7 days) did not protect ipsilateral NBM cholinergic neurons (see Table VIII). These results concur with those obtained by Di Patre and collaborators (1989), who found that GM1 i.p. or NGF i.c.v. partially compensated for the anterograde losses of cortical choline uptake sites or ChAT activity after ibotenic acid lesions of the NBM. The combined use of NGF with GM1 (at effective or ineffective doses)

Table VII

Effect of β-NGF Administered in Combination with an Effective Dose of GM1[a] on ChAT Activity in the NBM and Cortex of Mature Rats[b,c]

		Ipsilateral NBM		Ipsilateral cortex	
Group	*n*[d]	ChAT activity[e]	Percentage of control	ChAT activity[e]	Percentage of control
Control	6	57.67 ± 3.86	—	35.81 ± 2.39	—
Lesion + vehicle	6	31.16 ± 3.17	54*	35.85 ± 1.74	100
Lesion + GM1	5	61.94 ± 6.55	107	50.70 ± 2.44	142*
Lesion + NGF	5	50.94 ± 3.75	88	47.63 ± 3.12	132*
Lesion + GM1 + NGF	5	69.41 ± 1.06	120*	84.82 ± 10.42	237*

[a] 5 mg/kg/day/7 days, beginning immediately post-operatively.
[b] Rats were sacrificed 30 days following unilateral decortication.
[c] From Cuello *et al.* (1989).
[d] *n* indicates number of cases.
[e] Values for ChAT activity are the mean ± SEM, and expressed as n*M* ACh/mg protein/hr.
* Significantly different from control at $p < 0.01$, ANOVA followed by a posthoc Dunnett's test.

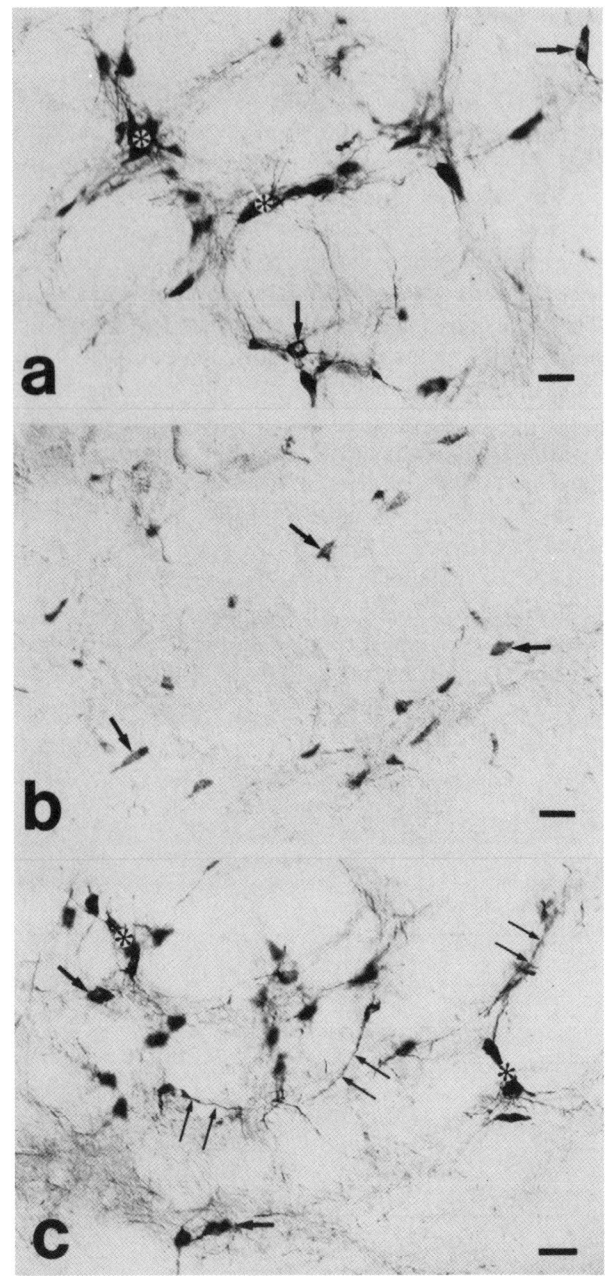

Fig. 14 Appearance of ChAT-immunoreactive neurons in NBM in control (a), lesioned (b), and lesioned, GM1/β-NGF-treated (c) rats. Clustered (asterisks) and isolated (arrows) cholinergic cell bodies are indicated. Thinner, paired arrows in *c* indicate immunoreactive processes. Note that cell shrinkage is prevented in factor-treated rats. Interference contrast optics; bar, 25 μm (Cuello *et al.*, 1989).

Table VIII

Effect of β-NGF Administered in Combination with an Ineffective Dose of GM1[a] on ChAT Activity in the NBM and Cortex of Mature Rats[b,c]

		Ipsilateral NBM		Ipsilateral cortex	
Group	*n*[d]	ChAT activity[e]	Percentage of control[f]	ChAT activity[e]	Percentage of control
Control	6	69.06 ± 4.67	—	39.20 ± 3.77	—
Lesion + vehicle	6	44.87 ± 6.60	65*	38.20 ± 4.69	97
Lesion + GM1	5	46.92 ± 2.80	68*	36.93 ± 2.80	94
Lesion + NGF	5	73.07 ± 3.30	109	59.06 ± 2.90	151*
Lesion + GM1 + NGF	5	83.87 ± 6.56	121*	72.98 ± 4.08	186*

[a] 0.5 mg/kg/day/7 days, beginning immediately post-operatively.
[b] Rats were sacrificed 30 days following unilateral decortication.
[c] From Cuello *et al.* (1989).
[d] *n* indicates number of cases.
[e] Values for ChAT activity are the mean ± SEM, and expressed as n*M* ACh/mg protein/hr.
* Significantly different from control at $p < 0.01$, ANOVA followed by a posthoc Dunnett's test.

potentiated NGF effects by restoring the two cholinergic markers to control levels.

4. Gangliosides in Cerebral Ischemia

Cerebral ischemia offers an opportunity for gangliosides to exert their putative reparative actions because there is no immediate neuronal loss in this pathology. This opportunity has been recognized clinically and, in fact, initial therapeutic trials using gangliosides in stroke patients have been undertaken, with some encouraging results (Bassi *et al.*, 1986; Battistin, 1987). As in the case for diabetic neuropathy, results from more extensive and well-controlled clinical trials are awaited.

Information on ganglioside effects in animal models of cerebral ischemia is rapidly accumulating. Karpiak and Mahadik (1984) and Cahn and co-workers (1986) agree that the application of gangliosides reduces the cerebral edema resulting from ischemia. It is this effect of GM1 or AGF2 which has been considered pivotal to the improved learning and retention in animals having suffered transient cerebral ischemia (Cahn *et al.*, 1986) or to the reduced mortality in animals suffering either focal or global ischemia (Karpiak *et al.*, 1987a,b, 1988). It has been speculated that these effects are due to the ability of gangliosides to insert into the plasma membranes, with resultant membrane stabilization and maintenance of Na^+,K^+-ATPase activity (Cahn *et al.*, 1986; Karpiak *et al.*, 1987a,b, 1988). Indeed, gangliosides have been shown to activate

ATPases directly (Caputto *et al.*, 1977; Leon *et al.*, 1981). Karpiak and coworkers (1988) found a significant loss in ATPase activity in homogenates from cortex and hippocampus of gerbils subjected to global ischemia. These losses were less evident in animals treated with AGF2 than those receiving GM1.

Focal ischemia in cats, produced by the transient occlusion of the middle cerebral artery, results in marked depression of electrocortical activity and changes in blood flow, glucose metabolism, and redox state. In this experimental model, a single dose of GM1 did not produce obvious beneficial short-term effects (Tanaka *et al.*, 1986). Hogan and colleagues (1988), using a novel rat model of cerebral ischemia based on the time-dependent clamping of the common carotid artery, also found no significant benefit when GM1 was applied immediately before insult, either in the extent of infarction or the degree of edema. These aforementioned conflicting results remain unresolved, although it should be noted that long-term effects of continuous ganglioside treatment merit examination. Some of these aspects have been more comprehensively reviewed by Karpiak and Mahadik (1989).

5. Permissive Conditions for *in Vivo* Reparative Effects of Gangliosides

It has become obvious that gangliosides require specific conditions to show their putative trophic effects *in vivo* or *in vitro*. These have been referred to as "permissive conditions" for the *in vivo* effects (Stephens *et al.*, 1987; Cuello *et al.*, 1989) or a "window of opportunity" for the *in vitro* effects (Varon *et al.*, 1986). It is conceivable that, under certain circumstances, the availability of endogenous trophic factors alters the ability of cells to respond to gangliosides. In the *in vivo* NBM cholinergic model, early initiation of ganglioside treatment is essential for the protection of the neurons (Stephens *et al.*, 1987). Thus, we have observed that a delay of 10 days renders gangliosides ineffective in preventing retrograde cholinergic degeneration (Stephens *et al.*, 1987). An analogous observation has been made for the anterograde degeneration of nigral dopaminergic neurons in the MPTP model (Hadjiconstantinou and Neff, 1988). These observations are consistent with findings that the injured brain produces endogenous trophic factors, but in low amounts, immediately after the insult (Nieto-Sampedro *et al.*, 1983). Therefore, in instances of extensive neural lesions, cells are likely to be in an extremely vulnerable state which could result in irreversible anterograde and retrograde cellular damage. In central cholinergic neurons, retrograde degenerative changes can be partially reversed with the timely administration of NGF (Hefti, 1986; Kromer, 1987; Williams *et al.*, 1986) as long as 21 days after injury (Hagg *et al.*, 1988). Therefore, it can be proposed that the *in vivo* administration of gangliosides prevents neuronal degeneration in the CNS cholinergic system by potentiating the actions of the low amounts of endogenous trophic factors produced in the first few days after a lesion. The lack of protection offered by exogenous gangliosides on cholinergic neurons in lesioned aged rats (Stephens *et al.*, 1987) can be explained in the same manner, since aging is accompanied by an apparent loss of NGF receptors (Koh and Loy, 1988) and a diminished production of endogenous factors after injury (Needles *et al.*, 1985). Another component of the "permissive conditions" which should be considered is the duration of ganglioside administration. In the cholinergic system, 7 days of i.c.v. administration of GM1 is adequate for protection against retrograde damage, the effect persisting at least 23 days beyond the cessation of treatment (Stephens *et al.*, 1987). However, a more prolonged treatment seems to be required for protection of cortical noradrenergic fibers affected by 6-OH-DA (Kojima *et al.*, 1984) and of dopaminergic neurons in the nigrostriatal system after MPTP lesioning (Hadjiconstantinou *et al.*, 1986; Hadjiconstantinou and Neff, 1988).

VI. Mechanisms of Actions

A. Gangliosides in Cell Receptor Mechanisms

Although many hypotheses have been advanced, the mechanism(s) of action through which gangliosides exert their protective or reparative effects remain(s) unclear. From the pharmacological viewpoint, one of the difficulties is that glycosphingolipids cannot, at least until now, be viewed in the orthodox context of drug–receptor interactions. One group, however, has proposed the existence of specific ganglioside receptors (Yasuda *et al.*, 1988). These authors employed classical ligand binding techniques using constructed protein–sugar complexes of which the sugar moiety is equivalent to that of the different gangliosides. The resultant complexes are referred to as "neoganglioproteins." When radiolabeled neoganglioproteins were incubated in the presence of immobilized rat brain membranes, a saturable binding was found in the nanomolar range which was displaced with different potencies by series of gangliosides. These results suggest that the primary biological effects of gangliosides depend on cell-to-cell interactions which would be mediated by the extramembranous component of the glycosphingolipid.

An important finding, in historical terms, is that membrane-bound gangliosides can themselves act as receptor molecules. Thus, gangliosides have been recognized as the prime binding target for a number of toxins, including cholera, tetanus (Van Heyningen, 1974), and botulinum (Kozaki *et al.*, 1984) toxins. In addition, Van Heyningen (1974) also proposed gangliosides as the receptor site for serotonin. Of these toxins, cholera toxin remains the best studied model for the role of membrane gangliosides as receptors (Cuatrecasas, 1973). For example, Fishman and colleagues (1978), and Fishman (1982) have proposed an elegant model for the internalization of the cholera toxin α-subunit. A number of glycoproteins, notably thyroid-stimulating hormone (TSH), are known to bind to a variety of gangliosides (Fishman and Brady, 1976). These findings suggest that gangliosides may act as a point of entry for molecular signals. In the context of neural repair, the receptor role of gangliosides could explain the activation or inhibition of cell growth through cell-to-cell recognition as well as the internalization of putative stimulatory or inhibitory trophic factors. In view of the above, clustering of surface GM1 by the β-subunit of cholera toxin can induce proliferation of thymocytes (Spiegel *et al.*, 1985) or bimodal (stimulatory or inhibitory) responses in the 3T3 fibroblast cell line (Spiegel and Fishman, 1987). The cholera toxin responses were found to depend on the state of growth of the cell line, such that stimulation of growth (and even potentiation of growth factor activity) occurred in quiescent, nontransformed cells, while growth was inhibited in a *ras*-transformed proliferating 3T3 cell line.

Whether gangliosides can effectively bind growth factors remains to be accurately determined. However, it is an attractive idea that endogenous as well as exogenous gangliosides (and glycosphingolipids in general) might modulate the state of receptors. The density and type of membrane gangliosides should influence membrane proteins and, in particular, their extracellular components. The membrane-bound gangliosides could in that manner alter receptor affinity, clustering, or internalization. These are hypothetical possibilities for trophic factor–ganglioside interactions. Moreover, Cheresh and collaborators, in a series of ingenious experiments, utilized the immunogold detection of gangliosides to show that the accumulation of GD2 ganglioside near the vitronectin receptor can alter the state of the receptor (Cheresh and Klier, 1986; Cheresh *et al.*, 1987). In turn, many of the ganglioside–receptor interactions or ganglioside–kinase interactions (see Section VI,C) may be affected by the ability of gangliosides to form complexes with Ca^{2+} (Rahman *et al.*, 1988).

B. Modulation of cAMP Levels

Some of the *in vitro* effects of gangliosides are apparently related to cAMP levels. In cortical membranes, gangliosides can elevate the activities of both adenylate cyclase and 3′,5′-cyclic nucleotide phosphodiesterase (Partington and Daly, 1979; Davis and Daly, 1980). By using extracts from rabbit sciatic nerve membranes. Yates and co-workers (1989) have recently found biochemical evidence that gangliosides can modulate cAMP levels by direct inhibition of cAMP kinase as well as via activation of phosphodiesterases. In relation to neural trauma, it remains to be seen how the modulation of cAMP levels is, if at all, related to ganglioside effects.

C. Modulation of the Activity of Protein Kinases

Another possibility is that glycosphingolipids in general, and gangliosides in particular, alter directly or indirectly the activities of protein kinases (PKs) which are crucial to cell repair. These interactions, which have been the subject of a recent review (Dawson and Vartanian, 1988) are illustrated in Fig. 15. Exogenous gangliosides stimulate in a calcium-dependent manner the phosphorylation of several proteins, in a pattern similar to that seen with calmodulin (Goldenring *et al.*, 1985). In this situation, it is not clear whether the ganglioside effects are due to the modulation of calmodulin or Ca^{2+}. Gangliosides have also been shown to inhibit protein phosphorylation of myelin basic protein (MBP), probably via a PK-C mechanism (Kim *et al.*, 1986). This inhibition did not take place when entire gangliosides were substituted with ceramide, the asialo-GM1 derivative, or NeuNAc. A potency rank order for these glycosphingolipids was as follows: GT1b > GD1b > GD1a > GM1 (Kim *et al.*, 1986). More direct evidence for an inhibitory influence on PK-C has been observed by using partially purified preparations of this PK from brain and nonneural cells (Kreutter *et al.*, 1986). Although the ganglioside modulatory effects on the degree of phosphorylation of MBP have been confirmed, whether this is PK-C dependent remains controversial (Chan, 1987). Needless to say, this field continues to evolve rapidly.

Some of the most compelling evidence for ganglioside modulation of PKs controlling growth activities comes from studies with nonneural cells. Bremer and Hakomori (1982) found that growth of a hamster fibroblast cell line (BHK) becomes refractory to the stimulatory effects of fibroblast growth factor (FGF) following preincubation with the ganglioside GM3 (Bremer and Hakomori,

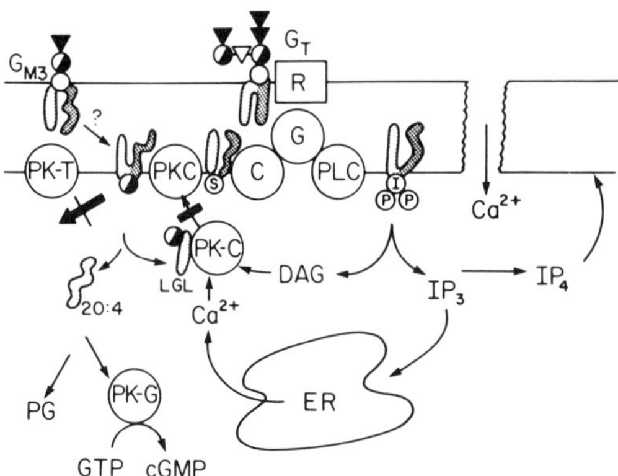

Fig. 15 Proposed scheme for gangliosides as modulators and source of second messengers. Glycosphingolipids generate lysoglycosphingolipids (LGL) to compete with diacylglycerol (DAG) for PK-C activation and 20 : 4 fatty acid to activate PK-G or generate prostanoids. R, Receptor protein; G, GTP binding protein; C, adenylate cyclase; PK-C, protein kinase C activated by diacylglycerol (DAG), calcium (Ca^{2+}), and phosphatidylserine (S); PK-T, tyrosine protein kinase inhibited by GM3 or lysoglycosphingolipid (LGL); IP_3, inositol-1,4,5 triphosphate; PK-G, cGMP-dependent kinase; 20 : 4, arachidonic acid; PG, prostanoids; ER, endoplasmic reticulum (Dawson and Vartanian, 1988).

1982). These effects were not dependent on a direct ganglioside–receptor interaction. The investigators also found that the increased affinity of the platelet-derived growth factor (PDGF) receptor to its ligand, which was induced by GM1 and GM3, paralleled the inhibition of PDGF-induced protein phosphorylation of the receptor protein (Bremer *et al.*, 1986). Similarly, gangliosides can decrease the EGF-stimulated phosphorylation of its receptor protein in epidermoid carcinoma cells without affecting receptor affinity. These effects may vary according to the micellar state of glycosphingolipids. This group has recently reported that sialyl paraglobosides, but not lacto- or ganglio- series glycosphingolipids, inhibited insulin-related cell growth and an associated receptor kinase (Hakomori, 1989).

Other studies have shown that the gangliosides GM1 and GT1b can inhibit the translocation and activation of PK-C evoked by glutamate in primary cultures of rat cerebellar granule cells. It has been suggested, therefore, that via this mechanism gangliosides may limit the neurotoxic actions of excitatory amino acids (Vaccarino *et al.*, 1987).

It should also be noted that at least some of the actions of gangliosides on PKs could be due to their metabolites. In particular, it has been seen that sphingosine can competitively displace diacyl glycerol or phorbol esters, thus preventing the formation of activated lipid–enzyme complexes (Hannun *et al.*, 1986).

D. Modulation of Trophic Factor Effects

Examples of ganglioside–trophic factor interactions have been discussed in the sections on ganglioside effects *in vitro* (Section IV,A) and *in vivo* (Section V,B,3). Ganglioside modulation of trophic factor effects can indeed take place with either positive or negative cooperativity for different sets of trophic substances, i.e., by influencing their corresponding receptor or any of the many secondary or tertiary mechanisms of cell signaling. Various examples of such possibilities have been discussed in Sections VI,A and C.

VII. Conclusions

Glycosphingolipids in general, and gangliosides in particular, are at present valuable and exciting research tools for the study of neural repair. Their mechanisms of action remain elusive. It is probable that they act in a specific, though multifactorial fashion. The combined application of molecular and cell biology methodologies to the *in vivo* models of neuronal injury and degeneration will provide the necessary clues to understanding their remarkable effects in experimental animals. Whether these compounds will find a wider therapeutic application in humans will depend on the research underway in a multitude of laboratories, as well as on the results of pilot clinical trials.

Acknowledgments

I would like to acknowledge the indefatigable secretarial expertise provided by Diane Leggett and word-processing assistance of Rosa Maria Greco. I would like to thank all members of my research group for sharing the excitement of investigating novel, pharmacological approaches to neural repair and especially my colleagues Erik P. Pioro and Lorella Garofalo for painstaking editing of the manuscript. Financial support from the Medical Research Council (Canada), Dean's Office, Faculty of Medicine (McGill University), FIDIA Research Laboratories (Italy), and Medicorp (Canada) is gratefully appreciated, as is the technical and photographic assistance from Sylvain Coté and Alan Forster. Finally, thanks go to Martha and Paula Cuello for their search for references. This review is dedicated to the memory of my father, Juan Andres Cuello Freyre.

References

Agnati, L. F., Fuxe, K., Benfenati, F., Battistini, N., Zini, I., and Toffano, G. (1983a). Chronic ganglioside treatment counteracts the biochemical signs of dopamine receptor supersensitivity induced by chronic haloperidol treatment. *Neurosci. Lett.* **40,** 293–297.

Agnati, L. F., Fuxe, K., Calza, L., Benfenati, F., Cavicchioli, L., Toffano, G., and Goldstein, M. (1983b). Gangliosides increase the survival of lesioned nigra dopamine neurons and favour the recovery of dopaminergic synaptic function in striatum of rats by collateral sprouting. *Acta Physiol. Scand.* **119,** 347–363.

Aguayo, A. J. (1985). Axonal regeneration from injured neurons in the adult mammalian central nervous system. *In* "Synaptic Plasticity" (C. W. Cotman, ed.), pp. 457–484. Guilford, Press, New York.

Aldino, C., Valenti, G., Savoini, G. E., Kirschner, G., Agnati, L. F., and Toffano, G. (1984). Monosialoganglioside internal ester stimulates the dopaminergic reinnervation of the striatum after unilateral hemitransection in rat. *J. Dev. Neurosci.* **2,** 267–275.

Appel, S. H. (1981). A unifying hypothesis for the cause of amyotrophic lateral sclerosis, Parkinsonism, and Alzheimer's disease. *Ann. Neurol.* **10,** 499–505.

Aquino, D. A., Bisby, M. A., and Ledeen, R. W. (1987). Bidirectional transport of gangliosides, glycoproteins and neutral glycosphingolipids in the sensory neurons of rat sciatic nerve. *Neuroscience* **20,** 1023–1029.

Arce, A., Maccioni, H. J. F., and Caputto, R. (1971). The biosynthesis of gangliosides. The incorporation of galactose, *N*-acetyl galactosamine and *N*-acetyl neuraminic acid into endogenous acceptors of subcellular particles from rat brain in vitro. *Biochem. J.* **121,** 483–493.

Baker, H. J., Lindsey, J. R., McKhann, G. M., and Farrell, P. F. (1971). Neuronal GM1 gangliosidosis in a siamese cat with β-galactosidase deficiency. *Science* **174,** 838–839.

Baker, H. J., Mole, J. A., Lindsey, J. R., and Creel, R. M. (1976). Animal models of human ganglioside and storage diseases. *Fed. Proc., Fed. Am. Soc. Exp. Biol.* **35,** 1193–1201.

Ballard, P. A., Tetrud, J. W., and Langstron, J. W. (1985). Permanent human Parkinsonism due to 1-methyl-4-phenyl-1,2,3,6-tetra-hydropyridine (MPTP): Seven cases. *Neurology* **35,** 949–956.

Bassi, S., Albizzati, M., Sbacchi, M., Grattola, L., and Massarotti, M. (1986). Subacute phase of stroke treated with ganglioside GM1. *In* "Gangliosides and Neuronal Plasticity" (G. Tettamanti, R. W. Ledeen, K. Sandhoff, Y. Nagai, and G. Toffano, eds.), pp. 461–464. Liviana Press, Padova/Springer-Verlag, Berlin.

Basu, S., Kaufman, B., and Roseman, S. (1973). Enzymatic synthesis of glucocerebroside by a glucosyltransferase from embryonic chicken brain. *J. Biol. Chem.* **248,** 1388–1394.

Battistin, L. (1987). A double bind evaluation of the effects of GM1-ganglioside in the subacute phase of cerebrovascular diseases. *In* "Neuroplasticity: A New Therapeutic Tool in the CNS Pathology" (R. L. Masland, A. Portera-Sanchez, and G. Toffano, eds.), Vol. 12. Liviana Press, Padova.

Bignami, A., Eng, L. F., Dahl, D., and Uyeda, C. T. (1972). Localization of the glial fibrillary acid protein in astrocytes by immunofluorescence. *Brain Res.* **43,** 429–435.

Björklund, A., and Stenevi, U. (1979). Regeneration of monoaminergic and cholinergic neurons in the mammalian central nervous system. *Physiol. Rev.* **59,** 62–100.

Björklund, A., Brundin, P., and Isacson, O. (1988). Neuronal replacement by intracerebral neural implants in animal models of neurodegenerative disease. *Adv. Neurol.* **47.**

Bowen, D. M., Smith, C. B., White, P., and Davidson, A. N. (1976). Neurotransmitter-related enzymes and indices of hypoxia in senile dementia and other abiotrophies. *Brain* **99,** 459–496.

Brady, R. O., and Barranger, J. A. (1981). Inborn lysosomal enzyme deficiencies. *In* "The Molecular Basis of Neuropathology" (Davison and R. H. S. Thompson, eds.), pp. 188–220. Edward Arnold, London.

Bremer, E. G., and Hakomori, S.-I. (1982). GM3 ganglioside induces hamster fibroblast growth inhibition in chemically-defined medium: Ganglioside may modulate growth factor receptor function. *Biochem. Biophys. Res. Commun.* **106,** 711–718.

Bremer, E. G., Schlessinger, J., and Hakomori, S.-I. (1986). Ganglioside-mediated modulation of cell growth. *J. Biol. Chem.* **261,** 2434–2440.

Burns, S. P., Chiueh, C. C., Markey, S. P., Ebert, M. H., Jacobowitz, D. M., and Kopin, I. J. (1983). A primate model of Parkinsonism: Selective destruction of dopaminergic neurons in the pars compacta of the substantia nigra by *N*-methyl-1,2,3,6-tetrahydropyridine. *Proc. Natl. Acad. Sci. U.S.A.* **80,** 4546–4550.

Byrne, M. C., Ledeen, R. W., Roisen, F. J., Yorke, G., and Sclafani, J. R. (1983). Ganglioside-induced neuritogenesis: Verification that gangliosides are the active agents, and comparison of molecular species. *J. Neurochem.* **41**(5), 1214–1222.

Caccia, M. F., Meola, G., Cerri, C., Frattola, L., Scarlato, G., and Aporti, F. (1979). Treatment of denervated muscle by gangliosides. *Muscle & Nerve* **2,** 382–389.

Cahn, J., Borzeix, M. G., and Toffano, G. (1986). Effect of GM1 ganglioside and of its inner ester derivative in a model of transient ischemia in the rat. *In* "Gangliosides and Neuronal Plasticity" (G. Tettamanti, R. W. Ledeen, K. Sandhoff, Y. Nagai, and G. Toffano, eds.), pp. 435–444. Liviana Press, Padova/Springer-Verlag, Berlin.

Caputto, R., Maccioni, H. J., Arce, A., and Cumar, R. F. A. (1976). Biosynthesis of brain gangliosides. *Adv. Exp. Med. Biol.* **71,** 27–44.

Caputto, R., Maccioni, A. H. R., and Caputto, B. I. (1977). Activation of deoxycholate solubilized adenosine triphosphatase by ganglioside and asialoganglioside preparations. *Biochem. Biophys. Res. Commun.* **74,** 1046–1052.

Carmignoto, G., Finesso, M., Siliprandi, R., and Gorio, A. (1983). Muscle reinnervation. I. Restoration of transmitter release mechanisms. *Neuroscience* **8,** 393–401.

Casamenti, F., Bracco, L., Bartolini, L., and Pepeu, G. (1985). Effects of ganglioside treatment in rats with a lesion of the cholinergic forebrain nuclei. *Brain Res.* **338,** 45–52.

Ceccarelli, B., Aporti, F., and Finesso, M. (1976). Effects of brain gangliosides on functional recovery in experimental regeneration and reinnervation. *In* "Ganglioside Function" (G. Porcellati, B. Ceccarelli, and G. Tettamanti, eds.), pp. 275–293. Plenum, New York.

Chen, K. F. J. (1987). Ganglioside-modulated protein phosphorylation in myelin. *J. Biol. Chem.* **262,** 2415–2422.

Cheramy, A., Leviel, V., and Glowinski, J. (1981). Dendritic release of dopamine in the substantia nigra. *Nature (London)* **289,** 537–542.

Cheresh, D. A., and Klier, F. G. (1986). Disialoganglioside GD2 distributes preferentially into substrate-associated microprocesses on human melanoma cells during their attachment to fibronectin. *J. Cell Biol.* **102,** 1887–1897.

Cheresh, D. A., Pytela, R., Pierschbacher, M. D., Klier, F. G., Ruoslahti, E., and Reisfeld, R. A. (1987). An Arg-Gly-Asp-directed receptor on the surface of human melanoma cells exists in a divalent cation-dependent functional complex with the disialoganglioside GD2. *J. Cell Biol.* **105,** 1160–1173.

Cohen, S. (1962). Isolation of a mouse submaxillary gland protein accelerating incisor eruption and eyelid opening in the newborn animal. *J. Biol. Chem.* **237,** 1555–1562.

Consolazione, A., and Toffano, G. (1988). Ganglioside role in functional recovery of damaged nervous system. *In* "New Trends in Ganglioside Research" (R. W. Ledeen, E. L. Hogan, G. Tettamanti, A. J. Yates, and R. K. Yu, eds.), pp. 523–533. Liviana Press, Padova; Springer–Verlag, Berlin.

Crome, L., and Stern, J. (1981). Inborn lysosomal enzyme deficiencies. *In* "Grenfield's Neuropathology" (W. Blackwood and J. N. Corsellis, eds.), 3rd ed., pp. 500–580. Edward Arnold, London.

Cuatrecasas, P. (1973). Gangliosides and membrane receptors for cholera toxin. *Biochemistry* **12,** 3558–3566.

Cuello, A. C., and Iversen, L. L. (1978). Interactions of dopamine with other neurotransmitters in the rat substantia nigra: A possible functional role of dendritic dopamine. *In* "Interactions between Putative Neurotransmitters in the Brain" (S. Garattinni, J. F. Pujol, and S. Samanin, eds.), pp. 127–147. Raven Press, New York.

Cuello, A. C., Stephens, P. H., Tagari, P. C., Sofroniew, M. V., and Pearson, R. C. A. (1986). Retrograde changes in the nucleus basalis of the rat, caused by cortical damage, are prevented by exogenous ganglioside GM1. *Brain Res.* **376,** 373–377.

Cuello, A. C., Maysinger, D., Garofalo, L., Tagari, P., Stephens, P. H., Pioro, E., and Piotte, M. (1987). Influence of gangliosides and nerve growth factor on plasticity of forebrain cholinergic neurons. *In* "Receptor-Receptor Interactions 1987" (K. Fuxe and L. F. Agnati, eds.), pp. 62–77. Macmillan, London.

Cuello, A. C., Garofalo, L., Kenigsberg, R. L., and Maysinger, D. (1989). Gangliosides potentiate *in vivo* and *in vitro* effects of nerve growth factor on central cholinergic neurons. *Proc. Natl. Acad. Sci. U.S.A.* **86,** 2056–2060.

Davies, P., and Maloney, A. J. F. (1976). Selective loss of central cholinergic neurons in Alzheimer's disease. *Lancet* **2,** 1403.

Davis, C. W., and Daly, J. W. (1980). Activation of rat cerebral cortical 3′,5′-cyclic nucleotide phosphodiesterase activity by gangliosides. *Mol. Pharmacol.* **17,** 206–211.

Dawson, G., and Vartanian, T. (1988). Glycolipids as the source and modulator of receptor-mediated second messengers. *In* "New Trends in Ganglioside Research" (R. W. Ledeen, E. L. Hogan, G. Tettamanti, A. J. Yates, and R. K. Yu, eds.), pp. 219–228. Liviana Press, Padova/Springer-Verlag, Berlin.

de Baecque, C. M., Duzuki, K., Rapin, I., Johnson, A. B., Whethers, D. L., and Suzuki, K. (1975). G_{M2}-gangliosidosis, AB variant: Clinico-pathological study of case. *Acta Neuropathol.* **33,** 207–226.

Dimpfel, W., Moller, W., and Mengs, O. (1981). Ganglioside-induced neurite formation in cultured neuroblastoma cells. *In* "Gangliosides in Neurological and Neuromuscular Function, Development and Repair" (M. Rapport and A. Gorio, eds.), Raven Press, New York.

Di Patre, P. L., Casamenti, F., Cenni, A., and Pepeu, G. (1989). Interaction between nerve growth factor and GM1 monosialoganglioside in preventing cortical choline acetyltransferase and high affinity choline uptake decrease after lesion of the nucleus basalis. *Brain Res.* **480,** 219–224.

Dodd, J., and Jessell, T. M. (1985). Lactoseries carboydrates specify subsets of dorsal root ganglion neurons projecting to the superficial dorsal horn of rat spinal cord. *J. Neurosci.* **5,** 3278–3294.

Doherty, P., and Walsh, F. S. (1987). Ganglioside GM_1 antibodies and B-cholera toxin bind specifically to embryonic chick dorsal root ganglion neurons but do not modulate neurite regeneration. *J. Neurochem.* **48,** 1237–1244.

Doherty, P., Dickson, J. G., Flanigan, T. P., and Walsh, F. S. (1985). Ganglioside GM1 does not initiate, but enhances neurite regeneration of nerve growth factor-dependent sensory neurones. *J. Neurochem.* **44,** 259–1265.

Drabkin, D. L. (1958). "Thudichum Chemist of the Brain." Univ. of Pennsylvania Press, Philadelphia.

Dunnett, S. B., Toniolo, G., Fine, A., Ryan, C. N., Björklund, A., and Iversen, S. D. (1985). Transplantation of embryonic ventral forebrain neurons to the neocortex of rats with lesions of nucleus basalis magnocellularis—II. Sensorimotor and learning impairments. *Neuroscience* **16,** 787–797.

Eckenstein, G., and Thoenen, H. (1982). Production of specific antisera and monoclonal antibodies in choline acetyltransferase. Characterization and use for identification of cholinergic neurons. *EMBO J.* **1,** 363–368.

Elliott, P., Garofalo, L., and Cuello, A. C. (1989). Limited neocortical devascularizing lesions causing deficits in memory retention and choline acetyltransferase activity—effects of the monosialoganglioside GM1. *Neuroscience* **31,** 63–76.

Facci, L., Leon, A., Toffano, G., Sonnino, S., Ghidoni, R., and Tettamanti, G. (1984). Promotion of neuritogenesis in mouse neuroblastoma cells by exogenous gangliosides. Relationship between the effect and the cell association of ganglioside GM1. *J. Neurochem.* **42,** 299–305.

Fass, B., and Ramirez, J. (1984). Effects of ganglioside treatments on lesion-induced behavioral impairment and sprouting in the CNS. *J. Neurosci. Res.* **12,** 445–458.

Ferrari, G., Fabris, M., and Gorio, A. (1983). Gangliosides enhance neurite outgrowth in PC12 cells. *Dev. Brain Res.* **8,** 215–22.

Ferrari, G., Soranzo, C., Callegaro, L., DalToso, R., Benvegnu, D., Toffano, G., and Leon, A. (1988). Characterization and purification of a striatal-derived neuronotrophic factor (SDNF). *In* "Neuronal Plasticity and Trophic Factors (Fidia Research Series, Symposia in Neuroscience VII)" (G. Biggio, P. F. Spano, G. Toffano, S. H. Appel, and G. L. Gessa, eds.), pp. 87–103. Liviana Press, Padova.

Ferretti, P., and Borroni, E. (1986). Putative cholinergic-specific gangliosides in guinea pig forebrain. *J. Neurochem.* **46,** 1888–1894.

Fine, A., Dunnett, S. B., Bjorklund, A., Clarke, D., and Iversen, S. D. (1985). Cholinergic ventral forebrain grafts into the neocortex improve passive avoidance memory in a rat model of Alzheimer's disease. *Proc. Natl. Acad. Sci. U.S.A.* **82,** 5227–5230.

Fisher, A., and Hanin, I. (1980). Minireview: Choline analogs as potential tools in developing selective animal models of central cholinergic hypofunction. *Life Sci.* **27,** 1615–1634.

Fishman, P. H. (1982). Role of membrane gangliosides in the binding and action of bacterial toxins. *J. Membr. Biol.* **69,** 85–97.

Fishman, P. H., and Brady, R. O. (1976). Biosynthesis and function of gangliosides. *Science* **194,** 906–915.

Fishman, P. H., Moss, J., and Osborne, J. C., Jr. (1978). Interaction of choleragen with the oligosaccharide of ganglioside GM1. Evidence for multiple oligosaccharide binding sites. *Biochemistry* **17,** 711–716.

Flicker, C., Dean, R. L., Watkins, D. L., Fisher, S. K., and Bartus, R. T. (1983). Behavioral and neurochemical effects following neurotoxic lesions of a major cholinergic input to the cerebral cortex in the rat. *Pharmacol., Biochem. Behav.* **18,** 973–981.

Florian, A., Casamenti, F., and Pepeu, G. (1987). Recovery of cortical acetylcholine output after ganglioside treatment in rats with lesion of the nucleus basalis. *Neurosci. Lett.* **75,** 313–316.

Freed, W. J. (1985). GM1 ganglioside does not stimulate reinnervation of the striatum by substantia nigra grafts. *Brain Res. Bull.* **14,** 91–95.

Geffen, L. B., Jessell, T. , Cuello, A. C., and Iversen, L. L. (1976). Release of dopamine from dendrites in rat substantia nigra. *Nature (London)* **260,** 358–360.

Gilad, G. M., and Reis, D. J. (1979). Collateral sprouting in cerebral mesolimbic dopamine neurons:

Biochemical and immunocytochemical evidence of changes in the activity and distribution of tyrosine hydroxylase in terminal fields and in cell bodies. *Brain Res.* **160,** 17–36.

Goins, B., Masserini, M., Barisas, B. G., and Freire, E. (1986). Lateral diffusion of ganglioside G_{M1} in phospholipid bilayer membranes. *Biophys. J.* **49,** 849–856.

Goldenring, J. R., Otis, L. C., Yu, R. K., and DeLorenzo, R. J. (1985). Calcium/ganglioside-dependent protein kinase activity in rat membrane. *J. Neurochem.* **44,** 1229–1234.

Gorio, A., Carmignoto, G., Facci, L., and Finesso, M. (1980). Motor nerve sprouting induced by ganglioside treatment. Possible implications for gangliosides in neuronal growth. *Brain Res.* **197,** 236–241.

Gorio, A., Carmignoto, G., Finesso, M., Polato, P., and Nunzi, M. G. (1983a). Muscle reinnervation. II. Sprouting, synapse formation and repression. *Neuroscience* **8,** 403–416.

Gorio, A., Marini, P., and Zanoni, R. (1983b). Muscle reinnervation. III. Motoneuron sprouting capacity, enhancement by exogenous gangliosides. *Neuroscience* **8,** 417–429.

Gorio, A., Di Giulio, A. M., Young, W., Gruner, J., Blight, A., De Crescito, V., Dona, M., Lazzaro, A., Figliomeni, B., Fusco, M., Hallman, H., Jonsson, G., Panozzo, C., Zanoni, R., and Vantini, G. (1986). GM1 effects on chemical traumatic and peripheral nerve induced lesions to the spinal cord. *In* "Development and Plasticity of the Mammalian Spinal Cord" (M. Goldberger, A. Gorio, and M. Murray, eds.), pp. 281–296. Liviana Press, Padova.

Gradkowska, M., Skup, M., Kiedrowski, L., Clzolari, S., and Oderfeld-Nowak, B. (1986). The effect of GM1 ganglioside on cholinergic and serotoninergic system in the rat hippocampus following partial denervation is dependent on the degree of fiber degeneration. *Brain Res.* **375,** 417–422.

Groves, P. M., Wilson, C. J., Young, S. J., and Rebec, G. V. (1975). Self-inhibition by dopaminergic neurones. *Science* **190,** 552–529.

Hadjiconstantinou, M., and Neff, N. A. (1988). Treatment with GM1 ganglioside restores striatal dopamine in the 1-methyl-4-phenyl-1,2,3,6-tetrahydropyridine treated mouse. *J. Neurochem.* **51,** 1190–1196.

Hadjiconstantinou, M., Rossetti, Z. L., Pazton, R. C., and Neff, N. H. (1986). Administration of GM1 ganglioside restores the dopamine content in striatum after chronic treatment with MPTP. *Neuropharmacology* **25,** 1075–1077.

Hagg, T., Manthorpe, M., Vahlsing, H. L., and Varon, S. (1988). Delayed treatment with NGF reverses the apparent loss of cholinergic neurons after acute brain damage. *Exp. Neurol.* **101,** 303–312.

Hakomori, S. (1986). Glycosphingolipids. *Sci. Am.* **254,** 44–53.

Hakomori, S. (1989). Glycosphingolipids as modulators of growth factor receptors. *In* "Trophic Factors and the Nervous System," Satellite to the 20th Annual Meeting of the American Society for Neurochemistry, Abstr., p. 11.

Hannun, Y. A., Loomis, C. R., and Bell, R. L. (1986). Protein kinase C activation in mixed micelles. Mechanistic implications of phospholipids, diacylglycerol and calcium interdependencies. *J. Biol. Chem.* **261,** 7184–7190.

Hatanaka, H., and Tsukui, H. (1986). Differential effects of nerve-growth factor and glioma-conditioned medium on neurons cultured from various regions of fetal rat central nervous system. *Dev. Brain Res.* **30,** 47–56.

Hefti, F. (1983). Is Alzheimer's disease caused by a lack of nerve growth factor? *Ann. Neurol.* **13,** 109–110.

Hefti, F. (1986). Nerve growth factor promotes survival of septal cholinergic neurons after fimbrial transections. *J. Neurosci.* **6,** 2155–2162.

Hefti, F., Dravid, A., and Hartikka, J. (1984). Chronic intraventricular injections of NGF elevate hippocampal ChAT activity in adult rats with partial septo-hippocampal lesions. *Brain Res.* **293,** 305–311.

Hefti, F., Hartikka, J., and Frick, W. (1985a). Gangliosides alter morphology and growth of astrocytes and increase the activity of choline acetyltransferase in cultures of dissociated septal cells. *J. Neurosci.* **5,** 2086–2094.

Hefti, F., Hartikka, J., Eckenstein, F., Gnahn, H., Heumann, R., and Schwab, M. E. (1985b). Nerve growth factor increases choline acetyltransferase but not survival or fibre outgrowth of cultured foetal septal cholinergic neurones. *Neuroscience* **14,** 55–68.

Hefti, F., Hartikka, J., and Knusel, B. (1989). Function of neurotrophic factors in the adult and aging brain and their possible use in the treatment of neurodegenerative diseases. *Neurobiol. Aging* **10,** 515–533.

Heikkila, R. E., Hess, A., and Duvoisin, R. C. (1984). Dopaminergic neurotoxicity of 1-methyl-4-phenyl-1,2,5,6-tetrahydropyridine in mice. *Science* **224,** 1451–1453.

Hogan, E. L., Hsu, C. Y., Liu, T. H., Leskawa, K. C., Xu, J., and Dasgupta, S. (1988). Ganglioside modification of nervous system disease. *In* "New Trends in Ganglioside Research" (R. W. Ledeen, E. L. Hogan, G. Tettamanti, A. J. Yates, and R. K. Yu, eds.), pp. 647–654. Liviana Press, Padova/Springer-Verlag, Berlin.

Horowitz, S. H. (1986). Ganglioside therapy in diabetic neuropathy. *Muscle & Nerve* **9,** 531–536.

Ilyas, A. A., Quarles, R. H., Dalakas, M. C., and Brady, R. O. (1985a). Polyneuropathy with monoclonal gammopathy: Glycoplipids are frequently antigens for IgM paraproteins. *Proc. Natl. Acad. Sci. U.S.A.* **82,** 6697–6700.

Ilyas, A. A., Quarles, R. H., Dalakas, M. C., Fishman, P. H., and Brady, R. O. (1985b). Monoclonal IgM in a patient with paraproteinemic polyneuropathy binds to gangliosides containing disalosyl groups. *Ann. Neurol.* **18,** 655–659.

Ilyas, A. A., Willison, H. J., Quarles, R. H., Jungalwala, F. B., Cornblath, D. R., Trapp, B. D., Griffin, D. E., Griffin, J. W., and McKhann, G. M. (1988). Serum antibodies to gangliosides in Guillain-Barre syndrome. *Ann. Neurol.* **23,** 440–447.

Jancso, G., Kiraly, E., and Jancso-Gabor, A. (1977). Pharmacologically induced selective degeneration of chemisensitive primary sensory neurons. *Nature (London)* **270,** 741–743.

Jessell, T. M., Iversen, L. L., and Cuello, A. C. (1978). Capsaicin-induced depletion of substance P from primary sensory neurones. *Brain Res.* **152,** 183–188.

Johnson, G. V. W., Simonato, M., and Jope, R. S. (1988). Dose- and time-dependent hippocampal cholinergic lesions induced by ethylcholine mustard aziridinium ion: Effects of nerve growth factor, GM_1 ganglioside, and vitamin E. *Neurochem. Res.* **13,** 685–692.

Johnston, M. V., McKinney, M., and Coyle, J. T. (1981). Neocortical cholinergic innervation: A description of extrinsic and intrinsic components in the rat. *Brain Res.* **43,** 159–172.

Jonsson, G., Gorio, A., Hallman, H., Kojima, H., Janigro, D., Luthman, J., and Zanoni, R. (1984). Effects of GM_1 ganglioside on developing and mature serotonin and noradraline neurons lesioned by selective neurotoxins. *J. Neurosci. Res.* **12**(2–3), 459–476.

Karpiak, S. E. (1983). Ganglioside treatment improves recovery of alteration behavior after unilateral entorhinal cortical lesion. *Exp. Neurol.* **81,** 330–339.

Karpiak, S. E., and Mahadik, S. P. (1984). Reduction of cerebral edema with GM1 ganglioside. *J. Neurosci. Res.* **12,** 485–492.

Karpiak, S. E., and Mahadik, S. P. (1990). Ganglioside reduction of CNS ischemic injury. *CRC Crit. Rev. Neurobiol.* (in press).

Karpiak, S. E., Li, Y. S., and Mahadik, S. P. (1987a). Gangliosides (GM1 & AGF2) reduce mortality due to ischemia. *Stroke* **18,** 184–187.

Karpiak, S. E., Li, Y. S., and Mahadik, S. P. (1987b). Ganglioside treatment: Reduction of CNS injury and facilitation of functional recovery. *Brain Injury* **1,** 141–170.

Karpiak, S. E., Li, Y. S., and Mahadik, S. P. (1988). Ischemic injury reduced by GM1 ganglioside. *In* "New Trends in Ganglioside Research" (R. W. Ledeen, E. L. Hogan, G. Tettamanti, A. J. Yates, and R. K. Yu, eds.), pp. 549–556. Liviana Press, Padova/Springer-Verlag, Berlin.

Katoh-Semba, R., Skaper, S. D., and Varon, S. (1984). Interaction of GM1 ganglioside with PC12 pheochromocytoma cells: Serum and NGF-dependent effects on neuritic growth (and proliferation). *J. Neurosci. Res.* **12,** 299–310.

Kim, J. Y. H., Goldenring, J. R., DeLorenzo, R. J., and Yu, R. K. (1986). Gangliosides inhibit phospholipid-sensitive Ca^{2+} dependent kinase phosphorylation of rat myelin basic proteins. *J. Neurosci. Res.* **15,** 159–166.

Kleinebeckel, D. (1982). Acceleration of muscle reinnervation in rats by ganglioside treatment: An electromyographic study. *Eur. J. Pharmacol.* **80,** 243–245.

Koh, S., and Loy, R. (1988). Age-related loss of nerve growth factor sensitivity in rat basal forebrain neurons. *Brain Res.* **440,** 396–401.

Kojima, H., Gorio, A., Janigro, D., and Jonsson, G. (1984). GM1 ganglioside enhances regrowth of noradrenaline nerve terminals in rat cerebral cortex lesioned by the neurotoxin 6-hydroxydopamine. *Neuroscience* **13,** 1011–1022.

Korf, J., Zieleman, M., and Westerink, B. H. G. (1976). Dopamine release in substantia nigra? *Nature (London)* **260,** 257.

Korsching, S., Auberger, G., Heumann, R., Scott, J., and Thoenen, H. (1985). Levels of nerve growth factor and its messenger RNA in the central nervous system of the rat correlate with cholinergic innervations. EMBO J. **4,** 1389–1393.

Kozaki, S., Sakaguchi, G., Nishimura, M., Iwamori, M., and Nagai, Y. (1984). Inhibitory effect of ganglioside GT1b on the activities of *Clostridium botulinum* toxins. *FEMS Microbiol. Lett.* **21,** 219–223.

Kreutter, D., Kim, J. Y. H., Goldenring, J. R., Rasmussen, H., Ukomadu, C., DeLorenzo, R. J., and Yu, R. K. (1986). Regulation of protein kinase C activity by gangliosides. *J. Biol. Chem.* **262,** 1633–1637.

Kromer, L. F. (1987). Nerve growth factor treatment after brain injury prevents neuronal death. *Science* **235,** 214–216.

Kromer, L. F. (1989). Effects of nerve growth factor, fibroblast growth factor, and GM1 ganglioside on the survival of axotomized septal cholinergic neurons. *In* "Molecular and Cellular Mechanisms of Neuronal Plasticity in Aging and Alzheimer's Disease." National Institute on Aging.

Lang, W. (1981). Pharmacokinetic studies with ^{3}H-labeled exogenous gangliosides injected intramuscularly into rats. *In* "Gangliosides in Neurological and Neuromuscular Function, Development and Repair" (M. Rapport and A. Gorio, eds.), pp. 241–252. Raven Press, New York.

Langston, J. W., Ballar, P., Tetrud, J. W., and Irwin, I. (1983). Chronic Parkinsonism in humans due to a product of meperidine-analog synthesis. *Science* **219,** 979–980.

Langston, J. W., Irwin, I., Langston, E. B., and Forno, L. S. (1984). Pargyline prevents MPTP-induced Parkinsonism in primates. *Science* **225,** 1480–1482.

Latov, N., Hays, A. P., Donofrio, P. D., Liao, J., Ito, H., McGinnis, S., Manoussos, K., Freddo, L., Shy, M. E., Sherman, W. H., Chang, H. W., Greenberg, H. S., Albers, J. W., Alessi, A. G., Keren, D., Yu, R. K., Rowland, L. P., and Kabat, E. A. (1988). Monoclonal IgM with unique specificity to gangliosides GM_1 and GD_{1b} and to lacto-*N*-tetraose associated with human motor neuron disease. *Neurology* **38,** 763–768.

Lehman, J., Nagy, J. I., Almadja, S., and Fibiger, H. C. (1982). The nucleus basalis magnocellularis; the origin of a cholinergic projection to the neocortex in the rat. *Neuroscience* **5,** 1161–1174.

Leon, A., Facci, L., Toffano, G., Sonnino, S., and Tettamanti, G. (1981). Activation of (Na^+,K^+)-ATPase by nanomolar concentrations of GM1 ganglioside. *J. Neurochem.* **37,** 350–357.

Leon, A., Facci, L., Benvegnu, D., and Toffano, G. (1982). Morphological and biochemical effects of gangliosides in neuroblastoma cells. *Dev. Neurosci.* **5,** 108–114.

Levi-Montalcini, R., and Aloe, R. (1985). Differentiating effects of murine nerve growth factor in the peripheral and central nervous system of Xenopus laevis tadpoles. *Proc. Natl. Acad. Sci. U.S.A.* **82,** 7111–7115.

Levi-Montalcini, R., and Calissano, P. (1986). Nerve growth factor as a paradigm for other polypeptide growth factors. *Trends Neurosci.* **9,** 473–477.

Liu, C.-N. (1955). Time pattern in retrograde degeneration after trauma of central nervous system of mammals. *In* "Regeneration in the Central Nervous System" (W. F. Windle, ed.), pp. 84–93. Thomas, Springfield, Illinois.

Maggio, B., Monferran, C. G., Montich, G. G., and Bianco, I. D. (1988). Effect of gangliosides and related glycosphingolipids on the molecular organization and physical properties of lipid–protein systems. *In* "New Trends in Ganglioside Research" (R. W. Ledeen, E. L. Hogan, G. Tattamanti, A. J. Yates, and R. K. Yu, eds.), pp. 105–120. Liviana Press, Padova/Springer-Verlag, Berlin.

Maier, C. E., and Singer, M. (1984). Gangliosides stimulate protein synthesis, growth and axon number of regenerating limb bud. *J. Comp. Neurol.* **230,** 459–464.

Marini, P., Vitadello, M., Bianchi, R., Triban, C., and Gorio, A. (1986). Impaired axonal transport of acetylcholinesterase in the sciatic nerve of alloxan-diabetic rats: Effect of ganglioside treatment. *Diabetologia* **29,** 154–258.

Maysinger, D., Herrera-Marschitz, M., Carlsson, A., Garofalo, L., Cuello, A. C., and Ungerstedt, U. (1988). Striatal and cortical acetylcholine release in vivo in rats with unilateral decortication: Effects of treatment with monosialoganglioside GM1. *Brain Res.* **461,** 355–360.

Maysinger, D., Garofalo, L., Jalsenjak, I., and Cuello, A. C. (1989). Effects of microencapsulated monosialoganglioside GM1 on cholinergic neurons. *Brain Res.* **496,** 165–172.

Menessini Chen, M. G., Chen, J. S., Calissano, P., and Levi-Montalcini, R. (1977). Nerve growth factor prevents vinblastine destructive effects on sympathetic ganglia in newborn mice. *Proc. Natl. Acad. Sci. U.S.A.* **74,** 5555–5563.

Mengs, U., and Stotzen, C. D. (1987). Ganglioside treatment and nerve regeneration: A morphological study after nerve crush in rats. *Eur. J. Pharmacol.* **142,** 419–424.

Mengs, U., Schmidt, K. F., Wolfe, H. G., Goldschmidt, R., and Tullner, H.-U. (1984). Effects of gangliosides on nerve regeneration in rats. *Arch. Int. Pharmacodyn. Ther.* **271,** 315–323.

Mengs, U., Goldschmidt, R., and Tullner, H.-U. (1986). Effect of ganglioside treatment on number of nerve fibres after nerve crush in rats. *Arch. Int. Pharmacodyn. Ther.* **283,** 229–236.

Mesulam, M., Mufson, E. J., and Wainer, B. H. (1986). Three dimensional representation and cortical projection topography of the nucleus basalis (Ch4) in the macque: Concurrent demonstration of choline acetyltransferase and retrograde transport with a stabilised tetramethyl-benzidine method for horseradish peroxidase. *Brain Res.* **367,** 301–308.

Morgan, J. I., and Seifert, W. (1979). Growth factors and gangliosides: A possible new perspective in neuronal growth control. *J. Supramol. Struct.* **10,** 111–124.

Nagai, Y., Momoi, T., Saito, M., Mitsuzawa, E., and Ohtani, S. (1976). Ganglioside syndrome, a new autoimmune neurologic disorder experimentally induced with brain gangliosides. *Neurosci. Lett.* **2,** 107–111.

Needles, D., Nieto-Sampedro, M., Scott, R. W., and Cotman, C. W. (1985). Neuronotrophic activity for ciliary ganglion neurons. Induction following injury to the brain of neonatal, adult, and aged rats. *Dev. Brain Res.* **18,** 275–284.

Nieoullon, A., Cheramy, A., and Glowinski, J. (1977). Release of dopamine *in vivo* from cat substantia nigra. *Nature (London)* **266,** 375–377.

Nieto-Sampedro, M., Manthorpe, M., Barbin, G., Varon, S., and Cotman, C. W. (1983). Injury-induced neuronotrophic activity in adult rat brain: Correlation with survival of delayed implants in the wound cavity. *J. Neurosci.* **3,** 2219–2229.

Norido, F., Canella, R., Zanoni, R., and Gorio, A. (1984). The development of diabetic neuropathy in the C57BL/Ks (db/db) mouse and its treatment with gangliosides. *Exp. Neurol.* **83,** 221–232.

Obata, K., Oide, M., and Handa, S. (1977). Effects of glycolipids on *in vitro* development of neuromuscular junction. *Nature (London)* **266,** 369–371.

Oderfeld-Nowak, B., Skup, M., Ulas, J., Jezierska, M., Gradknowska, R., and Zaremba, M.

(1984). Effect of GM1 ganglioside treatment on post lesion responses of cholinergic neurons in rat hippocampus after various partial deafferentations. *J. Neurosci. Res.* **12,** 409–420.

Orlando, P., Cocciante, G., Ippolito, G., Massari, P., Roberti, S., and Tettamanti, G. (1979). The fate of tritium labelled GM1 ganglioside injected in mice. *Pharmacol. Res. Commun.* **11,** 759–773.

Otten, U., Lorez, H. P., and Businger, F. (1983). Nerve growth factor antagonizes the neurotoxic action of capsaicin on primary sensory neurons. *Nature (London)* **301,** 515–517.

Partington, C. R., and Daly, J. W. (1979). Effect of gangliosides on adenylate cyclase activity in rat cerebral cortical membranes. *Mol. Pharmacol.* **15,** 484–491.

Pedata, F., Giovanelli, L., and Pepeu, G. (1984). GM1 ganglioside facilitates the recovery of high-affinity choline uptake in the cerebral cortex of rats with a lesion of the nucleus basalis magnocellularis. *J. Neurosci. Res.* **12,** 421–427.

Pestronk, A., Adams, R. N., Cornblath, D., Kuncl, R. W., Drachman, D. B., and Clawson, L. (1989). Patterns of serum IgM antibodies to GM1 and GD1a gangliosides in amyotrophic lateral sclerosis. *Ann. Neurol.* **25,** 98–102.

Purpura, D. P. (1978). Ectopic dendritic growth in mature pyramidal neurones in human ganglioside storage disease. *Nature (London)* **276,** 520–521.

Purpura, D. P., and Baker, H. J. (1977). Neurite induction in mature cortical neurons in feline G_{M1}-ganglioside storage disease. *Nature (London)* **266,** 553–554.

Purpura, D. P., and Baker, H. J. (1978). Meganeurites and other aberrant processes of neurons in feline GM_1-gangliosidosis: A Golgi study. *Brain Res.* **143**(1), 13–26.

Purpura, D. P., and Suzuki, K. (1976). Distortion of neuronal geometry and formation of aberrant synapses in neuronal storage disease. *Brain Res.* **116,** 1–21.

Purpura, D. P., Pappas, G. D., and Baker, H. J. (1978). Fine structure of meganeurites and secondary growth processes in feline GM_1-gangliosidosis. *Brain Res.* **143**(1), 1–12.

Quarles, R. H., Ilyas, A. A., and Willison, H. J. (1986). Antibodies to glycolipids in demyelinating disease of the human peripheral nervous system. *Chem. Phys. Lipids* **42,** 235–248.

Rahman, H., Kötje, K. H., Probst, W., Beitinger, H., Möius, D., and Ficker, E. (1988). Calcium, gangliosides and neuronal modulation. *In* "New Trends in Ganglioside Research" (R. W. Ledeen, E. L. Hogan, G. Tettamanti, A. J. Yates, and R. K. Yu, eds.), pp. 549–556. Liviana Press, Padova/Springer-Verlag, Berlin.

Raiteri, M., Versace, P., and Marchi, M. (1985). GM1 monosialoganglioside inner ester induces early recovery of striatal dopamine uptake in rats with unilateral nigrostriatal lesion. *Eur. J. Pharmacol.* **118,** 347–350.

Ramirez, J. J., Fass, B., Karpiak, S. E., and Steward, O. (1987). Ganglioside treatments reduce locomotor hyperactivity after bilateral lesions of the entorhinal cortex. *Neurosci. Lett.* **75,** 283–287.

Ramón y Cajal, S. (1928). Degeneration and regeneration of the nervous system. *In* (R. M. May, ed.), Vol. 2. Hafner, New York.

Reis, D. J., Gilad, G., Pickel, V. M., and Joh, T. H. (1978). Reversible changes in the activities and amounts of tyrosine hydroxylase in dopamine neurons of the substantia nigra in response to axonal injury as studied by immunohistochemical and immunocytochemical methods. *Brain Res.* **144,** 325–342.

Robb, G. A., and Keynes, R. J. (1984). Stimulation of nodal and terminal sprouting of mouse motor nerves by gangliosides. *Brain Res.* **295,** 368–371.

Roisen, F. J., Bartfeld, H., Nagele, R., and Yorke, G. (1981a). Ganglioside stimulation of axonal sprouting in vitro. *Science* **214,** 577–578.

Roisen, F. J., Bartfeld, H., and Rapport, M. M. (1981b). Ganglioside mediation of *in vitro* neuronal maturation. *In* "Gangliosides in Neurological and Neuromuscular Function, Development and Repair" (M. M. Rapport and A. Gorio, eds.), pp. 135–150. Raven Press, New York.

Roisen, F. J., Spero, D. A., Held, S. J., Yorke, G., and Bartfeld, H. (1984). Ganglioside induced surface activity and neurite formation of Neuro-2a neuroblastoma cells. *In* "Ganglioside Structure, Function, and Biomedical Potential" (R. W. Ledeen, R. K. Yu, M. M. Rapport, and K. Suzuki, eds.), pp. 499–511. Plenum, New York.

Roseman, S. (1970). Synthesis of complex carbohydrates by multiglycosyltransferase systems and their potential function in intercellular adhesion. *Chem. Phys. Lipids* **5,** 270–297.

Sabel, B. A., Slavin, M. D., and Stein, D. G. (1984). GM1 ganglioside treatment facilitates behavioural recovery from bilateral brain damage. *Science* **225,** 340–342.

Sabel, B. A., Dunbar, G. L., Butler, W. M., and Stein, D. G. (1985). GM1 gangliosides stimulate neuronal reorganization and reduce rotational asymmetry after hemitransections of the nigrostriatal pathway. *Exp. Brain Res.* **60,** 27–37.

Scheel, G., Schwarzmann, G., Hoffman-Bleihauer, P., and Sandhoff, K. (1985). The influence of ganglioside insertion into brain membranes on the rate of ganglioside degradation by membrane-bound sialidase. *Eur. J. Biochem.* **153,** 29, 35.

Schwab, M. E., Otten, U., Agid, Y., and Thoenen, H. (1979). Nerve growth factor (NGF) in the rat CNS: Absence of specific retrograde axonal transport and tyrosine hydroxylase induction in locus coeruleus and substantia nigra. *Brain Res.* **168,** 473–483.

Schwartz, M., and Spirman, N. (1982). Sprouting from chicken embryo dorsal root ganglia induced by nerve growth factor is specifically inhibited by affinity-purified antiganglioside antibodies. *Proc. Natl. Acad. Sci. U.S.A.* **79,** 6080–6083.

Seifert, W. (1981). Gangliosides in nerve cell cultures. *In* "Gangliosides in Neurological and Neuromuscular Function, Development and Repair" (M. M. Rapport and A. Gorio, eds.), pp. 99–117. Raven Press, New York.

Skaper, S. D., and Varon, S. (1985). Ganglioside GM1 overcomes serum inhibition of neuritic outgrowth. *Int. J. Dev. Neurosci.* **3,** 187–198.

Skaper, S. D., Katoh-Semba, R., and Varon, S. (1985). GM1 ganglioside accelerates neurite outgrowth from primary peripheral and central neurons under selective culture conditions. *Dev. Brain Res.* **23,** 19–26.

Skup, M., Gradkowska, M., Ulas, J., and Oderfeld-Nowak, B. (1987). Analysis of the time course of GM1 ganglioside effect on changes in choline acetyltransferase activity in partially denervated rat hippocampus. *Acta Neurobiol. Exp.* **47,** 199–211.

Sofroniew, M. V., and Isacson, O. (1988). Distribution of degeneration of cholinergic neurons in the septum following axotomy in different portions of the fimbria-fornix: A correlation between degree of cell loss and proximity of neuronal somata to the lesion. *J. Chem. Neuronat.* **1,** 327–337.

Sofroniew, M. V., Pearson, R. C. A., Eckenstein, F., Cuello, A. C., and Powell, R. (1983). Retrograde changes in cholinergic neurons in the basal forebrain of the rat following cortical damage. *Brain Res.* **289,** 370–374.

Sofroniew, M. V., Pearson, R. C. A., Cuello, A. C., Tagari, P. C., and Stephens, P. H. (1986). Parenterally administered GM1 ganglioside prevents retrograde degeneration of cholinergic cells of the rat basal forebrain. *Brain Res.* **398,** 393–396.

Sparrow, J. R., McGuinness, C., Schwartz, M., and Grafstein, B. (1984). Antibodies to gangliosides inhibit goldfish optic nerve regeneration *in vivo*. *J. Neurosci. Res.* **12,** 233–243.

Spero, D. A., and Roisen, F. J. (1984). Ganglioside-mediated enhancement of the cytoskeletal organization and activity in Neuro-2a neuroblastoma cells. *Dev. Brain Res.* **13,** 37–48.

Spiegel, S., and Fishman, P. H. (1987). Gangliosides as bimodal regulators of cell growth. *Proc. Natl. Acad. Sci. U.S.A.* **84,** 141–145.

Spiegel, S., Fishman, P. H., and Weber, R. J. (1985). Direct evidence that endogenous ganglioside GM1 can mediate thymocyte proliferation. *Science* **230,** 1283–1287.

Spirman, N., Sela, B. A., and Schwartz, M. (1982). Antiganglioside antibodies inhibit neuritic outgrowth from regenerating goldfish retinal explants. *J. Neurochem.* **39,** 874–877.

Spoerri, P. E., and Roisen, F. J. (1988). Ganglioside potentiation of NGF-independent conditioned medium enhancement of neuritic outgrowth from spinal cord and ciliary ganglia explants. *Int. J. Dev. Neurosci.* **6,** 223–232.

Stephens, P. H., Cuello, A. C., Sofroniew, M. V., Pearson, R. C. A., and Tagari, P. (1985). The effects of unilateral decortication upon choline acetyltransferase and glutamate decarboxylase activities in the nucleus basalis and other areas of the rat brain. *J. Neurochem.* **45,** 1021–1026.

Stephens, P. H., Tagari, P. C., Garofalo, L., Maysinger, D., Piotte, M., and Cuello, A. C. (1987). Neural plasticity of basal forebrain cholinergic neurons: Effects of gangliosides. *Neurosci. Lett.* **80,** 80–84.

Stephens, P. H., Tagari, P. C., and Cuello, A. C. (1988). Retrograde degeneration of basal forebrain cholinergic neurons after neurotoxin lesions of the neocortex: Application of ganglioside GM_1. *Neurochem. Int.* **12,** 475–481.

Svennerholm, L. (1980). Ganglioside designation. *Adv. Exp. Med. Biol.* **125,** 11.

Tanaka, K., Dora, E., Urbanics, R., Greenberg, J. H., Toffano, G., and Reivich, M. (1986). Effect of the ganglioside GM1 on cerebral metabolism, microcirculation, recovery kinetics of ECoG and histology, during the recovery period following focal ischemia in cats. *Stroke* **17,** 1170–1178.

Terry, R. D., and Weiss, M. (1963). Studies in Tay-Sachs disease. I. Ultrastructure of cerebrum. *J. Neuropathol. Exp. Neurol.* **22,** 18–55.

Tettamanti, G. (1988). Towards the understanding of the physiological role of gangliosides. *In* "New Trends in Ganglioside Research" (R. W. Ledeen, E. L. Hogan, G. Tettamanti, A. J. Yates, and R. K. Yu, eds.), pp. 625–646. Liviana Press, Padova; Springer–Verlag, Berlin.

Tettamanti, G., Venerando, B., Robert, S., Lhigorno, V., Sonnino, S., Ghidoni, R., Orlando, P., and Massari, P. (1981). The fate of exogenously administered brain development, and repair. *In* "Gangliosides in Neurological and Neuromuscular Function, Development and Repair" (M. Rapport and A. Gorio, eds.), pp. 225–239. Raven Press, New York.

Thoenen, H., Bandtlow, C., and Heumann, R. (1987). The physiological function of nerve growth factor in the central nervous system: Comparison with the periphery. *Rev. Physiol. Biochem. Pharmacol.* **109,** 145–178.

Tilson, H. A., Harry, G. J., Nanry, K., Hudson, P. M., and Hong, J. S. (1988). Ganglioside interactions with the dopaminergic system of rats. *J. Neurosci. Res.* **19,** 88–93.

Toffano, G., Benvegnu, D., Bonetti, A. C., Facci, L., Leon, A., Orlando, P., Ghidoni, R., and Tettamanti, G. (1980). Interactions of G_{M1} ganglioside with crude rat brain neuronal membranes. *J. Neurochem.* **35,** 861–866.

Toffano, G., Savoini, G., Moroni, F., Lombardi, G., Calza, L., and Agnati, L. F. (1983). GM1 ganglioside stimulates the regeneration of dopaminergic neurons in the central nervous system. *Brain Res.* **261,** 163–166.

Toffano, G., Agnati, L. F., Fuxe, K., Aldino, G., Consolazione, A., Valenti, G., and Savoini, G. (1984). Effect of GM1 ganglioside treatment on the recovery of nigro-striatal neurons after different types of lesions. *Acta Physiol. Scand.* **122,** 313–321.

Tomozawa, Y., and Appel, S. H. (1986). Soluble striatal extracts enhance development of mesencephalic dopaminergic neurons *in vitro*. *Brain Res.* **399,** 111–124.

Tsuji, S., Yamashita, T., Tanaka, M., and Nagai, Y. (1988). Synthetic sialyl compounds as well as natural gangliosides induce neuritogenesis in a mouse neuroblastoma cell line (Neuro2a) *J. Neurochem.* **50,** 414–423.

Vaccarino, F., Guidotti, A., and Costa, E. (1987). Ganglioside inhibition of glutamate-mediated protein kinase C translocation in primary cultures of cerebellar neurons. *Proc. Natl. Acad. Sci. U.S.A.* **84,** 8707–8711.

Van Heyningen, W. E. (1974). Gangliosides as membrane receptors for tetanus toxin, cholera toxin and serotonin. *Nature (London)* **249,** 415–417.

Vantini, G., Fusco, M., Bigon, E., and Leon, A. (1988). GM1 ganglioside potentiates the effect of nerve growth factor in preventing vinblastine-induced sympathectomy in newborn rats. *Brain Res.* **448,** 252–258.

Varon, S., Skaper, S. D., and Katoh-Semba, R. (1986). Neuritic responses to GM1 ganglioside in several *in vitro* systems. *In* "Gangliosides and Neural Plasticity" (G. Tettamanti, R. Ledeen, K. Sandhoff, Y. Nagai, and G. Toffano, eds.), pp. 215–230. Liviana Press, Padova/Springer-Verlag, Berlin.

Vitadello, M., Couraud, J. Y., Hassig, R., Gorio, A., and Di Giamberardino, L. (1983). Axonal transport of acetylcholinesterase in the diabetic mutant mouse. *Exp. Neurol.* **82,** 143–147.

Walkley, S. U. (1987). Further studies on ectopic dendrite growth and other geometrical distortions of neurons in feline GM1 gangliosidosis. *Neuroscience* **21,** 313–331.

Walkley, S. U., and Baker, H. J. (1984). Sphingomyelin lipidosis in a cat. II. Golgi studies. *Acta Neuropathol.* **65,** 138–144.

Walkley, S. U., and Siegel, D. A. (1985). Ectopic dendritogenesis occurs on cortical pyramidal neurons in swainsonine-induced feline α-mannosidosis deul. *Dev. Brain Res.* **20,** 143–148.

Walkley, S. U., Wurzelmann, S., and Purpura, D. P. (1981). Ultrastructure of neurites and meganeurites on cortical pyramidal neurons in feline gangliosidosis as revealed by the combined Golgi-EM technique. *Brain Res.* **211,** 393–398.

Wenk, H., Bigl, V., and Meyer, U. (1980). Cholinergic projections from magnocellular nuclei of the basal forebrain to cortical areas in rats. *Brain Res. Rev.* **2,** 295–316.

Whitehouse, P. J., Price, D. L., Strubie, R. G., Clark, A. W., Coyle, J. T., and Delong M. R. (1982). Alzheimer's disease and senile dementia loss of neurons in the basal forebrain. *Science* **215,** 1237–1239.

Whittemore, S. R., and Seiger, A. (1987). The expression, localization and functional significance of β-nerve growth factor in the central nervous system. *Brain Res. Rev.* **12,** 439–464.

Williams, L., Varon, S., Peterson, G., Wictorin, K., Fischer, W., Björklund, A., and Gage, F. (1986). Continuous infusion of nerve growth factor prevents basal forebrain neuronal death after timbria fornix transection. *Proc. Natl. Acad. Sci. U.S.A.* **83,** 9231–9235.

Wojcik, M., Ulas, J., and Oderfeld-Nowak, B. (1982). The stimulating effect of ganglioside injections on the recovery of choline acetyltransferase and acetylcholinesterase activities in the hippocampus of the rat after septal lesions. *Neuroscience* **7,** 495–499.

Yasuda, Y., Tiemeyer, M., Blackburn, C. C., and Schnaar, R. L. (1988). Neuronal recognition of gangliosides: Evidence for a brain ganglioside receptor. *In* "New Trends in Ganglioside Research" (R. W. Ledeen, E. L. Hogan, G. Tettamanti, A. J. Yates, R. K., and Yu, eds.), pp. 230–243. Liviana Press, Padova/Springer-Verlag, Berlin.

Yates, A. J., Walters, J. D., Wood, C. L., and Johnson, J. D. (1989). Ganglioside modulation of c-AMP dependent protein kinase and cyclic nucleotide phosphodiesterase *in vitro*. *J. Neurochem.* **53,**162–167.

Yusuf, H. K. M., Pohlentz, G., and Sandhoff, K. (1983). Tunicamycin inhibits ganglioside biosynthesis in rat liver Golgi apparatus by blocking sugar nucleotide transport across the membrane vesicles. *Proc. Natl. Acad. Sci. U.S.A.* **80,** 7075–7079.

Zieher, L. M., and Jaim-Etcheverry, G. (1983). Different effects of neonatal vinblastine on peripheral and central noradrenaline neurons. *Eur. J. Pharmacol.* **93,** 101–106.

New Approaches to Vaccination

Charles Flexner

Departments of Medicine, and Pharmacology and Molecular Sciences
Division of Clinical Pharmacology
The Johns Hopkins University School of Medicine
Baltimore, Maryland 21205

I. Introduction

Vaccination is one of the most cost-effective forms of medicine. Often, a single inoculation costing pennies to prepare and administer can prevent devastating illness. The impact of infectious diseases on human suffering, loss of life, and health care expenditures is substantial. The impact of a single effective vaccine on public health and welfare can be equally great.

Smallpox had been responsible for epidemics and pandemics since the dawn of civilization, accounting for up to 10% of the annual mortality in some areas (see Hopkins, 1983). Today, this virus is extinct as the result of widespread vaccination. The total cost of the World Health Organization Campaign to Eradicate

Advances in Pharmacology, Volume 21

Smallpox was approximately 300 million dollars, a small fraction of today's annual international health budget. The annual savings resulting from the elimination of this single disease would now have to be counted in the billions of dollars.

Although some would argue that the exceptional features of smallpox—absence of an animal reservoir and an inexpensive, easily administered vaccine—made it uniquely susceptible to eradication, several other infectious diseases could be prevented or eliminated by vaccination. A World Health Organization campaign to eradicate polio is currently underway, and it is clear that the potential impact of vaccination on human health is barely being realized.

The emergence of human immunodeficiency virus (HIV) in this decade is a reminder that infectious diseases are an ever-present threat to public health. Viruses in particular retain the capacity to produce new epidemics. The possibility of an influenza pandemic as devastating as that of 1918 persists, despite the availability of influenza vaccines. Modern commerce has facilitated the spread of other pathogenic viruses such as dengue fever virus; a mosquito vector for dengue has been recently introduced into the United States. The introduction of delta hepatitis virus into areas where hepatitis B is widespread, such as China and Korea, could result in substantial mortality from fulminant delta hepatitis.

Attempts to develop specific antimicrobial chemotherapy for viral diseases have been confounded by similarities between the biochemistry of the pathogen and the host. In contrast, vaccines have been remarkably effective in controlling the spread of a number of viruses, and could eradicate several major viral diseases within the next few decades. Nonetheless, the need for better vaccines remains acute. Outbreaks of measles (Markowitz *et al.*, 1989) and pertussis in this country and abroad, and the incomplete efficacy of influenza and pneumococcal vaccines highlight some of the problems with existing vaccines, and the need for improvements in vaccine technology.

Recent advances in our understanding of immunology and the pathophysiology of infectious diseases have created revolutionary new approaches to vaccine development. In addition, the success of vaccination as a means of controlling infectious diseases has encouraged the development of vaccines for other kinds of disease, including malignancy and autoimmune disease. Future vaccines may find their way into almost every branch of medicine. This review covers the current revolution in vaccine development, and focuses on changes brought about by molecular biology and immunology. Some of the techniques described are experimental; others are already finding application in veterinary and human vaccines.

This is not a comprehensive treatise on vaccination or immunology, although pertinent background information is provided. Interested readers are referred to chapters by Ada (1989) or Murphy and Chanock (1989) for a general overview of vaccines.

II. Fundamentals of Modern Vaccinology

An improved understanding of immunology has had a profound impact on experimental approaches to vaccination. A number of recent advances are reviewed here that are essential to understanding current vaccine research.

A. Definitions

The following definitions are provided for terms used in this text. An *antigen* is any unique molecular domain that is recognized as foreign and provokes an immune response. Antigens are most commonly proteins or complex carbohydrate moieties. An *epitope* is the quintessential region of an antigen responsible for antibody binding or lymphocyte recognition. An *immunogen* is any immunogenic epitope, i.e., any domain capable of activating a B and/or T cell response.

Humoral immunity refers to antigen-specific immunity in which serum immunoglobulin (antibody) is the effector. *Cell-mediated immunity* refers to antigen-specific immunity in which cells (T lymphocytes) are the effectors. For the purposes of this discussion, a *vaccine* is defined as any material which confers long-lasting immunity to a specific antigen or group of antigens following inoculation, and thus prevents or attenuates disease. Antigenic specificity and duration of immunity then distinguish vaccination from other prophylactic or therapeutic manipulations of the immune system.

Immunoprophylaxis refers to the induction of immunity for the purpose of preventing disease and thus encompasses vaccination; however, immunoprophylaxis is not necessarily antigen specific or long-lived. An example of nonspecific immunoprophylaxis is interferon administration to prevent virus infections (see Tyrell, 1987). *Immunotherapy* refers to the induction of immunity for amelioration of an established disease, for example, the use of interferon to treat hairy cell leukemia or Kaposi's sarcoma (Tyrell, 1987). Immunotherapy, unlike vaccination, requires neither antigen-specific responses nor long duration of effect. In some cases, however, the same material used for vaccination may be used for experimental immunotherapy, for example, the use of certain vaccine preparations to induce tumor regression (see Section V,A,4).

B. Immunologic Specificity

Immunity to a microorganism, tumor cell, large protein, or small peptide involves processes which are both antigen specific and nonspecific. Nonspecific immunity involves components of general inflammation; this includes the complement pathways, phagocytes such as macrophages and neutrophils, and cytokines, for example, interleukins, or cytotoxic proteins such as tumor necrosis factor or interferons. Although these nonspecific inflammatory responses are essential to control disease or eradicate microorganisms, they are not antigen-restricted. Furthermore, most of these responses are short-lived and self-limited in order to avoid self harm.

Antigen-specific immunity is of two types, humoral and cellular. Humoral immunity is mediated by immunoglobulins (Igs or antibodies) produced by B lymphocytes which are clonally specific for a particular domain (B cell epitope) of a foreign antigen. Cellular immunity is mediated by T lymphocytes which are clonally specific in their response to a particular portion (T cell epitope) of a foreign antigen. B cells recognize antigen after binding to immunoglobulin, whereas T cells recognize processed antigen on the surface of antigen presenting cells (APCs), which can be macrophages, Kupffer cells, dendritic cells, or B cells (see Fig. 1).

C. Components of the Immune Response and Implications for Vaccine Design

The stimulation of B and T lymphocyte responses involves complex interactions between a variety of surface proteins such as the lymphocyte CD3 (T3), CD4, and CD8 antigens and soluble factors such as lymphokines. The central mediator of antigen recognition is the T helper (T_H or CD4) cell, defined by possession of the CD4 surface protein. The T_H cell provides stimulation or "help" for further T cell responses, and also stimulates B cell proliferation through secretion of lymphokines. The T cell antigen receptor on the surface of this and other T lymphocytes recognizes polypeptide epitopes of proteolytically degraded foreign antigen which are bound to the antigen recognition site of a major histocompatability complex (MHC) molecule; this antigen/MHC complex is then transported to the surface of an APC for presentation to the T cell (see Fig. 1). The T cell receptor is a functional counterpart of surface immunoglobulin and is a member of the immunoglobulin supergene family (Kronenberg *et al.*, 1986).

The B cell "receptor" is immunoglobulin. However, helper T cells assist in the regulation and stimulation of B cell responses. It is this requirement which explains in part the need to conjugate small antigens (or haptens) to large, immunogenic carrier proteins containing T cell epitopes in order to optimize antibody production (see Section IV,B). B cell immunogens may be three-dimensionally complex. Immunoglobulin may bind to parts of a protein which are separated or discontinuous along the length of a folded polypeptide (see Fig. 1). If an epitope responsible for generating protective or neutralizing antibody involves complex tertiary (or possibly quaternary) conformation, an intact protein may be more likely to stimulate protective immunity than a short polypeptide (see Section IV,B).

In contrast to B cells, effector T cells recognize small, processed, linear

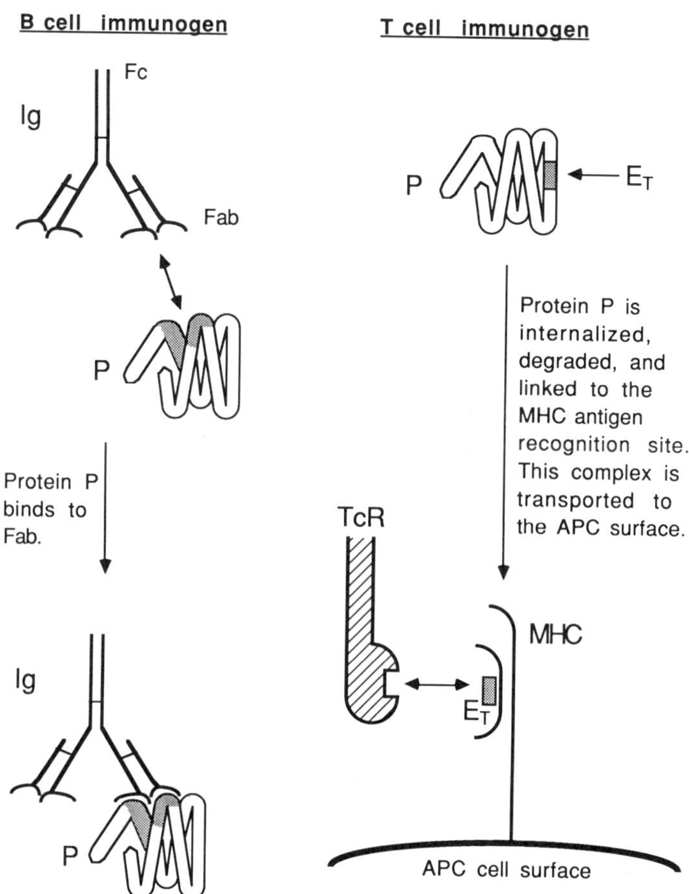

Fig. 1 Schematic representation of B and T cell immunogens. The left-hand side of the diagram shows recognition of a portion of a globular protein (P) by antibody. Heavy lines represent the heavy and light chains comprising the constant (Fc) and antibody binding (Fab) portions of immunoglobulin (Ig); short light lines represent interchain disulfide bridges. The right-hand side of the diagram shows a representative T cell epitope (E_t). The antigenic determinants of P are shaded in each case. Note that antigenic determinants for the B cell may be composed of discontinuous segments of P, whereas E_T is a short linear peptide which has been attached to the antigen recognition site of a major histocompatability (MHC) antigen after intracellular processing by the antigen presenting cell (APC) for recognition by the T cell receptor (TcR).

polypeptides. Some proliferating clones of lymphocytes are capable of lysing cells expressing particular foreign epitopes. Most cytotoxic T cells (Tc or CTLs) possess the CD8 surface marker. Cytotoxic $CD8^+$ cells recognize antigen linked to class I MHC molecules (HLA loci A, B, and C), which are expressed on the surface of most cells (see Townsend and Bodmer, 1989). Class I-restricted CTLs have been demonstrated following a number of viral infections in animals and man, and in several cases have demonstrated antiviral activity (see Section V,B,2). Passive infusion of $CD8^+$ CTLs can attenuate certain viral and parasitic infections experimentally, suggesting that these cells could play a protective role in immunity.

This arrangement has a number of implications important to the vaccinologist. First, a polypeptide of only a few amino acids in length could stimulate T-cell immunity. However, since T cells recognize peptides bound to a specific, autologous MHC antigen, effector T cell responses are genetically restricted. One peptide might only be recognized by a small percentage of the population—those possessing the appropriate HLA type. A vaccine dependent on T cell responses must contain as many T cell epitopes as would be needed to stimulate immunity in a target population of diverse HLA types. Second, since T cell recognition requires intracellular protein processing, vaccine preparations facilitating internalization and processing of antigen should generate a more effective immune response.

Investigation of the mechanisms of immunity in the past has focused on the humoral immune response, because antibody was easily measured and seemed to correlate well with recovery from a number of diseases. For some viral vaccines, antibody production correlated precisely with protection, but in most cases the precise mechanism by which vaccination prevents disease is still unknown. Cellular effectors, particularly antigen-specific CTLs, are now recognized as playing an important role in eradicating pathogens or infected cells. For example, protection from malaria may depend more on CTL activity than on specific antimalaria antibody production (Good *et al.*, 1988a). The ability to measure specific CTL activity in inbred mice and now in man (see Moss and Flexner, 1987; Townsend and Bodmer, 1989) may increasingly focus evaluation of vaccine responses on cell-mediated immunity. Some future vaccines could prevent disease without generating significant amounts of antibody (see section V,B).

Finally, when the immune system is exposed to a vaccine antigen, long-lived clones of antigen-specific B and T cells known as memory cells must also be generated. Antigen-laden APCs recruit B memory cells to form antibody-secreting cells and produce antibodies (see Ada, 1989). Long-lived APCs or networks of anti-idiotypic antibodies (see Section IV,C) may serve as an internal source of antigen for the life of the individual. Effective vaccination depends on the generation of long-lived, protective immunity to one or more antigens and requires effective antigen processing and presentation. The nature of the specific antigen and the duration of immunity then determine the efficacy of a vaccine.

D. Vaccine Targets

Protective immunity can target one or more steps in the complex life cycle of a microorganism (see Fig. 2). A vaccine may stimulate immunity to a pathogen before it enters a host cell, after it enters the cell, or may target a specific disease-causing molecule such as a toxin without having any direct effect on the pathogen. The tetanus toxoid vaccine, for example, targets immunity to this single

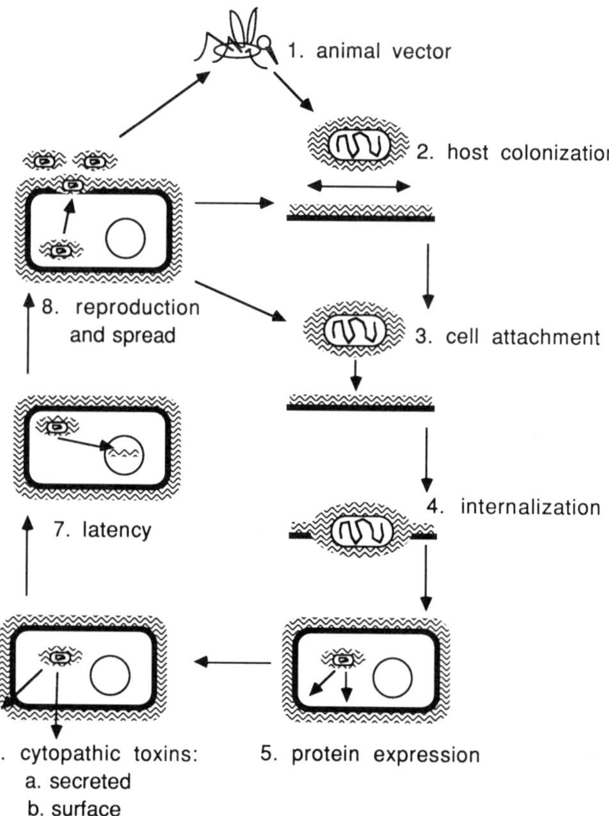

Fig. 2 Potential targets for vaccination. This diagram represents the life cycle of a prototypical pathogenic microorganism, in this case an intracellular pathogen. All numbered stages in the organism's life cycle are potential targets for vaccine-induced immunity (see text).

protein, preventing the disease tetanus without affecting colonization of the host by *Clostridium tetani* (Fig. 2, stage 6).

Bacterial vaccines may stimulate antibody to specific surface polysaccharides, and may prevent colonization with pathogenic bacteria or target bacteria for antibody and complement-mediated lysis or opsonization (Fig. 2, stage 2). Viral vaccines generally target surface proteins important for attachment to receptors on target cells, and thus prevent attachment or internalization (Fig. 2, stages 3 and 4). These same antibodies probably prevent spread of virus from infected cells by binding to new virions, but may also target infected cells for destruction by antibody binding to complement, or by antibody-dependent cytotoxic cells (ADCC).

CTLs can be targeted to lyse infected cells expressing either surface or internal antigens (Fig. 2, stage 5). Internal structural proteins and enzymes of viruses, bacteria, and parasites may be targets for both CTL and antibody production, but would not be expected to elicit neutralizing antibody. Vaccines based on the generation of CTLs reactive with internal virus antigens are experimental, but might be useful for controlling pathogens capable of establishing intracellular latency, such as retroviruses, or pathogens with highly variable surface proteins which readily escape neutralizing antibody (see Section V,B,2). An effective vaccine then does not necessarily have to prevent infection of host cells, but might target infected cells for destruction before disease becomes evident (Fig. 2, stages 5 and 7). This same principle would apply to vaccines directed against tumor cells.

Other novel vaccines might target the animal vector rather than the microorganism (Fig. 2, stage 1). For example, a vaccine preparation composed of intestinal antigens of the cattle tick *Boophilus microplus* elicits antibodies capable of killing ticks which ingest the blood of vaccinees (Johnston *et al.*, 1986; Opdebeek *et al.*, 1988). A tick-directed vaccine might prove practical for the prevention of Lyme disease and Rocky Mountain spotted fever in endemic areas, and since tick intestinal epithelial cells share cross-reactive antigens, a broad-spectrum antitick vaccine might be possible. This approach could be applied to other large blood-sucking parasites or arthropods which transmit diseases during blood meals.

Parasite vaccines might target different stages in the life cycle of the pathogen. For example, malaria vaccines might target the sporozoite stage of *plasmodia* and thereby prevent primary infection of hepatocytes. Should this prove impractical, vaccines could target later stages of the parasite (see Section V,A,2). Vaccines directed against the gametocyte (the last stage of development of *Plasmodium* in man) would prevent transmission of the gametocyte from man to mosquito. This would be of no direct benefit to the vaccinated host, but would break the cycle of transmission of malaria. Such altruistic vaccines might represent the only effective means of controlling the spread of some diseases.

III. Current Approaches to Immunization

A. Licensed Vaccines

Vaccines for 11 viral diseases are available for use in the United States (Table I). Although this seems an impressive number, only vaccines for measles, mumps, rubella, and polio are widely used in children, and only the inactivated influenza and hepatitis B virus vaccines are being widely used in targeted adult populations.

Of viral vaccines currently undergoing experimental trial, only the attenuated varicella zoster vaccine is at an advanced stage of development, and would be useful in targeted pediatric populations and, possibly, in immunocompromised hosts (see Ada, 1989). Other viral vaccines currently under development are replacements for suboptimal vaccines already in use, such as influenza, or are targeted to a specific group with a relatively unique exposure, such as dengue or Japanese B encephalitis. Vaccines would be useful for diseases caused by a number of other viruses, including respiratory syncytial virus, parainfluenza virus, cytomegalovirus, herpes simplex viruses, rotavirus, hepatitis A virus, and human immunodeficiency viruses. More efficacious vaccines are needed for influenza and sporadic tropical virus diseases such as dengue and Lassa fever.

Vaccines for 11 bacterial diseases are available in the United States (Table I). Only the diptheria/pertussis/tetanus (DPT) and *Haemophilus influenzae* type B vaccines are widely used in children; only the pneumococcal vaccine is being widely used in targeted adult populations. Of the other available vaccines, the Bacille Calmette-Guerin (BCG) strain of *Mycobacterium bovis* has fallen out of

Table I
Human Vaccines Currently Available

Virus vaccines	Bacterial vaccines
Adenovirus	Anthrax
Hepatitis B	BCG
Influenza (inactivated and split)	Diptheria
Japanese B encephalitis	*Haemophilus influenzae* type B
Measles	Meningococcus
Mumps	Pertussis
Polio (live and inactivated)	Plague
Rabies	Pneumococcus
Rubella	*Salmonella typhi*
Vaccinia	Tetanus
Yellow fever	*Vibrio cholerae*

favor in the United States because of controversy over its efficacy; the remaining bacterial vaccines (for *Vibrio cholerae* and *Salmonella typhi*) target travelers to underdeveloped areas, and are of partial or questionable efficacy.

Vaccines for five bacterial diseases are in the investigational stage in man (Ada, 1989). Only two of these—the leprosy and gonococcal vaccines—target diseases for which another vaccine is not already available. There are a number of bacterial diseases for which vaccines might have a beneficial impact, including gonorrhea, syphilis, group A and B streptococci, and pathogenic *Escherichia coli*. More efficacious vaccines are needed for cholera, salmonella, and other enteric pathogens, especially in underdeveloped countries. No human vaccines are currently available for fungal or parasitic diseases.

B. Types of Vaccines Currently Available

Contemporary vaccines fall into three categories: (1) subunit preparations of purified or partially purified bacterial polysaccharide (*Streptococcus pneumoniae, Meningococcus, haemophilus influenzae* type B), inactivated toxin (diphtheria, tetanus), or viral protein (hepatitis B); (2) killed (inactivated) bacteria (*Vibrio cholerae, Salmonella typhi*) or viruses (Salk polio, influenza, rabies); and (3) live attenuated bacteria (BCG) or viruses (Sabin polio, measles, mumps, rubella, yellow fever, vaccinia).

Many available vaccines suffer from inconstant or short-lived immunity, untoward toxicity, expense, or a combination of inadequacies. Subunit preparations are often difficult and expensive to prepare and may require chemical adjuvants or conjugation to carrier proteins to enhance immunity. Killed organisms may possess poor or inconstant immunogenicity; often, this is due to conformational alterations in antigenic molecules as a direct result of the chemical or thermal process used for inactivation. Furthermore, killed microorganisms may be less immunogenic, particularly with regard to cellular immunity, because of inefficient processing and presentation of antigens. The immune system seems better prepared to respond to live bacteria on mucosal surfaces or replicating viruses inside host cells than to protein or dead organisms. Unfortunately, live attenuated vaccines have the disadvantage of reversion to the virulent phenotype, and may themselves cause disease in immunocompromised individuals. Virulent revertants of polio virus, for example, can be isolated from the feces of children within a few days after receiving the Sabin vaccine (see Section IV,D,1). All vaccines possess potentially harmful side effects mediated by aberrant host immune responses, such as the neurotoxicity of the pertussis vaccine. Even without completely new approaches to vaccine development, there is a great need for improvement in available vaccines.

IV. New Approaches to Immunization

A. Adjuvant Systems

Chemical adjuvants have been successfully employed in vaccine formulations since the early days of immunology (reviewed by Warren *et al.*, 1986). The term adjuvant applies to any substance which can nonspecifically potentiate immunity. Given the complexity of immune responses, many steps can be targeted for enhancement. Accordingly, the mechanism of action of adjuvants is complex, and often poorly understood. Unfortunately, substances capable of nonspecifically activating immunity often elicit undesirable inflammatory or hypersensitivity reactions, and although the experimental promise of adjuvants has been great, their use in vaccines has been limited by toxicity. Alum remains the only accepted human vaccine adjuvant.

1. Chemical Vehicles

Chemical vehicles such as mineral oil or aluminum compounds appear to enhance antigenicity by facilitating antigen uptake and presentation. Oil emulsions and aluminum compounds also serve as a depot for antigen release, and are transported to lymph nodes, perhaps enhancing their proximity to the full repertoire of lymphocytes. Although these substances are effective in experimental animal models, they are very irritating, inducing local granulomas or cysts, and may be carcinogenic (Edelman, 1980). Problems with hypersensitivity, frequent failure to enhance immunogenicity of soluble antigens, and requirements for refrigeration of alum-containing preparations have prompted the search for other chemical means of improving antigen presentation. Artificial lipid membranes and polymers are replacing simple oil emulsions in experimental systems (see below), although aluminum compounds remain useful for vaccines intended for clinical application.

2. Peptide Adjuvants

The stimulation of immunity by mineral oil emulsions containing killed mycobacteria served as the foundation for all future adjuvants (Freund *et al.*, 1937). Complete Freund's adjuvant (CFA) remains the standard experimental carrier for inducing immunity in laboratory animals, but its toxicity—local irritation and granuloma formation—have hindered any applicability to human vaccines. In an attempt to define the quintessential immunostimulatory component of CFA, a group of investigators sequentially tested fractions of the tubercle bacillus for biological activity, and studied processed products of the immunogenic fractions. This work culminated in the discovery that a simple modified dipeptide,

N-acetylmuramyl-L-alanyl-D-isoglutamine (muramyl dipeptide or MDP), embodied nearly all of the adjuvant properties of CFA, without the attendant toxicities (Merser *et al.*, 1975). MDP experimentally enhances antibody production to a broad variety of antigens from viruses, bacteria, and parasites. Oil emulsion or incorporation into a liposome enhances MDP-mediated immunopotentiation of cellular immunity, especially if the dipeptide is chemically modified to a more lipophilic compound (Parant *et al.*, 1980). MDP is reported to enhance both B and T cell activation and proliferation, and to stimulate macrophages and granulocytes, prompting speculation that its action may be mediated by release of cytokines and/or lymphokines (see Section IV,A,3).

Although native MDP elicits a dramatic pyrogenic response, making it too toxic for use in man, the murabutide derivative (NAcMur-L-Ala-D-Gln-α-*n*-butyl ester) is nonpyrogenic. Early clinical studies with murabutide in man showed encouraging results, with enhancement of antibody responses to tetanus toxoid (Telzak *et al.*, 1986) and streptococcal M protein (Oberling *et al.*, 1985). In the former example, enhancement of antibody responses was dose dependent, with 6.2 mg of murabutide boosting antibody to tetanus toxoid by about twice as much as 3.1 mg. An adjuvant preparation combining threonyl MDP with Tween 80, squalene, and Pluronic 121 is apparently safe and effective and has been proposed for use in man (Byars and Allison, 1987). This adjuvant enhanced the antibody response to a variety of antigens in several animal species, including primates, and appears to enhance delayed type hypersensitivity (DTH) responses as well as antibody production, suggesting that such a combined adjuvant could stimulate both cellular and humoral immunity.

3. Lymphokines and Other Immunomodulators

The identification of monokines and lymphokines as regulators of inflammation and immunity produced a quantum advance in our understanding of immunology, and has to a great extent guided the development of immunopharmacology in this decade. Observations by Rosenberg and his colleagues of the antineoplastic properties of T cell-derived growth factor—later renamed interleukin-2 (IL-2)—were accompanied by studies on the antimicrobial activity of the same protein (reviewed by Rosenberg and Lotze, 1986). IL-2 protects animals from several experimental viral and bacterial infections, including herpes simplex (Weinberg *et al.*, 1987), rabies (Perrin *et al.*, 1988), and gram-negative septicemia (Weyand *et al.*, 1987), presumably due to stimulation of both B and T cell proliferation. Since antigen recognition *in vitro* is accompanied by IL-2 secretion from T_H cells, immune responses, including vaccination, might be augmented by IL-2.

In fact, IL-2 has been found to enhance antibody production in poorly responsive inbred mice, in whom antigen recognition is Ir gene-restricted (Kawamura *et al.*, 1985). IL-2 also enhanced antibody responses to a candidate malaria vaccine in nonresponder strains of mice (Good *et al.*, 1988b). More recently, IL-2 has been shown to enhance vaccination against herpes simplex virus in guinea pigs (Weinberg and Merigan, 1988), rabies virus in mice (Nunberg *et al.*, 1988), and *Haemophilus pleuropneumoniae* in swine (Nunberg *et al.*, 1988). IL-2 coexpression by a live recombinant virus boosted antibody titers to influenza antigens, but only when virus inoculum was very low (Flexner *et al.*, 1987). Exogenous lymphokine might then be ineffective, or possibly counterproductive, in situations where immunity is already optimal.

The potential use of IL-2 as a vaccine adjuvant has now been demonstrated in man. The majority of hemodialysis patients who were hepatitis B surface antigen (HBsAg) nonresponders showed a boosted anti-HBsAg response, with titers in the protective range, when vaccinated with commercial hepatitis B vaccine followed by 2.5×10^5 units of human IL-2. Antibody titers remained elevated for at least 15 weeks (Meuer *et al.*, 1989). This study substantiates findings that anti-HBsAg production could be enhanced *in vitro* with IL-2 in patients who were HBsAg nonresponders (Kakumu *et al.*, 1988), and suggests that exogenous IL-2 administration overcomes deficient IL-2 release in subsets of immunosuppressed patients. These encouraging results need to be followed by larger scale studies addressing duration of the IL-2 effect and possible application to others whose vaccine response is limited by compromised immunity or genetic restriction of antigen recognition.

Besides IL-2, other lymphokines are candidate adjuvants. A reliable adjuvant for boosting CTL responses would be useful, as would adjuvants for enhancing production of certain antibody classes. For example, IL-4 and IL-5, which appear to play a role in antibody class switching, might be used to enhance secretion of specific IgA to prevent infection or colonization of mucosal surfaces.

Chemicals other than lymphokines may also be used as immunomodulators. One such compound, diethylcarbamazine, appears to enhance opsonization of parasites, but may also enhance antibody production in viral infections, and could be used to enhance vaccination (Kitchen, 1988). Questions of toxicity must be foremost in the clinical development of immunomodulators, since nonspecific immune enhancement may lead to undesirable autoimmunity or hypersensitivity reactions.

4. Artificial Membranes

The human immune system has evolved to respond to antigen in the context of natural pathogenic microorganisms or cells. Thus, antigen incorporated into a lipid bilayer is more efficiently processed and is generally more immunogenic than antigen alone. This seems sensible given the evolution of immunity and the natural history of infectious diseases in man, and helps explain the poor immunogenicity of some subunit and peptide vaccines. The incorporation of protein or carbohydrate antigens into lipid bilayers is a powerful and widely applicable adjuvant system.

One experimental approach has been to incorporate antigen into lipid micelles or liposomes. Inclusion of diptheria toxoid in a liposome preparation is more immunogenic than free toxoid (Allison and Gregoriadis, 1974), and studies with other micelles have been equally encouraging. The incorporation of viral envelope protein into a micelle preparation created regular spheroids with the appearance of virions, but lacking structural proteins or nucleic acid (Morein and Simons, 1985); these so-called virosomes are highly immunogenic. The mechanism of liposome-mediated immune enhancement is controversial; evidence suggests that antigen incorporated into a liposome may mimic antigen presentation by a macrophage (Van Rooijen and Van Nieuwmegan, 1983), may enhance macrophage ingestion of antigen (Kramp *et al.*, 1982), or may simply serve as a depot from which antigen is slowly released.

A related system for antigen presentation is the use of nonionic polymers with surfactant properties. Copolymers of hydrophobic and hydrophilic pluronic polyol compounds have been shown to enhance antibody responses. The composition of the polymer seems to determine activity, with shorter polymers enhancing inflammatory responses, and alternating hydrophobic/hydrophilic polymers enhancing granuloma formation (Hunter and Bennett, 1984).

The toxicity of liposomes, disappointing immunogenicity, and occasional requirements for oil adjuvants led to approaches which incorporated antigen into artificial membranes along with matrix proteins with adjuvant properties. One particularly useful system takes advantage of the observation that a glycoside, Quil A, isolated from the bark of *Quillaja saponaria* molina, a tree found in the Chilean Andes, forms spherical particles of about 35 nm in diameter at concentrations above 0.03% when combined with lipid and amphipathic proteins (Morein *et al.*, 1984). Particles incorporating antigen, Quil A matrix, and lipid are known as immunostimulatory complexes (ISCOMs). Incorporation of antigen into an ISCOM often enhances antibody production and may be more immunogenic than either antigen plus CFA or antigen incorporated into a liposome. ISCOM-induced immunity is reported to mimic the natural course of immunity to antigen, with specific IgM production followed by IgG. ISCOMs can be administered intranasally or subcutaneously, and have been shown to stimulate specific CTL responses in rodents, and lymphocyte proliferative responses in primates. Finally, ISCOM vaccination has protected animals against experimental infection by at least five pathogenic viruses as well as toxoplasmosis (reviewed by Morein, 1988). Hepatitis B surface antigen incorporated into an ISCOM was much more immunogenic than the subunit alone in mice, and greatly boosted anti-HBsAg production in mice previously vaccinated with a subimmunogenic dose of HBsAG (Howard *et al.*, 1987), suggesting the utility of using ISCOMs as boosters for those having a poor antibody response to prior vaccination, or for those in whom boosting with a live vaccine would be unwise.

A similar approach substitutes a hydrophobic protein for lipid and glycoside to generate regular vesicles called proteosomes (Lowell *et al.*, 1988a). Proteosomes are composed of bacterial membrane proteins or porins to which antigenic proteins or peptides can be linked via interaction between hydrophobic domains; the model system described is composed of the outer membrane proteins of meningococci, although, theoretically, other suitable proteins could be substituted. The meningococcal membranes comprising proteosomes are not only highly immunogenic, serving as B cell mitogens, but should be safe for use in man, since similar preparations comprise the human meningococcal vaccine. Proteosomes containing trypanosome (Lowell *et al.*, 1988a) and malarial antigens (Lowell *et al.*, 1988b) are highly immunogenic and apparently safe in mice.

An even simpler method for cell-associated antigen presentation was recently reported. Antigen/antibody complexes can be bound to the surface of killed staphylococci and used directly for vaccination (Randall and Young, 1989). Neutralizing antibodies will bind to the Fc binding domain (protein A) on the surface of staphylococci. The resulting complex can be incubated with a mixture of proteins isolated from pathogenic viruses so that cell-associated Ig binds to the corresponding antigens. This solid matrix antibody/antigen (SMAA) complex, containing the appropriate antigens bound to antibody in a fixed array on the surface of bacteria, was highly immunogenic in mice, evoking high titer antibody responses to the predicted viral antigens (Randall and Young, 1989). This might be an economical means of preparing multivalent vaccines, offering many of the same advantages of ISCOMs or proteosomes without the required chemistry.

Concerns about the toxicity of artificial lipid/protein complexes have limited their clinical application. The major concern about ISCOM vaccines is the potential toxicity of Quil A. Intraperitoneal Quil A caused liver necrosis and death in mice, and toxicity was not reduced by incorporation into ISCOMs (Kersten *et al.*, 1988a). Unfortunately, the immunogenicity of ISCOMs seems to depend on the amount of Quil A in the preparation, possibly because of problems with micelle formation as the concentration is lowered (Kersten *et al.*, 1988b). One ISCOM vaccine for veterinary use has been licensed in Europe, but there has been little human experience with ISCOMs or proteosomes. SMAA vaccines might elicit hypersensitivity and possible inflammatory reactions to the staphylococcal carrier. Proteosome and SMAA vaccines may be less toxic than ISCOMs, but more extensive testing is required for both.

Artificial membranes such as ISCOMs and proteosomes may avoid the potential pathogenicity of live virus vaccines while retaining immunogenicity. In addition, they may prove useful for presenting subunits or peptides which are poorly immunogenic on their own. Finally, the potential for making polyvalent ISCOMs or proteosomes has not been addressed but deserves consideration.

B. Subunits and Synthetic Peptides

1. Background

Molecular biology has fostered a reductionist approach to therapeutics. In the area of vaccine development, this reductionism has been manifest in the search for the simplest molecules which might produce specific protective immunity. The definition at the molecular level of peptide epitopes responsible for immunity to infectious diseases in inbred animals has created interest in short peptides as vaccines components (reviewed by Rothbard, 1987). This approach is made possible by newly acquired facilities for producing large amounts of short polypeptides using recombinant DNA methodology or chemical protein synthesis. Synthetic peptide-based vaccines would contain one or more short linear epitopes, ranging in length from fewer than 15 to 100 or more amino acids. The theoretical advantage of peptide-based vaccines would be the generation of immunity with the least required immunogen. This avoids exposure to epitopes or proteins capable of eliciting unwanted toxicity, undesired hypersensitivity, or possessing immunosuppressive properties (see Kryzch, 1985). The peptide approach to vaccination is based on the success of working vaccines which are composed of a single protein or aggregate of closely related molecules, for example, the hepatitis B vaccine, which is composed of regular particles of hepatitis B surface antigen (HBsAg), or the diptheria and tetanus toxoid vaccines.

Peptide-based vaccines would be simple to formulate and, given expected improvements in facilities for mass-producing proteins, could be economical to manufacture. *De novo* synthesis of peptides would also have production advantages over inactivated, whole-microorganism vaccines or purified protein prepared from intact pathogenic microorganisms. Given the current ease with which microbial genes can be identified and sequenced, production of large amounts of protein using a recombinant DNA expression vector will often be cheaper and less time-consuming than purification of the same protein from large quantities of pathogen grown in culture, or obtained from infected animals or man. For example, recombinant yeast-expressed HBsAg will probably supplant its serum-derived counterpart if it retains clinical equivalency, because it bypasses human subjects, is easy to purify, and avoids potential exposure to pathogenic hepatitis virus.

Several immunological barriers limit the utility of peptide and subunit vaccines. First, pure polypeptides or carbohydrates tend to be weak immunogens; a strong B cell response to a subunit vaccine often requires a large carrier protein.

The current *Haemophilus influenzae* type B vaccine for example, contains capsular polysaccharide conjugated to diptheria toxoid, supplanting the previous unconjugated, poorly protective vaccine (Berkowitz *et al.*, 1987; Hendley *et al.*, 1987). In addition, simple peptides may also require a chemical adjuvant in order to be properly processed and efficiently presented to the immune system, and so the development of an optimal peptide vaccine requires concurrent development of an optimal adjuvant system (see Section IV,A).

The development of peptide vaccines may also be guided by naive assumptions about effective subunit vaccines. The success of the hepatitis B vaccine is almost certainly a result of the ability of this molecule to form regular aggregate particles, which are highly immunogenic. Most peptides, in contrast, would not be expected to aggregate into particles. Peptides in aqueous solution assume random secondary structures which may be quite different from the natural folding of the polypeptide in the intact protein. This may explain the variable and unpredictable immune response to some peptides (see Satterthwait *et al.*, 1988). Peptides are limited in their ability to generate B cell responses by the fact that immunoglobulin recognizes three-dimensional, often discontinuous epitopes, and a short linear peptide may be unlikely to mimic a three-dimensional, conformational domain. A small polypeptide might not then be sufficient to stimulate neutralizing antibody.

Short peptides might not contain sufficient T cell epitopes to protect an outbred population. A small polypeptide would only serve as a T cell epitope for a fraction of the population—those with the appropriate HLA type. An effective peptide vaccine might then have to contain a mixture of polypeptides to account for the fact that individuals of different HLA types may respond to distinct epitopes within the same protein.

2. Development of Peptides as Vaccines

Despite drawbacks, work with peptide vaccines against several experimental viral diseases has been encouraging. Mice immunized with peptides derived from herpes simplex virus (HSV) are protected from lethal challenge with HSV (Eisenberg *et al.*, 1985). Interestingly, protection from disease does not seem to correlate with neutralizing antibody production, suggesting that some other mechanism, perhaps CTL activity, was responsible for protection. Hepatitis B surface antigen peptides have also been studied. This protein is normally secreted after amino-terminal processing from a precursor known as large S. There has been a great deal of interest in the pre-S region at the amino terminus of large S, because the precursor is a better stimulator of both B and T cell immunity in experimental models than the processed antigen (Milich *et al.*, 1985), suggesting that T_H epitopes reside in the pre-S region. Chimpanzees vaccinated with peptides derived from the pre-S sequence produced antibodies sufficient to protect against infection. Human trials with a recombinant full-length HBsAg including the pre-S region (large S), are currently underway, but whether this will improve antibody production in man is unclear. There is also theoretical concern about correlation between antibodies to pre-S and the development of chronic active hepatitis.

Peptide subunits of bacterial antigens have been studied experimentally and would be expected to have many of the same advantages and disadvantages as peptide vaccines for viral diseases. Pilus proteins are responsible for the mucosal attachment and colonization of a number of pathogenic bacteria, including *Neisseria, E. coli,* and *Streptococcus.* Antibodies to pili block bacterial colonization and attachment (O'Hanley *et al.,* 1985; Rothbard *et al.,* 1985), and thus should be capable of preventing disease. Synthetic peptides mimicking the pilus protein subunits of a number of bacteria have been synthesized, and subunit vaccines containing synthetic pili have been shown to protect against experimental gonorrhea and invasive *E. coli* in laboratory animals (Tramont and Boslego, 1985; Schmidt *et al.,* 1988).

3. Enhancing Immunogenicity

A number of approaches are being investigated to enhance the immunogenicity of peptide vaccines. Certain proteins contain domains which seemed to be immunosuppressive in inbred mice (e.g., Kryzch *et al.,* 1985). Removal of immunosuppressive domains may enhance antibody responses to these proteins (Adorini *et al.,* 1979). The theoretical import of this experimental observation is apparent, though it has not yet been applied in practice to any human or veterinary vaccine.

Molecular manipulation of structure to mimic more closely natural three-dimensional conformation of a protein provides another approach to enhancing anbibody production. Peptides containing an intramolecular disulfide bond, for example, appear to be more immunogenic than those lacking cysteine residues (Dreesman *et al.,* 1982). A more elegant approach is to mimic tertiary or quaternary structure by inserting modified amino acids which can be covalently linked to produce the desired conformation. This has been achieved with a hydrazone–ethane link, or an intrapeptide ethylene bridge to mimic a normal α helix (Satterthwait *et al.,* 1988). One such peptide containing a covalent bridge between asparagine residues in a repeating epitope of the malaria circumsporozoite protein was reported to be highly immunogenic (Satterthwait *et al.,* 1988).

Fusion of peptides to known T cell epitopes may also improve immunogenicity. One example is the inclusion of pre-S in HBsAg peptides as described above. Another approach takes advantage of the observation that hepatitis B core protein (HBcAg) is a nearly universal stimulator of antibody production in individuals infected with hepatitis B virus. HBcAg contains epitopes recognized by T_H cells from all tested strains of inbred mice (Milich *et al.*, 1987). Like HBsAg, HBcAg forms regular aggregate particles in serum, a fact which probably contributes to its strong immunogenicity. A short peptide derived from the sequence of the neutralizing epitope of the viral capsid protein VP1 of foot-and-mouth disease virus (FMDV) produced a weak antibody response in cattle and pigs. However, fusion of the VP1 epitope to HBcAg as a carrier led to a dramatic increase in antibody titers to the peptide and greatly enhanced virus neutralization in vaccinated animals (Clark *et al.*, 1987). Fusion of helper T cell epitopes from inbred mice to FMDV or malaria polypeptides also led to greatly enhanced antibody production to FMDV (Francis *et al.*, 1987) and malarial antigens (Good *et al.*, 1987), presumably through enhanced recruitment and proliferation of B cells.

The search for "universal" T helper antigens, containing epitopes recognized by individuals of all HLA types, is underway. HBcAg could be one such carrier, although other molecules which are broadly immunogenic, such as tetanus and diptheria toxoids, could also be used. In theory, it should be possible to link multiple short peptides to HBcAg, and generate a particle which presents several different peptides simultaneously, arrayed on its surface. This may be a very effective way of producing a multivalent peptide vaccine.

C. Anti-Idiotypic Antibodies

1. Background

The near-infinite diversity of the variable (Fab) portions of human immunoglobulins led to the concept that the hypervariable region of a particular immunoglobulin (the idiotype, Ab_1) might serve as the target for a secondary antibody response, and thus generate an antibody (anti-idiotype, Ab_{2b}) reacting with it (see Jerne, 1974; UyteHaag *et al.*, 1986). Since the binding site of the anti-idiotype would have to fit precisely into the binding site of the idiotype, the anti-idiotype would then be a three-dimensional analog of the immunizing antigen (see Fig. 3). *In vivo,* idiotypes and anti-idiotypes might serve as part of a regulatory network for antibody production. In addition, anti-idiotypes, by providing an internal image of antigens, might continually stimulate host immunity and maintain memory cells.

Since the anti-idiotype provides an internal image of the antigen, it was also suggested that anti-idiotypic antibodies might be substituted for antigen in vaccination. Generation of anti-idiotypes involves immunizing an animal and isolating anti-idiotypes generated *in vivo,* or immunizing a second animal with Ab_1 to generate Ab_{2b}. Animals vaccinated with Ab_{2b} would then produce antibodies (Ab_3) capable of reacting with antigen in an identical manner to Ab_1 (Fig. 3).

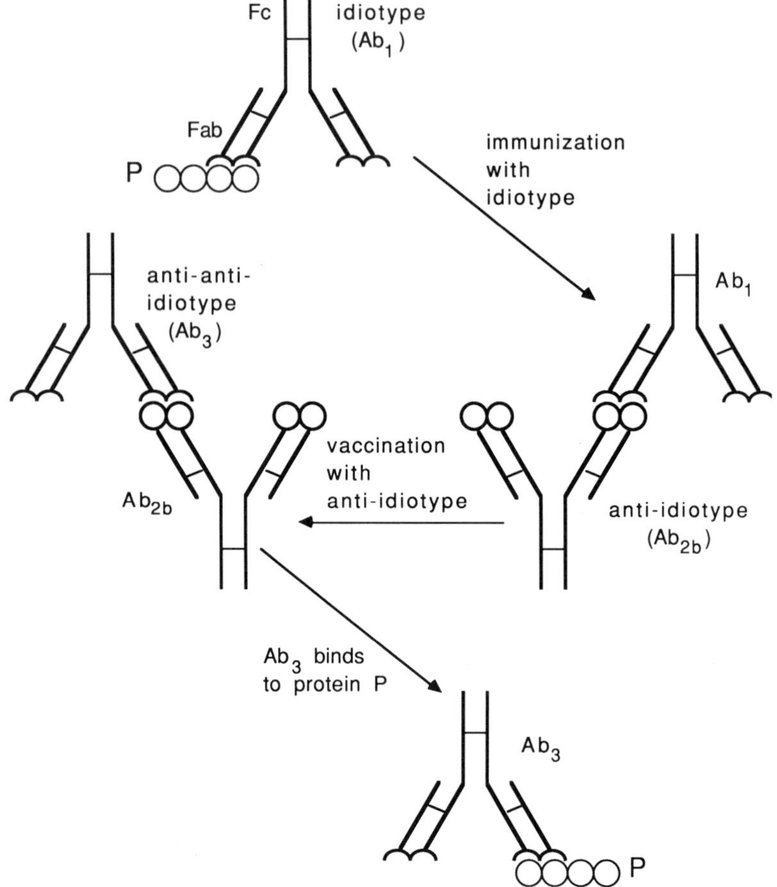

Fig. 3 Anti-idiotype vaccination. The idiotype (immunoglobulin Ab_1), specific for an antigenic determinant of a protein (P), is itself immunogenic. The anti-idiotype (Ab_2) recognizes the antigen binding site (Fab) of Ab_1 and serves as an internal image of the antigenic site on P. Vaccination with Ab_2 results in the production of an antibody (Ab_3) to the Fab of Ab_2. Ab_3 is thus an analog of Ab_1 and binds to the same antigenic determinant of P.

2. Development of Anti-Idiotype Vaccines

There is now a long list of immunogenic anti-idiotypic antibodies for a wide range of viral, bacterial, and parasitic antigens (reviewed by Finberg and Ertl, 1986; Ertl and Bona, 1988). In a few cases, these antibodies have generated a protective vaccine response in laboratory animals (Ertl and Bona, 1988). Anti-idiotypic antibodies are also capable of mimicking both carbohydrate and protein domains (Ward *et al.*, 1987).

The place of anti-idiotype vaccines in human disease remains unclear. It has been suggested that these antibodies would bypass the need for internalization, processing, and linkage to MHC molecules in generating immunity (Ertl and Bona, 1988), and would thus be particularly useful in certain immunocompromised hosts who normally generate poor vaccine responses. In addition, anti-idiotypes share the advantage of peptides in avoiding exposure to large quantities of pathogenic microbes during vaccine production. Such vaccines may also allow enhanced immunity in situations where there is a high frequency of mutation of neutralizing epitopes. All of this remains speculative, however.

Anti-idiotype vaccines would be encumbered by host antibody production against the Fc portion of immunoglobulin. This might severely curtail the utility of such vaccines if the Ig is derived from animal sources, and would limit the number of times an anti-idiotype might be administered. By analogy with available immune globulin preparations, large-scale production costs of such vaccines would probably be high, unless successful vaccination could be achieved with a small amount of protein. Finally, the ability of anti-idiotypic antibodies to stimulate specific CTL responses has not been clearly demonstrated, and anti-idiotypes might share with peptides and subunits the limitation of being good inducers of antibody but poor inducers of CTLs.

The most exciting potential for anti-idiotypes seems to be in immunotherapy. Anti-idiotypic antibodies prepared against human lymphomas have already been used successfully in treating advanced malignancy in animals (Campbell *et al.*, 1987) and man (Miller *et al.*, 1982), and the potential of anti-idiotypes in preventing allograft rejection is intriguing (Bluestone *et al.*, 1986).

D. Recombinant DNA Vectors

1. Attenuated Recombinant Microorganisms

About half of the viral vaccines currently in use are live attenuated microorganisms. Live vaccines appear to be more immunogenic than killed vaccines. In one of the few direct clinical comparisons published, live, cold-adapted influenza virus and live reassortant avian influenza virus vaccines elicited substantially higher antibody titers than their killed virus counterpart (Sears *et al.*, 1988). Live attenuated vaccines require the isolation of bacteria or viruses with the desired attenuation and immunogenicity, either as they arise in nature, or after serial passage of the parent microbe in tissue culture. Such vaccines are highly immunogenic since they mimic infection with the natural pathogen, but lack virulence factors responsible for causing disease. Unfortunately, live vaccines can cause disease in immunocompromised hosts, and can revert spontaneously to the virulent phenotype, causing disease in either primary vaccinees or contacts. Reversion is especially likely if the genetic differences between the virulent and attenuated strains are slight. The success of live virus vaccines, including polio, measles, mumps, rubella, and vaccinia, has generated interest in safer and more reliable means of attenuating pathogenic organisms to create vaccine strains.

Until recently, the attenuating genetic changes in live vaccines were not defined. Now, genetic changes responsible for attenuation in most live virus vaccines have been mapped, if not sequenced. Elucidation of the molecular genetics of the polio vaccine has been most instructive.

The live (Sabin) polio vaccine is a mixture of attenuated poliovirus types 1, 2, and 3. Rapid reversion to the virulent phenotype was long recognized clinicially in contact cases of polio, most often involving the type 3 strain of virus. Primary vaccinees may begin excreting virulent type 3 poliovirus as soon as a few days after vaccination, and continue to shed virus for several months (Minor *et al.*, 1986). In fact, the vaccine strain differs from wild type by only 10 point mutations (Westrop *et al.*, 1989), and only 2 of these appear to be responsible for attenuation of neurovirulence (Almond *et al.*, 1986; Westrop *et al.*, 1989). Frequent *in vivo* recombination between polio vaccine strains has been documented (Cammack *et al.*, 1988), and may account for rapid spontaneous reversion of the vaccine.

This dramatic exposition emphasizes the need for a new generation of live attenuated vaccines which retain immunogenicity but will not change phenotype or cause disease in immunocompromised hosts. Mutational analysis of viruses allows identification of virulence genes and lays the groundwork for attenuation through genetic manipulation. The elimination of a large piece of nonessential DNA, unlike a point mutation, greatly reduces the likelihood of a back-mutation or recombination which could restore virulence.

The pseudorabies virus (PRV) vaccine is an example of such an approach. Recognition of thymidine kinase as a virulence factor in herpes simplex virus infection prompted the search for a TK^- deletion mutant of PRV, an alphaherpesvirus which is the cause of Aujeszky's disease in livestock. Such a mutant was identified and was shown to be safe and efficacious as a PRV vaccine (Kit *et al.*, 1985). Furthermore, this mutant failed to revert to the TK^+ phenotype despite serial passage in selective media. Attempts to improve on the vaccine by deleting other nonessential PRV genes are underway (Kit *et al.*, 1987). Purposeful gene deletion through recombinant DNA techniques may eventually replace classical methodology for generating live vaccines.

Although we assume that the deletion of nonessential genes will attenuate a virus, this assumption may be naive. In fact, the deletion of a nonessential 19-kDa glycoprotein from the early region 3 of adenovirus type 5 resulted in enhanced virulence in laboratory animals (Ginsberg *et al.*, 1987). Experiments suggest that the normal function of this protein is to bind to class I MHC molecules and prevent transport of MHC–antigen complexes to the cell surface, thus blocking T cell recognition of adenovirus-infected cells and reducing the host immune response to adenovirus infection (Andersson *et al.*, 1985). This may explain why cotton rats infected with the deletion mutant develop more severe pneumonia and have a higher mortality than control animals infected with wild-type virus. Presumably, antigen presentation is enhanced in cells infected with the mutant, potentiating both the inflammatory response and immunopathology. Deletion mutants must therefore be evaluated with the same care as traditional live vaccines, since deletion will not necessarily result in attenuation, and genotype may give misleading information about *in vivo* phenotype.

In addition to passive attenuation by deletion or inactivation of genes, active attenuation may be achieved by incorporation of immunostimulatory elements such as lymphokine genes into recombinant viruses or bacteria. Insertion of the gene encoding interleukin-2 (IL-2) into live recombinant vaccinia virus protects immunodeficient athymic nude mice from lethal vaccinia virus infection, and significantly attenuates the virus in immunocompetent rodents (see Section IV,D,3a). The mechanism for attenuation is not clear, but presumably involves stimulation of antiviral immunity at an early stage after infection. Although not yet reported, incorporation of lymphokine genes such as IL-2 into other viruses or bacteria might improve the safety of other live vaccines. This approach could also be combined with the deletion of virulence genes.

2. Expression of Protein Subunits by Live Vectors

Gene transfer technology has made the expression of antigenic proteins by live recombinant microbial vectors routine. Bacteria, yeast, and cultured eukaryotic cell lines are all under development as protein expression systems. Proteins or polypeptides produced by live recombinant microorganisms share the same general features as polypeptides produced by conventional physicochemical processes (see Section IV,B). However, the intracellular processing of recombinant antigens may drastically alter the type and degree of immunity produced. In general, proteins expressed by homologous systems are the most immunogenic. Mimicry of natural infection remains a guiding principle.

Although recombinant bacteria such as *E. coli* are an economical and efficient means of generating simple proteins or polypeptides, complex mammalian proteins are not properly processed in bacterial cells, or may precipitate within the cell, making extraction difficult. This is especially critical with glycoproteins, since glycosylation does not occur faithfully in bacterial cells. The protective immunity generated by viral surface glycoproteins, particularly neutralizing antibody production, is felt to be critical for some viral vaccines. Bacteria may not be appropriate expression systems for viral antigens requiring posttranslational processing for full immunogenicity.

Recombinant yeast are another practical protein expression system. HBsAg produced by yeast is as immunogenic as the natural, virally encoded product (Jilg *et al.*, 1984), and a similar preparation has been licensed in the United States, representing the first human vaccine produced by recombinant DNA technology.

Live recombinant baculovirus is a second expression system utilizing lower eukaryotic cells. This insect virus directs expression of enormous quantities of a single protein, the polyhedrin, in infected insect cells. Foreign DNA inserted downstream from the polyhedrin promoter in recombinant baculovirus is likewise expressed in large quantities in insect cells infected with the recombinant. The envelope protein of HIV, gp160, purified from cultured insect cells infected with the recombinant virus, is immunogenic in man (Rusche *et al.*, 1987), and represents the first candidate HIV vaccine approved for experimental use in the United States. However, glycosylation in lower eukaryotic cells differs from that in mammalian cells. Consequently, the glycosylation of baculovirus-encoded viral glycoproteins differs slightly from the native configuration. This would be a major drawback for vaccines that rely on recognition of specifically glycosylated epitopes.

Recombinant protein expression in mammalian cells transfected with foreign DNA circumvents many of the disadvantages of viral antigen expression in bacteria, yeast, or insect cells. Expression of protein is directed by a known viral promoter, such as the SV40 late promoter, with attendant RNA processing signals. Foreign DNA can be inserted directly into chromosomal DNA using a retrovirus vector. This system offers the advantage of proper processing of complex glycoproteins, but unfortunately many mammalian cell systems do not produce large quantities of protein. Furthermore, recombinant mammalian cells may be unstable and lose the ability to express inserted DNA. Mammalian cells are also much more expensive to maintain in large cultures than bacteria or yeast. Finally, most mammalian cell lines used for protein production are derived from human tumors, and material may not be suitable for parenteral administration because of theoretical concerns about carcinogenesis due to contamination with oncogene products or latent viruses.

3. Live Recombinant Microorganisms as Vaccines

Major efforts in current vaccine research require expression of antigenic proteins in microbial vectors, in order to facilitate the study of protein function and immunogenicity. Several recombinant expression vectors are derived from microorganisms which readily infect man, such as *E. coli,* or have already been used as live vaccines, such as vaccinia. Some of these recombinants could be directly inoculated into an immunologically naive host, conferring immunity not only to the microbial vector, but also to any expressed foreign antigens. Vectors under consideration as possible live recombinant vaccines include mycobacteria, enteric bacteria, adenovirus, herpesviruses, poliovirus, and vaccinia virus (Table II).

This approach combines the advantages of both live and subunit vaccines. Advantages include authentic and immunogenic presentation of antigens, stimulation of both humoral and cell-mediated immunity, economic and facile administration of the vaccine, and the potential for multivalency. In addition, there is broad clinical experience with some of the vaccine vectors under consideration, including the Bacille Calmette-Guerin strain of *Mycobacterium bovis* (BCG), and vaccine strains of adenovirus, varicella zoster virus, and vaccinia virus.

Construction of live recombinant microorganisms is based on standard techniques. The expression of DNA encoding a foreign protein is controlled by host virus regulatory elements, including upstream promoter sequences and, where necessary, RNA processing signals. Consequently, antigen presentation mimics natural infection. The foreign protein is then expressed along with the proteins of the vector. Surface proteins, for example, are expressed in a manner indistinguishable from that seen in infection with the wild-type pathogen.

Different vectors could be used for different applications, depending on the

Table II

Organisms under Consideration as Live Recombinant Vaccine Vectors

Microorganism	Reference
Bacteria	
Enteric bacteria	
Escherichia coli	Charbit *et al.* (1987)
Salmonella	Baron *et al.* (1987), Clements *et al.* (1986)
Mycobacteria	Jacobs *et al.* (1987)
RNA viruses	
Poliovirus	Burke *et al.* (1988), Murray *et al.* (1988)
Avian influenza (reassortants)	Sears *et al.* (1988)
DNA viruses	
Adenovirus	Morin *et al.* (1987)
Herpesviruses	
Herpes simplex	Shih *et al.* (1984)
Herpes zoster	Lowe *et al.* (1987)
Poxviruses	
Fowlpox	Boyle and Coupar (1988), Taylor *et al.* (1988a)
Vaccinia	Moss and Flexner (1987)

characteristics of the microorganism. For example, enteric viruses or bacteria (e.g., adenovirus or *Salmonella*) would be optimal carriers for antigens from enteric pathogens, and would be expected to elicit strong mucosal immunity. The normal site of infection of a vector or route of inoculation would also be important for predicting immunogenicity.

The DNA viruses have been most actively developed as recombinant vaccines, largely because of familiarity with the attenuated versions of these viruses as live vaccines. Recombinant bacteria and RNA viruses are also being investigated. All hold great experimental promise as vaccines for certain diseases.

a. Recombinant Viruses Most viruses can be engineered for expression of foreign proteins or epitopes. As early as 1978, foreign DNA sequences were introduced into large DNA viruses through homologous recombination and marker rescue (reviewed by Roizman and Jenkins, 1985). Shortly thereafter, such recombinants were proposed as live vaccines. Although the technique was developed for herpes simplex virus, homologous recombination is useful for insertion of foreign DNA into other large DNA viruses, such as poxviruses (Moss and Flexner, 1987).

RNA viruses such as poliovirus have been used to express heterologous epitopes, but small RNA viruses are tightly packaged, contain few nonessential regions of DNA, and thus have limited capacity for foreign polypeptide expression. Smaller DNA viruses and RNA viruses may then be limited to expression of a single antigenic protein, or small polypeptides. Other virus vectors are widely used for protein expression, but their inability to replicate in mammalian hosts (e.g., baculovirus) or problems with constitutive protein expression and oncogenicity (e.g., retroviral vectors) precludes their consideration as vaccines.

i. Vaccinia The use of vaccinia as a live virus vaccine in the global campaign to eradicate smallpox made vaccinia an obvious choice for development as a live recombinant vaccine vector. Live recombinant vaccinia viruses expressing close to 100 different foreign proteins have been reported, and a number of these are effective experimental vaccines (reviewed by Moss and Flexner, 1987; Mackett and Smith, 1987). Vaccinia is particularly versatile as an expression vector because of its large genomic size, capability of accepting at least 25,000 base pairs of foreign DNA, and its ability to infect most eukaryotic cell types, including insect cells (ibid.). Unlike other DNA viruses, poxviruses replicate exclusively in the cytoplasm of infected cells, reducing the possibility of genetic exchange of recombinant viral DNA with the host chromosome. Recombinant vaccinia vectors have been shown to properly process and express proteins from a variety of sources including man, other mammals, parasites, RNA and DNA viruses, bacteria, and bacteriophage. The virus is capable of infecting most mammals, making it a useful vector for studying a broad range of human and animal diseases.

Recombinant vaccinia vaccines have been used to protect animals from a number of infectious diseases, including hepatitis B, influenza, rabies, measles, respiratory syncytial virus, and herpesviruses; in addition, vaccinia vectors expressing tumor antigens have been successfully used for the immunoprophylaxis and immunotherapy of animal tumors (Table III). Immunity is long-lived; mice vaccinated with a vaccinia recombinant expressing HSV glycoprotein D are fully protected from a lethal challenge with HSV up to 1 year after vaccination (Rooney *et al.*, 1988).

Live recombinant vaccinia viruses are capable of generating both humoral and cellular immunity. Although disease protection correlated with antibody titers in some cases, other recombinants appeared to protect by priming for Ig and effector lymphocyte responses. A vaccinia/HBsAg recombinant failed to stimulate protective titers of antibody in chimpanzees, but did protect against disease by priming animals for accelerated antibody production and possibly cell-mediated immunity (Moss *et al.*, 1984). Vaccinia recombinants expressing internal structural proteins or enzymes have also been protective in some cases, for example, with cytomegalovirus, Lassa fever, or influenza virus infections (see Table III). These vaccines almost certainly function by priming animals for CTLs which recognize and kill virally infected cells and thus attenuate disease (see Section V,B,2). A recombinant expressing the Friend murine leukemia virus envelope protein protected inbred mice with only certain MHC types from leukemia (Morrison *et al.*, 1987), suggesting Ir-restricted T_H or CTL activity.

The ubiquitous host range of the virus makes vaccinia an attractive vector for veterinary vaccines. Vaccinia/rabies glycoprotein recombinants can be administered orally, and are highly immunogenic in a range of wild and domestic animal species, including rodents, cattle, skunks, foxes, and raccoons (Rupprecht *et al.*, 1986; Moss and Flexner, 1987; Tolson *et al.*, 1987, 1988; Esposito *et al.*, 1988). Bait impregnated with live vaccinia virus is immunogenic when eaten, and can be air-dropped in areas where rabies is endemic; this strategy could be used to eradicate rabies in the wild (Johnston *et al.*, 1988). Such a system is currently being field-tested in open forestland in Europe (Newmark, 1988). Field trails of a vaccinia/rinderpest recombinant are also anticipated (Yilma *et al.*, 1988). Vaccinia is immunogenic in poultry, despite limited replication, and could be used to control outbreaks of avian influenza (Chambers *et al.*, 1988; De *et al.*, 1988).

Clinical experience with live recombinant vaccinia to date is limited. Vaccinia recombinants expressing the HIV envelope protein have been approved for investigational use as candidate acquired immunodeficiency syndrome (AIDS) vaccines in Zaire and the United States (Zagury *et al.*, 1987, 1988). The feasibility of using vaccinia in previously vaccinated individuals has been questioned, although revaccination was commonly practiced during the World Health Organization Campaign to Eradicate Smallpox (Galasso *et al.*, 1977). A handful of previously vaccinated individuals have been inoculated with live recombinants and have developed immunity to expressed foreign proteins (Jones *et al.*, 1986;

Zagury *et al.*, 1988). However, both of these examples involved the laboratory strain of vaccinia, designated WR, which is significantly more virulent than the Wyeth or Lister vaccine strains.

Because vaccinia has been perhaps the most widely used virus vaccine in history, its immunology, clinical efficacy, and side effects are rather well understood. Major side effects previously encountered include progressive or disseminated infection in infants or immunocompromised individuals; eczema vaccinatum, in which virus disseminated in areas of eczematous skin; vaccinia gangrenosum; and postvaccinal encephalopathy. Encephalopathy was a serious, and, fortunately, infrequent complication. Incidence was dependent on the vaccine strain employed, and ranged in frequency from 1 in 2,000, for the Copenhagen strain, to 1 in 200,000 or more for the Wyeth and Lister strains (Lane *et al.*, 1969; Johnson, 1982). Virulence therefore remains the overriding concern about renewed use of vaccinia as a vaccine vector. Since the virus replicates in the skin, there is also concern about contact spread of recombinants. Contact spread of vaccinia in man has occurred in the military (Baumgaertner *et al.*, 1985), the only group still routinely vaccinated. A single case of progressive vaccinia in a military recruit with AIDS has also been reported (Redfield *et al.*, 1987), and raises concerns about the vaccination of these and other immunocompromised hosts.

New techniques to attenuate recombinant viruses may dramatically enhance the safety of vaccinia and other live virus vectors. Inactivation of the vaccinia thymidine kinase (Buller *et al.*, 1985), vaccinia-encoded growth factor (Buller *et al.*, 1988), and fusion protein (Dallo and Esteban, 1987) greatly attenuates the virus in animals, and would also be expected to attenuate it in man. Active approaches to attenuation, in which host immunostimulatory proteins such as lymphokines are expressed by recombinant viruses (see Section III,A,4) are also promising. Human interleukin-2 (IL-2) expression prevents progressive vaccinia infection in immunodeficient athymic nude mice. This approach may reduce the danger of administering live viruses to other immunocompromised hosts (Flexner *et al.*, 1987; Ramshaw *et al.*, 1987). IL-2 expression also attenuates recombinant vaccinia in immunocompetent rodents (Flexner *et al.*, 1987) and primates (Flexner *et al.*, 1990) without significantly reducing immunogenicity, suggesting potential applicability to man.

Another approach to improving live vaccine safety is to select a virus vector which replicates so poorly in the vaccinated species that it is avirulent, for example, the use of avian influenza virus reassortants as human vaccines (Sears *et al.*, 1988, see below). The possibility of using host-range-restricted poxviruses is also under investigation. Fowlpox is an avipoxvirus which normally infects wildfowl; using the same techniques employed for recombinant vaccinia, two teams of investigators have constructed recombinant fowlpox vectors which express foreign proteins (Boyle and Coupar, 1988; Taylor *et al.*, 1988b). Recombinant fowlpox expressing the hemagglutinin of avian influenza virus protects poultry from lethal influenza (Taylor *et al.*, 1988b). In addition, a fowlpox/rabies glycoprotein recombinant is immunogenic and affords partial protection against lethal rabies in mice, cats, and dogs (Taylor *et al.*, 1988a). Recombinant fowlpox may then be immunogenic without the risks of contact spread of live virus or complications associated with virus replication, and could be useful in situations in which live vaccinia virus is undesirable, for example, in immunocompromised hosts (Taylor and Paoletti, 1988). However, the fowlpox/rabies glycoprotein recombinant produces a weaker immune response than a vaccinia/rabies glycoprotein recombinant. Although safer, recombinant fowlpox appears to be less immunogenic in mammals than recombinant vaccinia.

A number of approaches have been developed to improve the immunogenicity of live recombinant vaccinia vaccines. Since immunogenicity is largely dependent on the amount of foreign protein expressed, boosted levels of protein production would be desirable. This can be achieved through mutation of endogenous vaccinia promoters, or substitution of strong heterologous promoters (Fuerst *et al.*, 1986). Immunogenicity may also be enhanced by altering protein presentation on the surface of infected cells through membrane anchors (Langford *et al.*, 1986), or by incorporation of additional T cell epitopes in expressed antigens (Clark *et al.*, 1987; Good *et al.*, 1987).

The greatest potential impact of live recombinant vectors is in underdeveloped countries, where vaccination of infants and children could protect against the most serious infectious diseases. Two recent experiments suggest that maternal antibody may interfere with the immune response to recombinant vaccinia, as with other vaccines administered to children. Passive administration of antisera to respiratory syncytial virus (RSV) (Murphy *et al.*, 1988) or influenza (Johnson *et al.*, 1988) abrogates both the antibody response and disease protection mediated by vaccinia/RSV or vaccinia/influenza vaccines. Interestingly, replication and immunogenicity of vaccinia is apparently unaffected by antibodies to the influenza or RSV proteins. Passive blockade of antigen may be at least partially overcome by changing the route of inoculation, since intranasal administration of vaccinia/RSV vectors is significantly more immunogenic than dermal administration in cotton rats given anti-RSV antiserum parenterally (Murphy *et al.*, 1989).

ii. Other DNA viruses Herpesviruses, like poxviruses, have a large capacity for foreign DNA and have been proposed as vaccine vectors. Herpes simplex virus (HSV) can be readily engineered to express foreign antigens (Roizman and Jenkins, 1985; Shih *et al.*, 1984). However, HSV is a potential human pathogen and there is no clinical experience with live HSV as a vaccine vector. Since many people are already latently infected with HSV, the recombinant virus would probably have to be given in infancy or early childhood. Finally, since HSV establishes latency, there are questions about reactivation of the recombinant vector, genetic exchange with the host, and contact spread. Like vaccinia, TK^- HSV is greatly attenuated, and has a reduced capacity to establish latency in animal models (Meignier *et al.*, 1988). *In vivo* reactivation of recombinant HSV could be useful in some circumstances, for example, in gene replacement therapy, if foreign gene expression could be controlled.

Varicella-zoster virus (VZV), on the other hand, is a closely related herpesvirus which has been used as a human vaccine. The attenuated Oka strain of VZV has been used extensively in Japan with few adverse reactions, and is under investigation in this country for use in the immunocompromised. Like HSV, attenuated VZV has a reduced capacity for latency, although reactivation of the Oka vaccine in man has been reported. VZV can function as a vector for expression of foreign genes (Lowe *et al.*, 1987). One problem in the development of recombinant VZV is its restricted host range, with few animal models in which to test candidate vaccines. A primate host for VZV has recently been reported (Provost *et al.*, 1987).

One theoretical advantage of both HSV and VZV as live vaccine vectors is the availability of antiviral chemotherapy with acyclovir if immunocompromised vaccinees or contacts develop infectious complications. Effective chemotherapy is not currently available for the other DNA viruses under development as live vaccines.

Adenovirus has been used as a live vaccine by the military for several decades. It is also feasible to use adenovirus as a recombinant expression vector (Davis *et al.*, 1985). Adenovirus recombinants expressing HBsAg (Morin *et al.*, 1987) and HIV envelope protein (Dewar *et al.*, 1989) are immunogenic in animals, and have been proposed for use in man. Adenovirus is an attractive vaccine vector because of its clinical safety and efficacy via the oral route, making it especially attractive for the Third World. The oral route of inoculation makes adenovirus suitable for enteric pathogens and diseases in which mucosal immunity is desired. However, the adenovirus genome is tightly packaged and has a limited capacity for foreign DNA. Since immunity to adenovirus is ubiquitous and type specific, a recombinant vaccine would have to use an adenovirus strain to which vaccinees had not been previously exposed.

iii. Live recombinant RNA virus vaccines The avian influenza viruses replicate poorly in man, but are immunogenic (Sears *et al.*, 1988). Since the genomic organization of avian influenza virus is very similar to human influenza virus, virions isolated from cells infected with both human and avian influenza will consist of various reassortants carrying both human and avian virus genes. Selected reassortants carrying human hemagglutinin and neuraminidase genes, but with the remainder being avian genes, are immunogenic in man, and carry promise as live influenza vaccines (Sears *et al.*, 1988). Because these viruses replicate poorly in man, they should be safe in the immunocompromised.

Live recombinant poliovirus vectors have also been developed, involving replacement of immunogenic epitopes of the surface protein VP1 with the corresponding epitope from a different poliovirus strain (Burke *et al.*, 1988; Murray *et al.*, 1988). Chimeric polioviruses in which epitopes from more virulent strains are inserted into the capsid proteins of more attenuated strains might be safer live vaccines. In addition, poliovirus can be engineered to include neutralizing epitopes from other viruses such as HIV (Evans *et al.*, 1989). However, the limited capacity of poliovirus for heterologous DNA and constraints on VP1 processing may limit the application of this approach.

b. Recombinant Bacteria Live bacterial vaccines such as BCG have been used extensively. Plasmids containing foreign genes for expression can be engineered for many bacteria, and the direct inoculation of live recombinant bacteria follows logically.

Techniques for the expression of foreign immunogens in BCG, *S. typhi* vaccine strains, and *E. coli* have been reported (see Table II). Recombinant bacteria would be useful vaccines for bacterial diseases, although more complex

Table III

Disease Prevention by Vaccinia Virus Recombinants

Disease	Reference
Infections	
Cytomegalovirus	Jonjic *et al.* (1988)
Hepatitis B virus	Moss *et al.* (1984)
Herpes simplex virus type 1	Moss and Flexner (1987)
Human T cell leukemia virus type 1	Shida *et al.* (1987)
Influenza A virus	Moss and Flexner (1987)
Lassa fever virus	Clegg and Lloyd (1987), Fisher-Hoch *et al.* (1989)
Measles virus	Drillien *et al.* (1988)
Parainfluenza virus type 3	Spriggs *et al.* (1988)
Pseudorabies virus	Marchioli *et al.* (1987)
Rabies virus	Moss and Flexner (1987)
Respiratory syncytial virus	Moss and Flexner (1987)
Rinderpest virus	Yilma *et al.* (1988)
Simian virus 5	Paterson *et al.* (1987)
Venezuelan equine encephalitis virus	Kinney *et al.* (1988)
Vesicular stomatitis virus	Moss and Flexner (1987)
Malignancies	
Epstein-Barr virus lymphoma	Morgan *et al.* (1988)
Friend murine leukemia virus leukemia	Moss and Flexner (1987)
Melanoma	Estin *et al.* (1988)
Polyoma virus-induced tumor	Lathe *et al.* (1987)
Rat neu oncogene tumor	Bernards *et al.* (1987)

eukaryotic antigens, particularly glycoproteins, would not be properly processed (see Section IV,D,2). Enteric bacteria could be administered orally, and should be useful for enteric pathogens.

However, the stability of plasmids in bacterial vectors would have to be addressed, and chromosomal expression vectors should be further developed. Furthermore, recombinant enteric bacteria could be spread via the fecal–oral route, and could colonize the intestinal tract of some vaccinees, establishing a carrier state.

c. Revaccination and Polyvalency The decision to produce and use a vaccine is guided by a number of factors, including efficacy, safety, cost, and the gravity of the disease for which the vaccine has been developed. Advances in molecular biology have accelerated vaccine development, but also added complexity to questions about clinical vaccine use. This is particularly true for live recombinant vectors, where concerns about vector virulence, altered tissue tropism, and fear of release of live recombinant DNA organisms have brought controversy. Opposition to the use of the pseudorabies virus vaccines (see Kit *et al.*, 1985), a virus which probably differs little from naturally occurring mutants, points out public misunderstandings about recombinant DNA technology. Not surprisingly, initial field work with live recombinant vaccinia virus has also been accompanied by a great deal of controversy; an initial field trial of a vaccinia/rabies vaccine in Argentina was halted because of government concern about possible infection of animal handlers by the vector (Palca, 1988).

Since risk–benefit analysis of any vaccine would favor use if the vaccine were polyvalent, future vaccine development should concentrate on those systems which lend themselves to polyvalency. Polyvalent vaccines, such as live recombinant vectors expressing multiple protective antigens, or ISCOMs containing multiple protective epitopes, would be more economical and more acceptable, especially in the Third World. The capacity of DNA viruses for large amounts of foreign DNA suggests the possibility of constructing single live recombinant vaccines that express multiple foreign antigens. Single recombinant vaccinia viruses expressing up to three foreign proteins have been constructed (Perkus *et al.*, 1985; Flexner *et al.*, 1987, 1988).

A theoretical obstacle to the use of live recombinant vaccines is immune-mediated destruction of the vector in individuals who had already been exposed to the parent microorganism. For example, closely spaced inoculations with vaccinia resulted in a reduced vaccine "take," reflecting diminished virus replication; humans maintained a high level of immunity to vaccinia for at least 3 years (Galasso *et al.*, 1977). Experimentally, immunization with a vaccinia recombinant expressing HBsAg reduces the immune response to a different vaccinia recombinant expressing HSVgD when administered within 3 months of the original vaccination (Rooney *et al.*, 1988). It is likely that closely spaced inoculations with different live recombinant vaccinia vectors would result in reduced immunogenicity in man. Polyvalency would circumvent the reduction in immunogenicity of live vectors accompanying revaccination.

Existing immunity to one of the foreign antigens expressed by a polyvalent recombinant also might restrict replication of the vector, curtail expression of all antigens, and reduce the immune response to the vaccine. This could limit the application of any polyvalent recombinant live vaccine that contained an antigen to which a significant portion of the target population had preexisting immunity. Experiments with a polyvalent live vaccinia virus, however, suggest that preexisting immunity to one of the foreign antigens expressed by a polyvalent recombinant will not necessarily limit the efficacy of vaccination. A vaccinia recombinant expressing both influenza and HSV antigens was not less immunogenic than single recombinants in mice already immune to influenza virus or HSV (Flexner *et al.*, 1988).

V. Future Directions in Vaccine Research

Molecular biology has dominated vaccine development for the past decade. The ability to identify protective antigens, even epitopes, responsible for neutralizing antibody production and CTL activity has allowed scientists to target quickly particular polypeptides or oligosaccharides for inclusion in experimental vaccines. Identified antigens can be genetically mapped, sequenced, and expressed in short order. Candidate vaccines can be quickly assembled and tested in animal models.

Although molecular biology may greatly facilitate vaccine development, it has not fundamentally altered our approach to vaccination. Prophylactic inoculation with antigen, in a more or less purified state, is still the basic vaccine design. Nonetheless, the list of safe, effective vaccines remains short. This has led some to the conclusion that scientists are struggling with a group of diseases which are not amenable to vaccination. Recent difficulties in the development of an effective HIV vaccine have brought these shortcomings into the public limelight. Although some of the obstacles to vaccine development are technical, others are conceptual, requiring new ways of thought about what constitutes vaccination and how the immune system can be manipulated to prevent disease. This section summarizes some of the scientific horizons, as well as important socioeconomic factors, which will guide vaccine development in the near future.

Several experimental vaccines may soon have substantial impact on important areas of human health. At the same time, these vaccines emphasize several obstacles to vaccine development.

A. Targeted Diseases

1. Human Immunodeficiency Virus/Acquired Immunodeficiency Syndrome

Candidate vaccines were developed more rapidly for AIDS than for perhaps any disease in history. Within 3 years of the identification of the causative agent of this disease, a vaccine was generated, characterized, and tested in the only available animal model, the chimpanzee (Hu *et al.*, 1987). The failure of a live recombinant vaccinia virus expressing HIV envelope protein to protect against infection despite the production of both neutralizing antibodies (Hu *et al.*, 1987) and specific CTLs in vaccinated animals (Zarling *et al.*, 1987) was discouraging. Subsequent killed virus and subunit vaccines have also failed to protect chimpanzees from HIV infection. Nonetheless, a vaccinia/HIV envelope recombinant is being tested in man for safety and immunogenicity (Zagury *et al.*, 1987, 1988).

HIV possesses many features which make it resistant to eradication through vaccination, including great variability in surface proteins, chronicity of infection, cell-to-cell transmission of virus, and targeting of immune cells for destruction (reviewed by Ada, 1988). Perhaps the most ominous feature of this disease in terms of vaccine development is that, unlike most other viral diseases, the presence of both antibody and cell-mediated immunity appears to have no effect on disease progression, and may in certain instances be detrimental. Partial protection of macaques from simian immunodeficiency virus (SIV) infection and disease by killed virus preparations provide some encouragement that an effective HIV vaccine may be developed, although substantial difficulties remain (Desrosiers *et al.*, 1989; Murphey-Corb *et al.*, 1989).

2. Malaria

Malaria is one of the leading cause of mortality worldwide, accounting for over a million deaths annually, mostly in Africa. An effective malaria vaccine would be a major advance in public health. Success with human vaccination using irradiated sporozoites (the initial stage of *plasmodia*) decades ago raised hopes that an effective vaccine would be forthcoming. Initial vaccines were based on the stimulation of humoral immunity to the sporozoite or its major protein, the circumsporozoite protein (CSP) (Good *et al.*, 1988a). These vaccines have largely failed to protect in animal malaria models and in man, due to a combination of two factors. First, CSP contains a regularly repeating four amino acid motif which appears to be weakly immunogenic. Second, data acquired over the past decade suggest that cell-mediated immunity may correlate better than antibody with protection from infection in murine malaria models and man (Good *et al.*, 1988a). Current efforts are focusing on candidate vaccines which are good stimulators of cellular immunity. However, since T cell epitopes are HLA-restricted, simple peptide vaccines are not likely to be practical for malaria. Furthermore, data suggest that just as organisms change their B cell epitopes to evade neutralizing antibody, plasmodia may change their T cell epitopes to evade CTLs, since the major T cell epitopes of CSP are in a variable portion of the protein (Miller and Good, 1988).

3. Fertility Vaccines

Overpopulation, although not a disease, remains a major obstacle to human health and prosperity, particularly in underdeveloped regions. The failure of behavior modification or contraceptives to slow population growth in the Third World has led to research into immunization as a means of controlling fertility (Aitken and Paterson, 1988; Talwar and Raghupathy, 1989). Although a number of stages of fertilization and implantation have been targeted, the most advanced experimental vaccine to date is the β subunit of human chorionic gonadotropin (β-HCG). Although the intact subunit has significant homology to luteinizing hormone (LH), the carboxy-terminal polypeptide apparently has no close molecular relatives in man, so that antibodies to this molecule would not be expected to cross-react with other self proteins.

Efficacy studies with candidate β-HCG peptides in baboons have demonstrated no adverse reactions from the immunization and efficacy as great as that of oral contraceptives. Furthermore, "immunity" to conception correlates precisely with the level of anti-βHCG antibody produced. Once immunity has waned below the protective threshold, usually within 2 years, animals again become fertile. Such a vaccine could then produce a transient sterility, lasting for only a few years. At best, this vaccine should function as a long-acting contraceptive, rather than as a sterilization procedure. Phase I trials of β-HCG subunits in women of child-bearing age have now been completed in Australia and India, demonstrating both safety and induction of antibody titers which would be capable of preventing pregnancy (Talwar and Raghupathy, 1989). Phase II trials are planned in the same two countries.

There has been some concern over those vaccines employing intact β-HCG because of the potential for autoantibodies to LH. In addition, ethical objections have been raised to β-HCG vaccination because immunity is directed against implantation of the recently fertilized ovum. The vaccine might then be viewed as an early abortifacient. Although fertility vaccines seem practical, ethical and cultural considerations may prove more difficult to circumvent than human physiology.

4. Antineoplastic Vaccines

The use of vaccines to prevent viral illnesses associated with malignancy could have an enormous impact on the incidence of cancer worldwide. Hepatitis B vaccination appears to have already reduced the incidence of hepatocellular carcinoma in Taiwan. Widespread vaccination in southeast Asia, where hepatitis B and hepatoma are common, would be greatly beneficial. Similarly, development of an effective Epstein-Barr virus vaccine might have a major impact on the incidence of nasopharyngeal carcinoma and some B cell lymphomas (Epstein, 1987).

The importance of the immune system in suppressing tumor induction, controlling tumor growth, and inducing tumor regression is only now being fully appreciated. This has led to the use of immunomodulatory substances such as interferons (Tyrell, 1987) and IL-2 (Rosenberg and Lotze, 1986) as primary or adjunctive cancer therapy.

The observation that some solid tumor antigens invoked antitumor immunity fostered the notion that vaccination with tumor antigens might prevent malignancy. This concept was tested experimentally in the 1970s, demonstrating the ability of vaccination to prevent tumor growth in animal models and, in some cases, to induce regression of established tumors. This approach could be particularly beneficial in tumors with a high frequency of spontaneous regression, such as melanoma; these malignancies seem most susceptible to active immunotherapy (Rosenberg and Lotze, 1986). Unfortunately, most reported animal models suffer from the fact that established tumors were either derived from different species or from virally transformed cells, raising doubts about their relevance to solid tumors in man.

Vaccinia virus recombinants expressing tumor antigens from three different solid tumors have been shown to protect animals from tumor development and, in some cases, to stimulate regression of established tumors (see Table III). Given some suggestions of nonspecific antitumor activity of vaccinia virus cell lysates in man (Mitchell, 1989), vaccinia could be a promising carrier for antigens for tumor vaccines or adjuvant immunotherapy.

A third approach to prevention of malignancy involves stimulation of antibodies capable of "neutralizing" chemical carcinogens. An animal model was recently reported in which intestinal administration of cholera toxin conjugated to 2-acetylaminofluorene induced specific IgA capable of binding to this carcinogenic molecule (Silbart and Keren, 1989). Antibodies impaired intestinal absorption of the free carcinogen, and would presumably reduce the chance of neoplastic transformation. It is conceivable that similar vaccines could be developed for selected carcinogens or environmental toxins.

B. Novel Approaches to Immunization

1. Prevention of Virus Attachment to Cellular Receptors

The identification and molecular characterization of virus receptors have led to attempts to block infectivity by preventing virus–receptor interaction. Two approaches have been employed. The first is to synthesize large quantities of synthetic receptor which bind to virus envelope proteins and thus prevent envelope–receptor binding. This concept has been most recently applied with soluble CD4, the HIV receptor used to block the infectivity of HIV (see Capon *et al.*, 1989). The second approach is to administer antibodies passively to the cell surface receptor to block virus envelope protein from binding to receptor. One recent example is based on the observation that antibodies which neutralize rhinovirus prevent the attachment of the viral capsid protein to a specific cell surface receptor (Colonno *et al.*, 1989), recently identified as intercellular adhesion molecule 1 (ICAM-1; Tomassini *et al.*, 1989). Administration of a murine monoclonal antibody to ICAM-1 appears to be safe and nontoxic in laboratory animals, and a small human trial with this monoclonal administered intranasally demonstrated some efficacy in delaying the onset and reducing the severity of cold symptoms following challenge with rhinovirus (Hayden *et al.*, 1988).

Anti-idiotypic antibodies mimicking virus receptor proteins could be used as prophylaxis or treatment for established infections, and might offer certain advantages over either soluble receptor or receptor antibody. Anti-idiotypic antibodies to the monoclonal antibody OKT4a, which binds to the HIV attachment site on the CD4 receptor and prevents HIV infection of $CD4^+$ cells, block infection of cells by HIV (Dagleish *et al.*, 1987). Theoretically, such a preparation could also be used to prevent HIV infection in man.

One drawback to therapeutic receptor blockade, either with polypeptide or with immunoglobulin, is that the blocking molecule must be present in high concentrations at all times in order to be effective. This may be impractical for viruses causing prolonged systemic infection, such as HIV, but may be useful for viruses causing local infections, such as rhinovirus, where blocking antibody could be administered intranasally when needed. Vaccine-induced antibodies to epitopes of cellular virus receptors, or anti-idiotype vaccines mimicking soluble receptor, might provide long-lived systemic protection. However, by definition, such antibodies would require an autoimmune response which might be difficult or impossible to sustain, and might interfere with normal cellular functions.

2. Vaccines Targeting Internal Antigens

Because neutralizing antibody responses are directed against surface proteins of microbial pathogens, vaccine development has focused largely on envelope or outer membrane proteins and polysaccharides. The recognition that CTL responses in mice and humans are often directed against internal, rather than surface proteins (see Townsend and Bodmer, 1989) has created interest in internal antigens as possible vaccine targets.

A major CTL target following influenza A virus infection in inbred mice is the nucleoprotein (NP) (Townsend and Bodmer, 1989). Mice vaccinated with purified NP (Wraith *et al.*, 1987) or vaccinia/NP recombinants (Andrew *et al.*, 1986; Flexner *et al.*, 1987) are protected from lethal challenge with influenza A virus; infection is not prevented in these animals, instead they develop attenuated disease and recover from an otherwise lethal inoculum of virus. Protection correlates with CTL activity, and although anti-NP antibodies are generated, they appear to play no role in recovery. Predictably, mouse strains lacking anti-NP CTL responses are not protected after NP vaccination (Flexner *et al.*, 1987), supporting the notion that CTL activity mediates the attenuation of disease.

This initial observation has now been followed by reports that internal proteins of other viruses can be used as vaccine antigens. Vaccination with Lassa fever nucleoprotein (Clegg and Lloyd, 1987), dengue virus (Schlesinger *et al.*, 1987) and other flavivirus nonstructural antigens (Gibson *et al.*, 1988), and a cytomegalovirus immediate early antigen (Jonjic *et al.*, 1988) attenuate disease and protect animals from otherwise lethal infections. In the latter example, protection was proven to be CTL dependent (Reddehase *et al.*, 1987).

Because internal antigens are relatively conserved compared to surface proteins, their inclusion might reduce concerns about antigenic drift and produce cross-reactive immunity to related proteins from other pathogens. The nucleoprotein of influenza, for example, has varied by only a few amino acids over the past 50 years, despite enormous variability in the hemagglutinin and neuraminidase surface proteins (see Wraith *et al.*, 1987). Since internal antigens seem to induce protection via specific CTL activity, this approach might prove particularly useful for intracellular pathogens, or organisms capable of establishing latency, including herpesviruses and retroviruses.

Vaccines which depend on a CTL response must contain sufficient T cell epitopes to cover the full range of HLA types in the target population (see Section II,C). In addition, since CTLs recognize processed antigen and are only stimulated after cells have been infected with virus, these vaccines would not likely prevent infection, but would prime the host for boosted cellular immunity. This strategy might not then block the transmission of respiratory viruses, and might be undesirable for pathogens which are capable of quickly establishing latency and "hiding" from the immune system, such as HIV. Although neutralizing antibody persists for months or years, substantial CTL activity persists for only a few days in animal models of acute infection (see Ada, 1989). A "protective" CTL response might then persist for only a short time after vaccination, and might require extended antigenic stimulation, such as antigen release from an internal depot, in order to produce longer-lived protection.

3. T Cell Vaccination

Passively administered immunoglobulin and anti-idiotype antibodies have been used for experimental prophylaxis of infectious diseases (see Section IV,C).

Passively administered T lymphocytes are now under study as experimental vaccines for autoimmune diseases. Immunity to myelin basic protein (MBP) produces experimental autoimmune encephalomyelitis (EAE) in rats. Passive infusion of MBP-reactive T lymphocytes prevents the development of EAE after challenge with antigen (Lider *et al.*, 1988). Data suggest that the infused lymphocytes stimulate an anti-idiotypic network of T cells, which suppress the pathogenic anti-MBP cellular response.

T cell vaccination prevents several other experimental autoimmune diseases (Lider *et al.*, 1988), and presumably could be applied to any disease in which immunity to alloantigens is pathogenic, including transplantation. Clinical application of this technique seems remote at present. *In vivo* stimulation of suppressor T cell activity without infusion of autologous lymphocytes might make T cell vaccination more practical.

C. Principles Guiding Future Vaccine Development

Despite their relative cost-effectiveness and potential for disease eradication, the development of vaccines has proceeded slowly compared to other pharmaceuticals. In recent years, vaccine production and use in the developed world have been heavily influenced by issues of liability and profitability. The cost of the DPT vaccine, for example, has increased 100-fold in this decade because of litigation or the perceived threat of litigation (Kolata, 1986), and other vaccines have been similarly affected. The number of manufacturers of DPT in the United States dwindled at one point to a single company, with attendant short supply (Kolata, 1986). Misgivings about vaccine toxicity have led many parents to leave their children unvaccinated (Zimmerman *et al.*, 1987). Continued outbreaks of measles and pertussis in the United States and Europe are reminders of the fact that vaccines not used are not effective. Product liability limitation, tort reform, and uniform compensation for adverse reactions have been proposed as possible solutions to this problem, but must be accompanied by continued efforts to improve vaccine safety and efficacy.

Finally, since vaccination's greatest potential impact on longevity is in countries with limited health budgets, financial and logistical considerations must weigh heavily in vaccine design if the full benefit of new vaccines is to be realized. The utility of an expensive recombinant peptide vaccine, for example, will be lost in countries where total annual per capita health expenditures are less than 10 dollars.

Modern approaches to the definition of protective epitopes and identification of harmful components of vaccines should help to improve existing vaccines. Advances in immunology, microbiology, and molecular biology should continue to provide the basis for the next generation of safe and effective vaccines.

Acknowledgment

The author would like to thank Gordon Ada for helpful discussions during the preparation of this manuscript.

References

Ada, G. L. (1988). Prospects for HIV vaccines. *J. Acquired Immune Deficiency Syndromes* **1,** 295–303.

Ada, G. L. (1989). Vaccines. *In* "Fundamental Immunology" (W. Paul, ed.), 2nd ed. pp. 985–1032. Raven Press, New York.

Adorini, L., Harvey, M. A., Miller, A., and Sercarz, E. E. (1979). Fine specificity of regulatory T cells. II. Suppressor and helper T cells are induced by different regions of hen egg-white lysozyme in a genetically non-responder mouse strain. *J. Exp. Med.* **150,** 293–306.

Aitken, R. J., and Paterson, M. (1988). New horizons in contraception. *Nature (London)* **335,** 492–493.

Allison, A. C., and Gregoriadis, G. (1974). Liposomes as immunological adjuvants. *Nature (London)* **252,** 252.

Almond, J. W., Westrop, G. D., Evans, D. M. A., Dunn, G., Minor, P. D., Magrath, D., and Schild, G. C. (1986). Studies on the attenuation of the Sabin type 3 oral polio vaccine. *J. Virol. Methods* **17,** 183–189.

Andersson, M., Paabo, S., Nilsson, T., and Peterson, P. A. (1985). Impaired intracellular transport of class I MHC antigens as a possible means for adenoviruses to evade immune surveillance. *Cell (Cambridge, Mass.)* **43,** 215.

Andrew, M. E., Coupar, B. E. H., Ada, G. L., and Boyle, D. B. (1986). Cell-mediated immune response to influenza virus antigens expressed by vaccinia virus recombinants. *Microb. Pathog.* **1,** 443–452.

Baron, L. S., Kopecko, D. J., Formal, S. B., Seid, R., Guerry, P., and Powell, C. (1987). Introduction of Shigella flexneri 2a type and group antigen genes into oral typhoid vaccine strain Salmonella typhi Ty21a. *Infect. Immun.* **55,** 2797–2801.

Baumgaertner, J. C., Hogan, R., Born, C., Berg, J., and Davis, J. P. (1985). Contact spread of vaccinia from a National Guard vaccinee. *JAMA, J. Am. Med. Assoc.* **253,** 2348.

Berkowitz, C. D., Ward, J. I., Meier, K., Hendley, J. O., Brunell, P. A., Barkin, R. A., Zahradnik, J. M., Samuelson, J., and Gordon, L. (1987). Safety and immunogenicity of Haemophilus influenzae type B polysaccharide and polysaccharide diptheria toxoid conjugate vaccines in children 15 to 24 months of age. *J. Pediatr.* **110,** 509–514.

Bernards, R., Destree, A., McKenzie, S., Gordon, E., Weinberg, R. A., and Panicali, D. (1987). Effective tumor immunotherapy directed against an oncogene-encoded product using a vaccinia virus vector. *Proc. Natl. Acad. Sci. U.S.A.* **84,** 6854–6858.

Bluestone, J. A., Leo, O., Epstein, S. L., and Sachs, D. H. (1986). Idiotypic manipulation of the immune response to transplantation antigens. *Immunol. Rev.* **90,** 5–27.

Boyle, D. B., and Coupar, E. H. (1988). Construction of recombinant fowlpox viruses as vectors for poultry vaccines. *Virus Res.* **10,** 343–356.

Buller, R. M. L., Smith, G. L., Cremer, K., Notkins, A. L., and Moss, B. (1985). Decreased virulence of recombinant vaccinia virus vectors is associated with a thymidine kinase-negative phenotype. *Nature (London)* **317,** 813–815.

Buller, R. M. L., Chakrabarti, S., Cooper, J. A., Twardzik, D. R., and Moss, B. (1988). Deletion of the vaccinia virus growth factor gene reduces virus virulence. *J. Virol.* **62,** 866–874.

Burke, K. L., Dunn, G., Ferguson, M., Minor, P. D., and Almond, J. W. (1988). Antigen chimaeras of poliovirus as potential new vaccines. *Nature (London)* **332,** 81–82.

Byars, N. E., and Allison, A. C. (1987). Adjuvant formulation for use in vaccines to elicit both cell-mediated and humoral immunity. *Vaccine* **5,** 223–228.

Cammack, N., Phillips, A., Dunn, G., Patel, V., and Minor, P. D. (1988). Intertypic genomic rearrangements of poliovirus strains in vaccinees. *Virology* **167,** 507–514.

Campbell, M. J., Caroll, W., Kon, S., Thielemans, K., Rothbard, J., Levy, S., and Levy, R. (1987). Idiotype vaccination against murine B cell lymphoma. *J. Immunol.* **139,** 2825–2833.

Capon, D. J., Chamow, S. M., Mordenti, J., Marsters, S. A., Gregory, T., Mitsuya, H., Byrn, R. A., Lucas, C., Wurm, F. M., Groopman, J. E., Broder, S., and Smith, D. H. (1989). Designing CD4 immunoadhesins for AIDS therapy. *Nature (London)* **337,** 525–531.

Chambers, T. M., Kawaoka, Y., and Webster, R. G. (1988). Protection of chickens from lethal influenza infection by vaccinia-expressed hemagglutinin. *Virology* **167,** 414–421.

Charbit, A., Sobczak, E., Michel, M.-L., Molla, A., Tiollais, P., and Hofnung, M. (1987). Presentation of two epitopes of the preS2 region of hepatitis B virus on live recombinant bacteria. *J. Immunol.* **139,** 1658–1664.

Clark, B. E., Newton, S. E., Carroll, A. R., Francis, M. J., Appleyard, G., Syred, A. D., Highfield, P. E., Rowlands, D. J., and Brown, F. (1987). Improved immunogenicity of a peptide after fusion to hepatitis B core protein. *Nature (London)* **330,** 381–384.

Clegg, J. C. S., and Lloyd, G. (1987). Vaccinia recombinant expressing Lassa-virus internal nucleocapsid protein protects guinea pigs against Lassa fever. *Lancet* **2,** 186–188.

Clements, J. D., Lyon, F. L., Lowe, K. L., Farrand, A. L., and El-Morshidy, S. (1986). Oral immunization of mice with attenuated Salmonella enteritidis containing a recombinant plasmid which codes for production of the B subunit of heat-labile Escherichia coli enterotoxin. *Infect. Immun.* **53,** 685–692.

Colonno, R. J., Callahan, P. L., Leippe, D. M., Rueckert, R. R., and Tomassini, J. E. (1989). Inhibition of rhinovirus attachment by neutralizing monoclonal antibodies and their Fab fragments. *J. Virol.* **63,** 36–42.

Dagleish, A. G., Thomson, B. J., Chanh, T. C., Malkovsky, M., and Kennedy, R. C. (1987). Neutralization of HIV isolates by anti-idiotypic antibodies which mimic the T4 (CD4) epitope: A potential AIDS vaccine. *Lancet* **2,** 1047–1050.

Dallo, S., and Esteban, M. (1987). Isolation and characterization of attenuated mutants of vaccinia virus. *Virology* **159,** 408–422.

Davis, A. R., Kostek, B., Mason, B. B., Hsiao, C. L., Morin, J., Dheer, S. K., and Hung, P. P. (1985). Expression of hepatitis B surface antigen with a recombinant adenovirus. *Proc. Natl. Acad. Sci. U.S.A.* **82,** 7560–7564.

De, B. K., Shaw, M. W., Rota, P. A., Harmon, M. W., Esposito, J. J., Rott, R., Cox, N. J., and Kendal, A. P. (1988). Protection against virulent H5 avian influenza virus infection in chickens by an inactivated vaccine produced with recombinant vaccinia virus. *Vaccine* **6,** 257–261.

Desrosiers, R. C., Wyand, M. S., Kodama, T., Ringler, D. J., Arthur, L. O., Sehgal, P. K., Letvin, N. L., King, N. W., and Daniel, M. D. (1989). Vaccine protection against simian immunodeficiency virus infection. *Proc. Natl. Acad. Sci. U.S.A.* **86,** 6353–6357.

Dewar, R. L., Natarajan, V., Vasudevachari, M. B., and Salzman, N. (1989). Synthesis and processing of human immunodeficiency virus type 1 envelope proteins encoded by a recombinant human adenovirus. *J. Virol.* **63,** 129–136.

Dreesman, D. R., Sanchez, Y., Ionescu-Matin, I., Sparrow, J. T., Six, H. R., Peterson, D. L., Hollinger, F. B. and Melnick, J. L. (1982). Antibody to hepatitis B surface antigen after a single inoculation of uncoupled synthetic HBsAg peptides. *Nature (London)* **295,** 158–160.

Drillien, R., Spehner, D., Kirn, A., Giraudon, P., Buckland, R., Wild, F., and Lecocq, J.-P. (1988).

Protection of mice from fatal measles encephalitis by vaccination with vaccinia virus recombinants encoding either the hemagglutinin or the fusion protein. *Proc. Natl. Acad. Sci. U.S.A.* **85,** 1252–1256.

Edelman, R. (1980). Vaccine adjuvants. *Rev Infect. Dis.* **2,** 370.

Eisenberg, R., Cerini, C. P., Heilman, C. J., Joseph, A. D., Dietzschold, B., Golub, E., Long, D., de Leon, M. P., and Cohen, G. H. (1985). Synthetic glycoprotein D related peptides protect mice against herpes simplex challenge. *J. Virol.* **56,** 1014–1017.

Epstein, M. A. (1987). Vaccine prevention of virus-induced human cancers. *Proc. R. Soc. London, Ser. B* **230,** 147–161.

Ertl, H. C. J., and Bona, C. A. (1988). Criteria to define anti-idiotypic antibodies carrying the internal image of the antigens. *Vaccine* **6,** 80–84.

Esposito, J. J., Knight, J. C., Shaddock, J. H., Novembre, F. J., and Baer, G. M. (1988). Successful oral rabies vaccination of raccoons with raccoon poxvirus recombinants expressing rabies virus glycoprotein. *Virology* **165,** 313–316.

Estin, C. D., Stevenson, U. S., Plowman, G. D., Hu, S.-L., Sridhar, P., Hellström, I., Brown, J. P., and Hellström, K. E. (1988). Recombinant vaccinia virus vaccine against the human melanoma antigen p97 for use in immunotherapy. *Proc. Natl. Acad. Sci. U.S.A.* **85,** 1052–1056.

Evans, D. J., McKeating, J., Meredith, J. M., Burke, K. L., Katrak, K., John, A., Ferguson, M., Minor, P. D., Weiss, R. A., and Almond, J. W. (1989). An engineered poliovirus chimaera elicits broadly reactive HIV-1 neutralizing antibodies. *Nature* **339,** 385–388.

Finberg, R. W., and Ertl, H. C. J. (1986). The use of T-cell specific anti-idiotypes to immunize against viral infections. *Immunol. Rev.* **90,** 129–155.

Fisher-Hoch, S. P., McCormick, J. B., Auperin, D., Brown, B. G., Castor, M., Perez, G., Ruo, S., Conaty, A., Brammer, L., and Bauer, S. (1989). Protection of rhesus monkeys from fatal Lassa fever by vaccination with a recombinant vaccinia virus containing the Lassa virus glycoprotein gene. *Proc. Natl. Acad. Sci. U.S.A.* **86,** 317–321.

Flexner, C., Hugin, A., and Moss, B. (1987). Prevention of vaccinia virus infection in immunodeficient mice by vector-directed IL-2 expression. *Nature (London)* **330,** 259–262.

Flexner, C., Murphy, B. R., Rooney, J. F., Wohlenberg, C., Yuferov, V., Notkins, A. L., and Moss, B. (1988). Successful vaccination with a polyvalent live vector despite existing immunity to an expressed antigen. *Nature (London)* **335,** 259–262.

Flexner, C., Moss, B., London, W. T., and Murphy, B. R. (1990). Attenuation and immunogenicity in primates of vaccinia virus recombinants expressing human interleukin-2. *Vaccine* (in press).

Francis, M. J., Hastings, G. Z., Syred, A. D., McGinn, B., Brown, F., and Rowlands, D. J. (1987). Non-responsiveness to a foot-and-mouth disease virus peptide overcome by addition of foreign helper T-cell determinants. *Nature (London)* **330,** 168–172.

Freund, J., Casals, J., and Hismer, E. P. (1937). Sensitization and antibody formation after injection of tubercle bacilli and paraffin oil. *Proc. Soc. Exp. Biol. Med.* **37,** 509.

Fuerst, T. R., Niles, E. G., Studier, F. W., and Moss, B. (1986). Eukaryotic transient expression system based on recombinant vaccinia virus that synthesizes bacteriophage T7 RNA polymerase. *Proc. Natl. Acad. Sci. U.S.A.* **83,** 8122–8126.

Galasso, G. J., Karzon, D. T., Katz, S. L., Krugman, S., Neff, J., and Robbins, F. C. (1977). Clinical and serologic study of four smallpox vaccines comparing variations of dose and route of administration. *J. Infect. Dis.* **135,** 131–185.

Gibson, C. A., Schlesinger, J. J., and Barrett, A. D. T. (1988). Prospects for a virus non-structural protein as a subunit vaccine. *Vaccine* **6,** 7–9.

Ginsberg, H., Valdesuso, J., Horswood, R., Chanock, R. M., and Prince, G. (1987). Adenovirus gene products affecting pathogenesis. *In* "Vaccines '87, Modern Approaches to New Vaccines" (R. M. Chanock R. A. Lerner, F. Brown, and H. Ginsberg, eds.), pp. 322–326. Cold Spring Harbor Lab., Cold Spring Harbor, New York.

Good, M. F., Maloy, W. L., Lunde, M. N., Margalit, H., Cornette, J. L., Smith, G. L., Moss, B., Miller, L. H., and Berzofsky, J. A. (1987). Construction of synthetic immunogen: Use of new T-helper epitope on malaria circumsporozoite protein. *Science* **235,** 1059–1062.

Good, M. F., Berzofsky, J. A., and Miller, L. H. (1988a). The T cell response to the malaria circumsporozoite protein: An immunological approach to vaccine development. *Annu. Rev. Immunol.* **6,** 663–688.

Good, M. F., Pombo, D., Lunde, M. N., Maloy, W. L., Halenbeck, R., Koths, K., Miller, L., and Berzofsky, J. A. (1988b). Recombinant human IL-2 overcomes genetic nonresponsiveness to malaria sporozoite peptides. *J. Immunol.* **141,** 972–977.

Hayden, F. G., Gwaltney, J. M., and Colonno, R. J. (1988). Modification of experimental rhinovirus colds by receptor blockade. *Antiviral Res.* **9,** 233–247.

Hendley, J. O., Wenzel, J. G., Ashe, K. M., and Samuelson, J. S. (1987). Immunogenicity of Haemophilus influenzae type B capsular polysaccharide vaccines in 18-month-old infants. *Pediatrics* **80,** 351–354.

Hopkins, D. R. (1983). "Princes and Peasants; Smallpox in History." Univ. of Chicago Press, Chicago, Illinois.

Howard, C. R., Sundquist, B., Allan, J., Brown, S. E., Chen, S.-H., and Morein, B. (1987). Preparation and properties of immune-stimulating complexes containing hepatitis B virus surface antigen. *J. Gen. Virol.* **68,** 2281–2289.

Hu, S.-L., Fultz, P. N., McClure, H. M., Eichberg, J. W., Thomas, E. K., Zarling, J., Singhal, M. C., Kosowski, S. G., Swenson, R. B., Anderson, D. C., and Todaro, G. (1987). Effect of immunization with a vaccinia-HIV env recombinant on HIV infection of chimpanzees. *Nature (London)* **328,** 721–723.

Hunter, R. L., and Bennett, B. (1984). The adjuvant activity of non-ionic block polymer surfactants. II. Antibody formation and inflammation related to the structure of triblock and octablock copolymers. *J. Immunol.* **133,** 3167.

Jacobs, W. R., Tuckman, M., and Bloom, B. R. (1987). Introduction of foreign DNA into mycobacteria using a shuttle phasmid. *Nature (London)* **327,** 532–535.

Jerne, N. K. (1974). Towards a network theory of the immune system. *Ann. Immunol. (Paris)* **125C,** 373.

Jilg, W., Schmidt, M., Zoulek, G., Larbeer, B., Wilske, B., and Deinhardt, F. (1984). Clinical evaluation of a recombinant hepatitis B vaccine. *Lancet* **2,** 1174–1175.

Johnson, M. P., Meitin, C. A., Bender, B. S., and Small, P. A. (1988). Passive immune serum inhibits antibody response to recombinant vaccinia virus. *In* "Vaccines '88, New Chemical and Genetic Approaches to Vaccination" (H. Ginsberg, F. Brown, R. A. Lerner, and R. M. Chanock, eds.), pp. 189–192. Cold Spring Harbor Lab., Cold Spring Harbor, New York.

Johnson, R. T. (1982). Parainfectious neurological syndromes. *In* "Viral Infections of the Nervous System," pp. 180–182. Raven Press, New York.

Johnston, D. H., Voigt, D. R., MacInnes, C. D., Bachman, P., Lawson, K. F., and Rupprecht, C. E. (1988). An aerial baiting system for the distribution of attenuated or recombinant rabies vaccines for foxes, raccoons, and skunks. *Rev. Infect. Dis.* **10** (Suppl. 4), S660–S664.

Johnston, L. A., Kemp, D. H., and Pearson, R. D. (1986). Immunization of cattle against Boophilus microplus using extracts derived from adult female ticks: Effects of induced immunity on tick populations. *Int. J. Parasitol.* **16,** 27–34.

Jones, L., Ristow, S., Yilma, T., and Moss, B. (1986). Accidental human vaccination with vaccinia virus expressing nucleoprotein gene. *Nature (London)* **319,** 543.

Jonjic, S., del Val, M., Keil, G. M., Reddehase, M. J., and Koszinowski, U. H. (1988). A nonstructural viral protein expressed by a recombinant vaccinia virus protects against lethal cytomegalovirus infection. *J. Virol.* **62,** 1653–1658.

Kakumu, S., Fuji, A., Tahara, H., Yoshioka, K., and Sakamoto, N. (1988). Enhancement of antibody production to hepatitis B surface antigen by interleukin 2. *J. Clin. Lab. Immunol.* **26,** 25–27.

Kawamura, H., Rosenberg, S. A., and Berzofsky, J. A. (1985). Immunization with antigen and interleukin 2 in vivo overcomes Ir gene low responsiveness. *J. Exp. Med.* **162,** 381–386.

Kersten, G. F. A., Teerlink, T., Derks, H. J. G. M., Verkleij, A. J., Van Wezel, T. L., Crommlein, D. J. A., and Beuvery, E. C. (1988a). Incorporation of the major outer membrane protein of Neisseria gonorrhoeae in saponin–lipid complexes (Iscoms): Chemical analysis, some structural features, and comparison of their immunogenicity with three other antigen delivery systems. *Infect. Immun.* **56,** 432–438.

Kersten, G. F. A., Van de Put, A.-M., Teerlink, T., Beuvery, E. C., and Crommlein, D. J. A. (1988b). Immunogenicity of liposomes and Iscoms containing the major outer membrane protein of Neisseria gonorrhoeae: Influence of protein content and liposomal bilayer composition. *Infect. Immun.* **56,** 1661–1664.

Kinney, R. M., Esposito, J. J., Mathews, J. H., Johnson, B. J. B., Roehrig, J. T., Barrett, A. D. T., and Trent, D. W. (1988). Recombinant vaccinia virus/Venezuelan equine encephalitis (VEE) virus protects mice from peripheral VEE virus challenge. *J. Virol.* **62,** 4697–4702.

Kit, S., Kit, M., and Pirtle, E. C. (1985). Attenuated properties of thymidine kinase-negative deletion mutant of pseudorabies virus. *Am. J. Vet. Res.* **46,** 1359–1367.

Kit, S., Sheppard, M., Ichimura, H., and Kit, M. (1987). Second-generation pseudorabies virus vaccine with deletions in thymidine kinase and glycoprotein genes. *Am. J. Vet. Res.* **48,** 780–793.

Kitchen, L. W. (1988). Effect of diethylcarbamazine on serum antibodies to feline infectious peritonitis in cats. *Vaccine* **6,** 10–11.

Kolata, G. (1986). Litigation causes huge price increases in childhood vaccines. *Science* **232,** 1339.

Kramp, W. J., Six, H. R., and Kasel, J. A. (1982). Post-immunization clearance of liposome-entrapped adenovirus type 5 Hexon. *Proc. Soc. Exp. Biol. Med.* **169,** 135–139.

Kronenberg, M., Siu, G., Hood, L. E., and Shastri, N. (1986). The molecular genetics of the T cell antigen receptor and T cell antigen recognition. *Annu. Rev. Immunol.* **4,** 529–591.

Krzych, U., Fowler, A. V., and Sercarz, E. E. (1985). Repertoires of T cells directed against a large antigen, beta-galactosidase. *J. Exp. Med.* **162,** 311–323.

Lane, J. M., Ruben, F. L., Neff, J. M., and Millar, J. D. (1969). Complications of smallpox vaccination, 1968. *N. Engl. J. Med.* **281,** 1201–1208.

Langford, C. J., Edwards, S. J., Smith, G. L., Moss, B., Kemp, D. J., Anders, R. F., and Mitchell, G. F. (1986). Anchoring a secreted plasmodium antigen on the surface of recombinant vaccinia virus-infected cells increases its immunogenicity. *Mol. Cell. Biol.* **6,** 3191–3199.

Lathe, R., Kieny, M. P., Gerlinger, P., Clertant, P., Guizani, I., Cuzin, F., and Chambon, P. (1987). Tumour prevention and rejection with recombinant vaccinia. *Nature (London)* **326,** 878–880.

Lider, O., Reshef, T., Beraud, E., Ben-Nun, A., and Cohen, I. R. (1988). Anti-idiotypic network induced by T cell vaccination against experimental autoimmune encephalomyelitis. *Science* **239,** 181–183.

Lowe, R. S., Keller, P. M., Keech, B. J., Davison, A. J., Whang, Y., Morgan, A. J., Kieff, E., and Ellis, R. W. (1987). Varicella-zoster virus as a live vector for the expression of foreign genes. *Proc. Natl. Acad. Sci. U.S.A.* **84,** 3896–3900.

Lowell, G. H., Smith, L. F., Seid, R. C., and Zollinger, W. D. (1988a). Peptides bound to proteosomes via hydrophobic feet become highly immunogenic without adjuvants. *J. Exp. Med.* **167,** 658–663.

Lowell, G. H., Ballou, W. R., Smith, L. F., Wirtz, R. A., Zollinger, W. D., and Hockmeyer, W. T. (1988b). Proteosome-lipopeptide vaccines: Enhancement of immunogenicity for malaria CS peptides. *Science* **240,** 800–802.

Marchioli, C. C., Yancey, R. J., Petrovskis, E. A., Timmins, J. G., and Post, L. E. (1987). Evaluation of pseudorabies virus glycoprotein gp50 as vaccine for Aujeszky's disease in mice and swine: Expression by vaccinia virus and Chinese hamster ovary cells. *J. Virol.* **61,** 3977–3982.

Markowitz, L. E., Preblud, S. R., Orenstein, W. A., Rovira, E. Z., Stat, M., Adams, N. C., Hawkins, C. E., and Hinman, A. R. (1989). Patterns of transmission in measles outbreaks in the United States, 1985–1986. *N. Engl. J. Med.* **320,** 75–81.

Meignier, B., Longnecker, R., and Roizman, B. (1988). R7017 and R7020 herpes simplex virus recombinant prototype vaccine strains: Animal studies. *In* "Vaccines '88, New Chemical and Genetic Approaches to Vaccination" (H. Ginsberg, F. Brown, R. A. Lerner, and R. M. Chanock, eds.), pp. 193–196. Cold Spring Harbor Lab., Cold Spring Harbor, New York.

Merser, C., Sinay, P., and Adam, A. (1975). Total synthesis and adjuvant activity of bacterial peptidoglycan derivatives. *Biochem. Biophys. Res. Commun.* **66,** 1316.

Meuer, S. C., Dumann, H., Meyer zum Buschenfelde, K.-H., and Kohler, H. (1989). Low-dose interleukin-2 induces systemic immune responses against HBsAg in immunodeficient non-responders to hepatitis B vaccination. *Lancet* **1,** 15–18.

Milich, D. R., Thornton, G. B., Neurath, A. B., Kent, S. B., Michel, M.-L., Tiollais, P., and Chisari, F. V. (1985). Enhanced immunogenicity of the pre-S region of hepatitis B surface antigen. *Science* **228,** 1195–1199.

Milich, D. R., McLachlan, A., Moriarty, A., and Thornton, G. B. (1987). Immune responses to hepatitis B core antigen (HBcAg): Localization of T cell recognition sites within HBcAg/HBeAg. *J. Immunol.* **139,** 1230–1231.

Miller, L. H., and Good, M. F. (1988). The main obstacle to a malaria vaccine: The malaria parasite. *Vaccine* **6,** 104–106.

Miller, R. A., Maloney, D. G., Warnke, R., and Levy, R. (1982). Treatment of B-cell lymphoma with monoclonal anti-idiotype antibody. *N. Engl. J. Med.* **306,** 517–522.

Minor, P. D., John, A., Ferguson, M., and Icenogle, J. P. (1986). Antigenic and molecular evolution of the vaccine strain of type 3 poliovirus during the period of excretion by a primary vaccinee. *J. Gen. Virol.* **67,** 693–706.

Mitchell, M. S. (1989). Active specific immunotherapy in the treatment of human cancers. *In* "Immunity to Cancer," Vol. 2, pp. 323–336. Liss, New York.

Morein, B. (1988). The iscom antigen-presenting system. *Nature (London)* **332,** 287–288.

Morein, B., and Simons, K. (1985). Subunit vaccines against enveloped viruses: Virosomes, micelles, and other protein complexes. *Vaccine* **3,** 83–93.

Morein, B., Sundquist, B., Hoglund, S., Dalsgaard, K., and Osterhaus, A. (1984). Iscom, a novel structure for antigenic presentation of membrane proteins from enveloped viruses. *Nature (London)* **308,** 457–460.

Morgan, A. J., Mackett, M., Finerty, S., Arrand, J. R., Scullion, F. T., and Epstein, M. A. (1988). Recombinant vaccinia virus expressing Epstein-Barr virus glycoprotein gp340 protects cottontop tamarins against EB virus-induced malignant lymphomas. *J. Med. Virol.* **25,** 189–195.

Morin, J. E., Lubeck, M. D., Barton, J. E., Conley, A. J., Davis, A. R., and Hung, P. (1987). Recombinant adenovirus induces antibody response to hepatitis B virus surface antigen in hamsters. *Proc. Natl. Acad. Sci. U.S.A.* **84,** 4626–4630.

Morrison, R. P., Earl, P. L., Nishio, J., Lodmell, D. L., Moss, B., and Chesebro, B. (1987). Different H-2 subregions influence immunization against retrovirus and immunosuppression. *Nature (London)* **329,** 729–732.

Moss, B., and Flexner, C. (1987). Vaccinia virus expression vectors. *Annu. Rev. Immunol.* **5,** 305–324.

Moss, B., Smith, G. L., Gerin, J. L., and Purcell, R. H. (1984). Live recombinant vaccinia virus protects chimpanzees against hepatitis B. *Nature (London)* **311,** 67–69.

Murphey-Corb, M. Martin, L. N., Davison-Fairburn, B., Montelaro, R. C., Miller, M., West, M., Ohkawa, S., Baskin, G. B., Zhang, J.-Y., Putney, S. D., Allison, A. C., and Eppstein, D. A.

(1989). A formalin-inactivated whole SIV vaccine confers protection in macaques. *Science* **246,** 1293–1297.

Murphy, B. R., and Chanock, R. M. (1989). Immunization against viruses. In "Virology" (B. N. Fields *et al.,* eds.), 2nd ed., pp. 469–502. Raven Press, New York.

Murphy, B. R., Olmsted, R. A., Collins, P. L., Chanock, R. M., and Prince, G. A. (1988). Passive transfer of respiratory syncytial virus (RSV) antiserum suppresses the immune response to the RSV fusion (F) and large (G) glycoproteins expressed by recombinant vaccinia viruses. *J. Virol.* **62,** 3907–3910.

Murphy, B. R., Collins, P. L., Chanock, R. M., and Prince, G. A. (1989). Intranasal immunization with vaccinia-RSV recombinant viruses is superior to intradermal immunization in animals with passively acquired RSV antibodies. *In* "Vaccines '89" (R. M. Chanock *et al.,* eds.). Cold Spring Harbor Lab., Cold Spring Harbor, New York (in press).

Murray, M. G., Kuhn, R. J., Arita, M., Kawamura, N., Nomoto, A., and Wimmer, E. (1988). Poliovirus type 1/type 3 antigenic hybrid virus constructed in vitro elicits type 1 and type 3 neutralizing antibodies in rabbits and monkeys. *Proc. Natl. Acad. Sci. U.S.A.* **85,** 3203–3207.

Newmark, P. (1988). New vaccine and initiative mean end of rabies in sight for Europe? *Nature (London)* **336,** 416.

Nunberg, J. H., Doyle, M. V., Newell, A. D., Anderson, G. A., and York, C. J. (1988). Interleukin-2 as an adjuvant to vaccination. *In* "Vaccines '88, New Chemical and Genetic Approaches to Vaccination" (H. Ginsberg, F. Brown, R. A. Lerner, and R. M. Chanock, eds.), pp. 247–251. Cold Spring Harbor Lab., Cold Spring Harbor, New York.

Oberling, F., Morin, A., Duclos, B., Lang, J. M., Beachey, E. H., and Chédid, L. (1985). Enhancement of antibody response to a natural fragment of streptococcal M protein by murabutide administered to healthy volunteers. *Int. J. Immunopharmacol.* **7,** 398.

O'Hanley, P., Lark, D., Falkow, S., and Schoolnik, G. (1985). Molecular basis of *Escherichia coli* colonization of the upper urinary tract in BALB/c mice. *J. Clin. Invest.* **75,** 347–360.

Opdebeek, J. P., Wong, J. Y. M., Jackson, L. A., and Dobson, C. (1988). Hereford cattle immunized and protected against *Boophilus microplus* with soluble and membrane-associated antigens from the mid gut of ticks. *Parasite Immunol.* **10,** 405.

Palca, J. (1988). Row over vaccine trial. *Nature (London)* **331,** 470.

Parant, M., Audibert, F., Chédid, L., Level, M., Lefrancier, P., Choay, J., and Lederer, E. (1980). Immunostimulant activities of a lipophilic muramyl dipeptide derivative and of desmuramyl peptidolipid analogs. *Infect. Immun.* **27,** 826.

Paterson, R. G., Lamb, R. A., Moss, B., and Murphy, B. R. (1987). Comparison of the relative roles of the F and HN surface glycoproteins of the paramyxovirus simian virus 5 in inducing protective immunity. *J. Virol.* **61,** 1972–1977.

Perkus, M. E., Piccini, A., Lipinskas, B. R., and Paoletti, E. (1985). Recombinant vaccinia virus: Immunization against multiple pathogens. *Science* **229,** 981–983.

Perrin, P., Joffret, M. L., Leclerc, C., Oth, D., Sureau, P., and Thibodeau, L. (1988). Interleukin 2 increases protection against experimental rabies. *Immunobiology* **177,** 199–209.

Provost, P. J., Keller, P. M., Banker, F. S., Keech, B. J., Klein, H. J., Lowe, R. S., Morton, D. H., Phelps, A. H., McAleer, W. J., and Ellis, R. W. (1987). Successful infection of the common marmoset (Callithrix jacchus) with human varicella-zoster virus. *J. Virol.* **61,** 2951–2955.

Ramshaw, I. A., Andrew, M. E., Phillips, S. M., Boyle, D. B., and Coupar, B. E. H. (1987). Recovery of immunodeficient mice from a vaccinia virus/IL-2 recombinant infection. *Nature (London)* **329,** 545–546.

Randall, R. E., and Young, D. F. (1989). Immunization against multiple viruses by using solid-matrix–antibody–antigen complexes. *J. Virol.* **63,** 1808–1810.

Reddehase, M. J., Mutter, W., Munch, K., Buhring, H.-J., and Koszinowski, U. H. (1987). CD-8 positive T lymphocytes specific for murine cytomegalovirus immediate-early antigens mediate protective immunity. *J. Virol.* **61,** 3102–3108.

Redfield, R. R., Wright, D. C., James, W. D., Jones, T. S., Brown, C., and Burke, D. S. (1987). Disseminated vaccinia in a military recruit with human immunodeficiency virus (HIV) disease. *N. Engl. J. Med.* **316,** 673–676.

Roizman, B., and Jenkins, F. J. (1985). Genetic engineering of novel genomes of large DNA viruses. *Science* **229,** 1208–1214.

Rooney, J. F., Wohlenberg, C., Cremer, K. J., Moss, B., and Notkins, A. L. (1988). Immunization with a vaccinia virus recombinant expressing herpex simplex virus type 1 glycoprotein D: Long-term protection and effect of revaccination. *J. Virol.* **62,** 1530–1534.

Rosenberg, S. A., and Lotze, M. T. (1986). Cancer immunotherapy using interleukin-2 and interleukin-2-activated lymphocytes. *Annu. Rev. Immunol.* **4,** 681–709.

Rothbard, J. B. (1987). Synthetic peptides as vaccines. *Nature (London)* **330,** 106–107.

Rothbard, J. B., Fernandez, R., Wang, L., Teng, N. N. H., and Schoolnik, G. K. (1985). Antibodies to peptides corresponding to a conserved sequence of gonococcal pilins block bacterial adhesion. *Proc. Natl. Acad. Sci. U.S.A.* **82,** 915–919.

Rupprecht, C. E., Wiktor, T. J., Johnston, D. H., Hamir, A. N., Dietzschold, B., Wunner, W. H., Glickman, L. T., and Koprowski, H. (1986). Oral immunization and protection of raccoons (*Procyon lotor*) with a vaccinia-rabies glycoprotein recombinant virus vaccine. *Proc. Natl. Acad. Sci. U.S.A.* **83,** 7947–7950.

Rusche, J. R., Lynn, D. L., Robert-Guroff, M., Langlois, A. J., Lyerly, H. K., Carson, H., Krohn, K., Ranki, A., Gallo, R. C., and Bolognesi, D. P. (1987). Humoral immune response to the entire human immunodeficiency virus envelope glycoprotein made in insect cells. *Proc. Natl. Acad. Sci. U.S.A.* **84,** 6924–6928.

Satterthwait, A. C., Arrhenius, T., Hagopian, R. A., Zavala, F., Nussensweig, V., and Lerner, R. A. (1988). Conformational restriction of peptidyl immunogens with covalent replacements for the hydrogen bond. *Vaccine* **6,** 99–103.

Schlesinger, J. J., Brandriss, M. W., and Walsh, E. E. (1987). Protection of mice against dengue 2 virus encephalitis by immunization with dengue 2 virus non-structural glycoprotein NS1. *J. Gen. Virol.* **68,** 853–857.

Schmidt, M. A., O'Hanley, P., Lark, D., and Schoolnik, G. K. (1988). Synthetic peptides corresponding to protective epitopes of *Escherichia coli* digalactoside-binding pilin prevent infection in a murine pyelonephritis model. *Proc. Natl. Acad. Sci. U.S.A.* **85,** 1247–1251.

Sears, S. D., Clements, M. L., Betts, R. B., Maasab, H. F., Murphy, B. R., and Snyder, M. H. (1988). Comparison of live, attenuated H1N1 and H3N2 cold-adapted and avian-human influenza A reassortant viruses and inactivated virus vaccine in adults. *J. Infect. Dis.* **158,** 1209–1219.

Shida, H., Tochikura, T., Sato, T., Konno, T., Hirayoshi, K., Seki, M., Ito, Y., Hatanaka, M., Hinuma, Y., Sugimoto, M., Takahashi-Nishimaki, F., Maruyama, T., Miki, K., Suzuki, K., Morita, M., Sashiyama, H., and Hayami, M. (1987). Effect of the recombinant vaccinia viruses that express HTLV-I envelope gene on HTLV-I infection. *EMBO J.* **6,** 3379–3384.

Shih, M.-F., Arsenakis, M., Tiollais, P., and Roizman, B. (1984). Expression of hepatitis B virus S gene by herpes simplex virus type 1 vectors carrying α- and β-regulated gene chimeras. *Proc. Natl. Acad. Sci. U.S.A.* **81,** 5867–5870.

Silbart, L. K., and Keren, D. F. (1989). Reduction of intestinal absorption by carcinogen-specific secretory immunity. *Science* **243,** 1462–1464.

Spriggs, M. K., Collins, P. L., Tierney, E., London, W. T., and Murphy, B. R. (1988). Immunization with vaccinia virus recombinants that express the surface glycoproteins of human parainfluenza virus type 3 (PIV3) protects patas monkeys against PIV3 infection. *J. Virol.* **62,** 1293–1296.

Talwar, G. P., and Raghupathy, R. (1989). Anti-fertility vaccines. *Vaccine* **7,** 97–101.

Taylor, J., and Paoletti, E. (1988). Fowlpox virus as a vector in non-avian species. *Vaccine* **6,** 466–468.

Taylor, J., Weinberg, R., Languet, B., Desmettre, P., and Paoletti, E. (1988a). Recombinant fowlpox virus inducing protective immunity in non-avian species. *Vaccine* **6,** 497–503.

Taylor, J., Weinberg, R., Kawaoka, Y., Webster, R. G., and Paoletti, E. (1988b). Protective immunity against avian influenza induced by a fowlpox recombinant. *Vaccine* **6,** 504–508.

Telzak, E., Wolff, S. M., Dinarello, C. A., Conlon, T., El Kholy, A. E., Bahr, G. M., Choay, J. P., Morin, A., and Chédid, L. (1986). Clinical evaluation of the immunoadjuvant murabutide, a derivative of MDP, administered with a tetanus toxoid vaccine. *J. Infect. Dis.* **153,** 628–633.

Tolson, N. D., Charlton, K. M., Stewart, R. B., Campbell, J. B., and Wiktor, T. J. (1987). Immune response in skunks to a vaccinia virus recombinant expressing the rabies virus glycoprotein. *Can. J. Vet. Res.* **51,** 363–366.

Tolson, N. D., Charlton, K. M., Casey, G. A., Knowles, M. K., Rupprecht, C. E., Lawson, K. F., and Campbell, J. B. (1988). Immunization of foxes against rabies with a vaccinia recombinant virus expressing the rabies glycoprotein. *Arch. Virol.* **102,** 297–301.

Tomassini, J. E., Maxson, T. R., and Colonno, R. J. (1989). Biochemical characterization of a glycoprotein required for rhinovirus attachment. *J. Biol. Chem.* **264,** 1656–1662.

Townsend, A., and Bodmer, H. (1989). Antigen recognition by class I restricted T lymphocytes. *Annu. Rev. Immunol.* **7,** 601–624.

Tramont, E. C., and Boslego, J. W. (1985). Pilus vaccines. *Vaccine* **3,** 3–10.

Tyrell, D. A. J. (1987). Interferons and their clinical value. *Rev. Infect. Dis.* **9,** 243–249.

UytdeHaag, F. G. C. M., Bunschoten, H., Weijer, K., and Osterhaus, A. D. M. E. (1986). From Jenner to Jerne: Towards idiotype vaccines. *Immunol. Rev.* **90,** 93–113.

Van Rooijen, N., and Van Nieuwmegan, R. (1983). Use of liposomes as biodegradable and harmless adjuvants. *In* "Methods in Enzymology" (J. J. Lengone and H. Van Vunakis, eds.), Vol. 93, p. 83. Academic Press, New York.

Ward, M. M., Ward, R. E., Huang, J.-H., and Kohler, H. (1987). Idiotype vaccine against Streptococcus pneumoniae. *J. Immunol.* **139,** 2775–2780.

Warren, H. S., Vogel, F. R., and Chédid, L. A. (1986). Current status of immunological adjuvants. *Annu. Rev. Immunol.* **4,** 369–388.

Weinberg, A., and Merigan, T. C. (1988). Recombinant interleukin 2 as an adjuvant for vaccine-induced protection: Immunization of guinea pigs with herpes simplex virus subunit vaccines. *J. Immunol.* **140,** 294–299.

Weinberg, A., Konrad, M., and Merigan, T. C. (1987). Regulation by interleukin-2 of protective immunity against recurrent herpes simplex virus type 2 genital infection in guinea pigs. *J. Virol.* **61,** 2120–2127.

Westrop, G. D., Wareham, K. A., Evans, D. M. A., Dunn, G., Minor, P. D., Magrath, D. I., Taffs, F., Marsden, S., Skinner, M. A., Schild, G. C., and Almond, J. W. (1989). Genetic basis of attenuation of the Sabin type 3 oral poliovirus vaccine. *J. Virol.* **63,** 1338–1344.

Weyand, C., Goronzy, J., Fathman, C. G., and O'Hanley, P. (1987). Administration in vivo of recombinant interleukin 2 protects mice against septic death. *J. Clin. Invest.* **79,** 1756–1763.

Wraith, D. C., Vessey, A. E., and Askonas, B. A. (1987). Purified influenza virus nucleoprotein protects mice from lethal infection. *J. Gen. Virol.* **68,** 433–440.

Yilma, T., Hsu, D., Jones, L., Owens, S., Grubman, M., Mebus, C., Yamanaka, M., and Dale, B. (1988). Protection of cattle against rinderpest with vaccinia virus recombinants expressing the HA or F gene. *Science* **242,** 1058–1061.

Zagury, D., Leonard, R., Fouchard, M., Reveil, B., Bernard, J., Ittele, D., Cattan, A., Zirimwabagabo, L., Kalmumbu, M., Justin, W., Salaun, J.-J., and Goussard, B. (1987). Immunization against AIDS in humans. *Nature (London)* **326,** 249.

Zagury, D., Bernard, J., Cheynier, R., Desportes, I., Leonard, R., Fouchard, M., Reveil, B., Ittele, D., Lurhuma, Z., Mbayo, K., Wane, J., Salaun, J.-J., Goussard, B., Dechazal, L., Burny, A., Nara, P., and Gallo, R. C. (1988). A group specific anamnestic immune reaction against HIV-1 induced by a candidate vaccine against AIDS. *Nature (London)* **332,** 728–731.

Zarling, J. M., Eichberg, J. W., Moran, P., McClure, J., Sridhar, P., and Hu, S.-L. (1987). Proliferative and cytotoxic T cells to AIDS virus glycoprotein in chimpanzees immunized with a recombinant vaccinia virus expressing AIDS virus envelope glycoprotein. *J. Immunol.* **139,** 988–990.

Zimmerman, B., Gold, R., and Lavi, S. (1987). Adverse effects of immunization. *Postgrad. Med.* **82,** 225–232.

Allosteric Modulation of N-Methyl-D-Aspartate Receptors

Ian J. Reynolds* and Richard J. Miller†

**Department of Pharmacology*
University of Pittsburgh
Pittsburgh, Pennsylvania 15261

†Department of Pharmacological and Physiological Sciences
University of Chicago
Chicago, Illinois 60637

I. Introduction

The last few years has seen an explosion of interest in excitatory amino acids and their receptors. The surge in interest is due, in large part, to the development of more effective pharmacological tools with which to probe the function of excitatory amino acid receptors. Much of our current understanding of the nature and function of excitatory amino acids has come from the use of natural products or newly synthesized agents that are not normally found endogenously. Using such tools, three subtypes of receptor for glutamate in the mammalian nervous system have been described, namely *N*-methyl-D-aspartate (NMDA), kainate, and quisqualate receptors, based on the selective agonist actions of these drugs (Watkins, 1984; Watkins and Olverman, 1987). All three types of receptor feature neurotransmitter recognition sites that are intimately coupled to cation-preferring ligand-gated ion channels that are more or less analogous to the nicotinic acetylcholine receptor (Mayer and Westbrook, 1987). A fourth type of receptor has recently been described. This receptor is sensitive to quisqualate and probably transduces information via G-protein-coupled activation of the inositol phosphate pathway (Nicoletti *et al.,* 1987; Sugiyama *et al.,* 1987; Murphy and Miller, 1988; Palmer *et al.,* 1988; Kushner *et al.,* 1988; Verdoorn and Dingledine, 1988).

This review focuses on the NMDA-preferring glutamate receptor. NMDA receptors are involved in a wide range of physiological and pathophysiological events, and this has resulted in a great deal of interest in the development of tools to probe and manipulate NMDA receptor function. Moreover, many studies have demonstrated that the activity of the NMDA receptor can be modulated by a wide range of endogenous agents, including glycine, Mg^{2+}, and Zn^{2+}. As NMDA receptors have a key role in so many synaptic events, understanding the nature of the modulation of the receptor is of paramount importance to understanding, in a holistic sense, NMDA receptor function. The purpose of this review, therefore, is to examine the actions of the known modulators of the receptor in terms of their binding sites, and to try to determine how these binding sites interact with each other. By understanding the interactions between the known modulators of this receptor it may be possible to comprehend better how the receptor may operate in different circumstances, and it may also be possible to target more accurately therapeutic agents to interrupt specific NMDA receptor-mediated events.

For the purposes of this review, the term "NMDA receptor" is used to describe the whole macromolecular complex, while "binding site" is the preferred term to describe the site of action of the various drugs that act at the receptor. The term "noncompetitive," as applied to antagonists, is not very useful in this context. Drugs which block the ion channel may be noncompetitive with respect to drugs acting at the NMDA binding site. However, these drugs will obviously be competitive with respect to other ion channel-blocking drugs of the same class. For this reason, every attempt will be made to classify drugs according to their probable site of action wherever this is possible.

II. Functional Aspects of *N*-Methyl-D-Aspartate Receptors

A. Physiology

At most glutamatergic synapses the fast postsynaptic events are believed to be mediated by non-NMDA glutamate receptor. This is implied by the lack of sensitivity to NMDA antagonists (Herron *et al.,* 1986; Collingridge *et al.,* 1988a), and the sensitivity of such responses to selective kainate/quisqualate antagonists such as the quinoxalinediones CNQX and DNQX (Fletcher *et al.*, 1988; Neuman *et al.*, 1988). However, various manipulations will reveal an NMDA-mediated component of the postsynaptic response. Thus, if the kainate/quisqualate response is blocked, a response remains that is sensitive to NMDA antagonists such as aminophosphonovalerate (AP5) (Fletcher *et al.*, 1988). Alternatively, if the synapse is stimulated by a train of pulses in close succession (Herron *et al.*, 1986; Collingridge *et al.*, 1988b; Thomson *et al.*, 1985), or if Mg^{2+} is removed from the bathing medium (Collingridge *et al.*, 1988a; Thomson *et al.*, 1985), the AP5-sensitive component is magnified. This latter phenomenon arises as a consequence of blockade of the NMDA-operated ion channel by Mg^{2+} that occurs at physiological Mg^{2+} concentrations. The location of the site of action of Mg^{2+} inside the channel is suggested by the voltage dependence of the Mg^{2+} block (Mayer *et al.*, 1984; Nowak *et al.*, 1984). Thus, when cells are depolarized, the Mg^{2+} block is relieved and the NMDA receptor can function. The precise localization of the Mg^{2+} site within the channel has not yet been determined (see Ascher and Nowak, 1988, for discussion).

Glycine modulates the NMDA receptor and may be an important factor controlling its activity *in vivo*. The effects of glycine were first demonstrated by Johnson and Ascher electrophysiologically (Johnson and Ascher, 1987). Glycine invariably modulates NMDA receptors expressed in oocytes (Kleckner and Dingledine, 1988; Verdoorn and Dingledine, 1988), suggesting that the glycine binding site is an integral part of the receptor molecule. It is not entirely clear at this time whether glycine is an absolute requirement for NMDA receptor activation. In simple paradigms, such as the *Xenopus* oocyte expression system, it is possible to reduce glycine concentrations to very low levels (Kleckner and Dingledine, 1988). Under these circumstances NMDA responses are virtually nonexistent, leading to the suggestion that glycine may be a cotransmitter, along with glutamate, in the brain. Putative glycine antagonists have also been used; these are discussed further below.

Ambient glycine concentrations in the cerebrospinal fluid are 1–10 μM, which implies that the glycine site may normally be fully saturated. This concept is also supported by observations in various isolated brain preparations. Glycine is rarely observed to have a direct effect in these preparations, although direct effects of glycine and D-serine have recently been reported (Thomson *et al.*, 1989; Salt, 1989). More consistent effects are seen if glycine antagonists are added, which depresses responses to NMDA. The subdued responses can then be restored by the subsequent addition of glycine (Fletcher and Lodge, 1988; Ransom and Deschenes, 1989). It is not clear whether isolated preparations closely resemble the *in vivo* state. If glial damage were to occur during tissue preparation significant glycine release may occur, as it has been suggested that glia are the source of the glycine that acts on NMDA receptors (Forsythe *et al.*, 1988). A recent report suggested that intrathecal injections of glycine could enhance strychnine-induced seizures (Larson and Beitz, 1988). This supports the notion that alteration of glycine availability may be a physiological option for modulating NMDA receptor function.

In addition to Mg^{2+} and glycine, Zn^{2+} may be an endogenous negative modulator of NMDA receptors. Concentrations of Zn^{2+} in the 1–10 μM range reversibly depress responses to NMDA while sparing kainate and quisqualate receptors (Peters *et al.*, 1987; Westbrook and Mayer, 1987). The actions of Zn^{2+} are not competitive with respect to NMDA or glycine, suggesting a different site of action. Moreover, the effects of Zn^{2+} are not voltage dependent to the same degree as those of Mg^{2+}, suggesting a different locus of action (Westbrook and Mayer, 1987; Mayer *et al.*, 1988). There is a heterogeneous distribution of Zn^{2+} in the mammalian central nervous system (Crawford and Connor, 1972; Perez Clausell and Danscher, 1985). It is localized in synaptic regions in the hippocampus, and may also be found in synaptic vesicles (Perez Clausell and Danscher, 1985). Potassium-stimulated release and high-affinity uptake of Zn^{2+} have been observed (Wensink *et al.*, 1988). Thus, Zn^{2+} fulfills many of the criteria of a neurotransmitter. However, as in the case of glycine, it is not absolutely clear that Zn^{2+} does function as either a cotransmitter, an "anti"-transmitter, or a modulator *in vivo*.

Although evidence exists for a contribution of an NMDA receptor component in synaptic transmission in several locations in the central nervous system, the function of that component remains unclear in most cases. One possible exception is the phenomenon of long-term potentiation (LTP), which is the sustained increase in the postsynaptic response that is seen following a rapid train of pulses presynaptically (Collingridge and Bliss, 1987; Nicoll *et al.*, 1988; Brown *et al.*, 1988). Although the increased response is carried by non-NMDA glutamate receptors (Muller *et al.*, 1988; Muller and Lynch, 1988) and may be mediated by pre- and postsynaptic mechanisms (Davies *et al.*, 1989), NMDA receptors are essential for the induction of LTP in both hippocampus and cortex (Collingridge and Bliss, 1987; Reymann *et al.*, 1989; Artola and Singer, 1987; Addae and Stone, 1987). The passage of Ca^{2+} through the NMDA receptor ionophore is a key event, as Ca^{2+} removal can prevent the induction of LTP (Mulkeen *et al.*, 1988), and the elevation of intracellular Ca^{2+} can, to some extent, mimic NMDA receptor activation (Malenka *et al.*, 1988; Mulkeen *et al.*, 1987). LTP is believed to be an *in vitro* model for the acquisition of memory. Although not all forms of LTP involve NMDA receptors (Nicoll *et al.*, 1988), these receptors clearly have a fundamental role in basic learning processes.

Some evidence suggests that NMDA receptors have a role in visual plasticity. The development of the visual cortex in vertebrates is associated with a segregation of the input from the retina into ocular dominance columns. The process can be interrupted by alteration of the visual sensory input by light deprivation, by applying tetrodotoxin to the retina to eliminate output, or by surgically closing one or both eyes. The involvement of NMDA receptors in this process is suggested by the finding that NMDA receptor antagonists prevent the segregation of the visual cortex in animals with normal retinal input (Cline *et al.*, 1987). Interestingly, the development of ocular dominance also requires the input of either adrenergic or cholinergic nerves (Gruel *et al.*, 1988), demonstrating the utility of this system as a good model of a classical Hebbian synapse. The interaction of adrenergic and cholinergic responses with NMDA receptor-mediated events also serves to illustrate the potential for physiological, as opposed to pharmacological, interactions between neurotransmitters. The mechanisms underlying such events remains largely unexplored at this time.

B. Pathophysiology

Much of the current interest in NMDA receptors stems from the potential use of exogenous NMDA receptor agonists and antagonists as therapeutic agents in a wide variety of neurological disorders (Choi, 1988). Evidence linking NMDA receptors to these disorders has come from a wide variety of *in vitro* and *in vivo* studies. During neuronal ischemia a massive release of glutamate has been observed (Benveniste *et al.*, 1984; Rothman, 1984), possibly due to the failure of ATP-dependent uptake of glutamate. The resultant excitotoxicity and cell death are due in part to the actions of glutamate on NMDA receptors, and are mediated by a substantial influx of Ca^{2+} associated with NMDA receptor activation (Simon *et al.*, 1984; Rappaport *et al.*, 1987; Deshpande *et al.*, 1987; Harris and Symon, 1984; Marcoux *et al.*, 1988). Moreover, significant protection against excitotoxic cell death occurs when NMDA receptor antagonists of various sorts are applied before or after the insult (Foster *et al.*, 1987; Boast *et al.*, 1988; Prince and Feeser, 1988; Gotti *et al.*, 1988). The prevention of excitotoxicity by postinsult antagonist treatment (Foster *et al.*, 1988) suggests that some form of ongoing glutamate action must be occurring, although the nature of this phenomenon remains unclear. Excitotoxicity has also been modeled in cell culture very effectively. Thus, hypoxia, ischemia, or NMDA treatment of monolayer cultures also results in cell death (Choi *et al.*, 1987; Rothman, 1984; Goldberg *et al.*, 1988; Marcoux *et al.*, 1988). This cell death is dependent on extracellular Ca^{2+} (Choi *et al.*, 1987), and is blocked by various NMDA receptor antagonists, including low concentrations of Zn^{2+} (Choi *et al.*, 1988; Rothman *et al.*, 1987; Goldberg *et al.*, 1987; Peters *et al.*, 1987). This model also demonstrates a peri-insult window during which cells can be rescued by the addition of NMDA antagonists (Choi *et al.*, 1988), thus underscoring the utility of the *in vitro* approach.

The demonstration that various endogenous neurotoxins can kill neurons *in vitro* as well as *in vivo* (Whetsell and Schwarcz, 1989; Kim *et al.*, 1987;

Rothman, 1984) has suggested that NMDA receptor-mediated excitotoxicity may be a fundamental pathological event in several neurological disorders, including Huntington's disease and Alzehimer's disease (Ellison *et al.*, 1987; Cowburn *et al.*, 1988). Clearly, therapeutically efficacious NMDA receptor antagonist that is suitably free of significant side effects could be extremely useful in treating these diseases.

Epilepsy may also involve inappropriate activation of NMDA receptors. This is suggested by several lines of evidence. First, mice with an inbred predisposition to seizures are protected from seizures by competitive NMDA antagonists (Croucher *et al.*, 1982). Second, several ion channel-blocking NMDA receptor antagonists are effective anticonvulasants (Bennett *et al.*, 1988; Sato *et al.*, 1988; Gilbert, 1988; Brady and Swann, 1986). Indeed, the most potent channel blocker, MK801, was discovered using a screening procedure for anticonvulsants (Clineschmidt, 1982). Finally, removal of Mg^{2+} from *in vitro* brain slice preparations results in epileptiform discharges of hippocampus or cortex that can be suppressed using a variety of NMDA receptor antagonists, including channel blockers and antagonists acting at the NMDA recognition site (Aram *et al.*, 1989). Moreover, NMDA antagonists can also reduce the epileptogenic effects of agents acting at other receptors, including pilocarpine, carbachol, bicuculline, and picrotoxin (Aram *et al.*, 1989; Millan *et al.*, 1988). Thus, NMDA receptors seem to have a central role in the initiation of seizure events.

III. Modulation of *N*-Methyl-D-Aspartate Receptors

The previous section illustrated the importance of NMDA receptor-mediated events in various physiological and pathophysiological states. In order to understand these processes more fully, both in terms of normal events and the possible therapy of pathophysiological states, it is clearly important to understand how the activity of the receptor is regulated by the many different ligand binding sites. The purpose of this section is to examine the characteristics of ligand binding to the various sites, and to describe, where possible, the interactions between the various sites. The site for the ion channel blockers is examined first, as it has been most intensively studied and has demonstrated the greatest utility with respect to analysis of drug actions at the other binding sites of the receptor.

A. The Phencyclidine Binding Site

The phencyclidine site was first labeled using [^{3}H]phencyclidine in an attempt to understand more fully the psychotomimetic effect of this widely abused drug (Vincent *et al.*, 1979; Zukin and Zukin, 1979). Early studies suggested that [^{3}H]phencyclidine bound to the σ-opiate receptor, based on the ability of a number of σ-opiate ligands including SKF 10,047, cyclazocine, and pentazocine, to displace binding in a stereospecific manner. It became clear that the designation "opiate" for the σ-receptor was inappropriate, as naloxone could not reverse the psychotomimetic effects of σ-receptor ligands. More recent studies using [^{3}H]thyienylphencyclidine ([^{3}H]TCP), a ligand with superior potency and specificity (Vignon *et al.*, 1982), demonstrated that the high-affinity phencyclidine site and the σ receptor were indeed distinct, both pharmacologically and anatomically (Largent *et al.*, 1986). It was clear, however, that certain ligands, such as phencyclidine and SKF 10,047, could bind to both sites (Largent *et al.*, 1986).

The connection between the phencyclidine site and the NMDA receptor was made by the pioneering studies of Lodge and co-workers (Anis *et al.*, 1983), who demonstrated that phencyclidine and ketamine could specifically inhibit NMDA-induced depolarization of spinal cord neurons. Subsequent studies demonstrated that a strong correlation existed between the ability of phencyclidine site ligands to displace [^{3}H]TCP binding and their ability to block NMDA responses in the spinal cord and cortex. Autoradiographic comparisons have also demonstrated almost perfect colocalization between ligand binding to NMDA and phencyclidine sites in rat brain (Maragos *et al.*, 1988; Bowery *et al.*, 1988; Monaghan *et al.*, 1988; Jarvis *et al.*, 1987). Moreover, a similar distribution of [^{3}H]glycine and [^{3}H]TCP binding sites has been observed in human hippocampus (Jansen *et al.*, 1989). The only discrepancy was found in the cerebellum, where NMDA-sensitive [^{3}H]glutamate binding was found in areas with very low [^{3}H]TCP binding (Maragos *et al.*, 1988; Jarvis *et al.*, 1987). The invariable coexistence of NMDA and phencyclidine sites in NMDA receptors expressed in oocytes (Kleckner and Dingledine, 1988; Verdoorn and Dingledine, 1988) also supports the contention that the sites are all an intergral part of a macromolecular receptor complex.

The proposed coidentity of the phencyclidine site and the NMDA receptor has led to many studies based on the known regulators of the NMDA receptor. These studies have been performed with both [^{3}H]TCP and [^{3}H]MK801, a novel ligand for the phencyclidine site that demonstrates higher affinity and specificity for the NMDA receptor than either phencyclidine or TCP (Wong *et al.*, 1986; Reynolds *et al.*, 1987). Based on the analogy between the NMDA and $GABA_A$ receptors, Loo and co-workers demonstrated that binding of [^{3}H]TCP was dependent on the presence of glutamate in the incubation medium (Loo *et al.*, 1986). Progressive washing reduced specific [^{3}H]TCP binding to low levels, and this inhibitory effect could be reversed by adding back glutamate in concentrations very similar to those which activate the receptor in intact systems. More recent studies have demonstrated a close correlation between the potency of ligands increasing [^{3}H]TCP or [^{3}H]MK801 binding and their ability to activate NMDA receptors (Foster and Wong, 1987; Fagg, 1987). Furthermore, NMDA receptor antagonists, such as AP5 and CPP, that act at the NMDA recognition site inhibit binding of $[^3H]$TCP and $[^3H]$MK801 (Reynolds *et al.*, 1987; Javitt *et al.*, 1987; Loo *et al.*, 1987; Lodge *et al.*, 1988; Reynolds *et al.*, 1989). These data suggest that phencyclidine site ligands preferentially bind to NMDA receptors that are in a state consistent with channel opening, while ligands bind less well to channels that cannot open.

This relationship was carried further following the discovery by Johnson and Ascher that glycine could promote the activation of the NMDA receptor by glutamate and NMDA (Johnson and Ascher, 1987). Several studies demonstrated that glutamate-stimulated binding of $[^3H]$MK801 and $[^3H]$TCP could be enhanced further by glycine and other glycine-mimetic amino acids (Reynolds *et al.*, 1987; Wong *et al.*, 1987; Snell *et al.*, 1987; Bonhaus *et al.*, 1987; Thomas *et al.*, 1988). The finding of additive effects of glycine on $[^3H]$MK801 binding indicated that glycine probably binds to a site distinct from glutamate (Reynolds *et al.*, 1987). Moreover, as the ability of glycine to enhance binding was not antagonized by strychnine, and as the glycine-mimetic abilities of other amino acids were different (Reynolds *et al.*, 1987; Wong *et al.*, 1987; Snell *et al.*, 1987; Bonhaus *et al.*, 1987; Thomas *et al.*, 1988), these studies confirmed the original suggestion of Johnson and Ascher that the glycine site associated with the NMDA receptor was distinct from the "classical" glycine receptor found predominantly in the spinal cord (Johnson and Ascher, 1987). Interestingly, a strychnine-insensitive glycine binding site had been previously demonstrated by several independent groups without clearly determining its identity (Bristow *et al.*, 1986; Kishimoto *et al.*, 1981).

A variety of electrophysiological studies have demonstrated that the actions of phencyclidine-like NMDA antagonists are both use- and voltage-dependent. The degree to which use dependence is manifested seems to vary widely between the various drugs acting at the phencyclidine site, and is most profound with MK-801 (Wong *et al.*, 1986; Huettner and Bean, 1988; MacDonald *et al.*, 1987). Block of the NMDA receptor by use-dependent ligands is only seen when agonists have been added. Similarly, recovery is observed only when the channel is activated (Wong *et al.*, 1986; Huettner and Bean, 1988; Kushner *et al.*, 1988; MacDonald *et al.*, 1987). A second non-use-dependent block of NMDA receptors has been proposed recently, in which phencyclidine and related compounds approach the receptor through the lipid phase (Javitt and Zukin, 1989). Receptor blockade, and the recovery from such blockade is then time, but not activation, dependent. This mechanism for channel block apparently accounts for a relatively small proportion of the block of the NMDA receptor by phencyclidine-like drugs (Javitt and Zukin, 1989). The action of some phencyclidine-site drugs is also voltage dependent in the same way as Mg^{2+} (Honey *et al.*, 1985). This was clearly demonstrated by MacDonald and co-workers (1987) using ketamine, but is much less apparent with MK801. However, the reversal of the action of MK-801 on the activated channel can be accelerated by depolarizing the membrane (Halliwell *et al.*, 1989; Mayer *et al.*, 1989b), indicating at least some voltage dependency of its effects.

The foregoing studies suggested that the site of action of phencyclidine-like ligands was located within the NMDA-operated ion channel. This represents a testable hypothesis from a biochemical standpoint. Initial analyses of the effects of glutamate and glycine on [^{3}H]MK-801 and [^{3}H]TCP binding suggested that channel activation apparently increased the affinity of the ligands for their binding site (Reynolds *et al.*, 1987). Subsequent studies examined the association and dissociation rate of phencyclidine-site ligands and found that, in the absence of agonists, the association of both [^{3}H]MK801 and [^{3}H]TCP was very slow such that many hours were required for equilibrium to be reached (Reynolds and Miller, 1988b; Kloog *et al.*, 1988a,b; Bonhaus and McNamara, 1988). The predominant effect of adding glutamate alone, or in combination with glycine, was a dramatic increase in the association rate. This was also accompanied by an increase in the dissociation rate. The effects of glutamate and glycine on the kinetics of ligand binding to the phencyclidine site have been modeled by Bonhaus and co-workers (Bonhaus and McNamara, 1988), based on a description of transiently accessible binding sites by Starmer and colleagues, who modeled local anesthetic action at voltage-dependent sodium channels (Starmer *et al.*, 1987). According to this model, glutamate and glycine do not change the actual affinity of the phencyclidine site for its ligands, as indicated by the kinetically derived dissociation constant (Bonhaus and McNamara, 1988). The change in apparent affinity that had been observed is a consequence of binding under nonequilibrium conditions (Starmer *et al.*, 1987). The change in rates of binding and dissociation that are observed presumably reflect an alteration in the fraction of the time that the binding site is accessible (Starmer *et al.*, 1987). As predicted from such models, the addition of antagonists acting at the NMDA recognition site results in the slowing of association and dissociation rates (Reynolds and Miller, 1988b; Kloog *et al.*, 1988b; Bonhaus and McNamara, 1988), as would be anticipated with binding to a site that allows ligand access for a smaller fraction of the time (Starmer *et al.*, 1987). A model of a transiently accessible binding site has also been proposed by Kloog and colleagues (1988a). These studies found, as predicted from the model, that if allowed to incubate for a sufficient period of time, similar levels of binding should be reached regardless of the state of channel activation (Kloog *et al.*, 1988b). Thus, as results from various binding studies can be explained by ligand binding to a transiently accessible site, with access to the site controlled by glutamate and glycine, these data clearly support the notion that the binding site is located within the channel.

It appears, therefore, that ligand binding at the phencyclidine site represents a good model to monitor drug effects on the state of channel activation *in vitro*. The studies described above show that, to demonstrate agonist effects on the binding of [^{3}H]MK801 or [^{3}H]TCP most effectively, it is necessary to use well-washed tissue preparations. Implicit in the above findings is the notion that agonist effects will be relatively larger at shorter incubation times, so that shorter incubations should be used to assay the effects of compounds which putatively activate the receptor. Conversely, if an estimation of the receptor density is the desired end point of a study, it is appropriate to activate maximally the receptor by saturating the glutamate and glycine sites and ensuring that equilibrium conditions are reached. This will prevent any artifacts arising from an inappropriate determination of ligand affinity.

B. The Glutamate/NMDA Binding Site

The binding of tritiated ligands to the glutamate recognition site represents the first method used to biochemically label the NMDA receptor. [^{3}H]Glutamate has been widely used for this purpose, and its use has been reviewed in depth (Foster and Fagg, 1984). NMDA-sensitive [^{3}H]glutamate remains the ligand of choice when trying to label the NMDA recognition site with an agonist due to its superior affinity compared to [^{3}H]NMDA (Foster and Fagg, 1987). The NMDA site has also been labeled with a variety of tritiated antagonists, including [^{3}H]D-AP5 (Olverman *et al.*, 1988; Foster and Fagg, 1987; Monaghan *et al.*, 1988), [^{3}H]CPP (Olverman *et al.*, 1986; Murphy *et al.*, 1987; Lodge *et al.*, 1988), and, most recently, [^{3}H]CGS-19755 (Maragos *et al.*, 1988). Comparisons between the binding of ligands to the agonist recognition site and the phencyclidine site generally show 4-6 times as many glutamate sites than, for example, [^{3}H]TCP sites (Maragos *et al.*, 1988). This suggests that there may be several neurotransmitter recognition sites per receptor molecule. It may be necessary to interpret such results cautiously when [^{3}H]glutamate is employed, as this ligand binds to several sites in neuronal membranes, including a glutamate transport site (Foster and Fagg, 1984). However, as stated above, the autoradiographic localization of the [^{3}H]TCP and NMDA-sensitive [^{3}H]glutamate binding are almost identical, supporting the coexistence of the sites.

The affinities of ligands for the NMDA recognition site, found using ligand binding to the NMDA site, are generally higher than those obtained from analogous experiments using [^{3}H]TCP or [^{3}H]MK801 as the ligand. This may be due to lower ambient glutamate concentrations, as ligand binding to the NMDA site is often performed in detergent-washed tissues to remove endogenous glutamate. However, it was recently suggested that two discrete states of the NMDA site exist, one of which preferentially binds agonists, and one which binds antagonists of the NMDA site. The suggestion was based on observations that indicated that agonists were consistently more potent against agonist binding, while antagonists were less potent against agonist binding and more potent against antagonist binding (Monaghan *et al.*, 1988). As a parallel to these observations, Fagg and co-workers recently proposed that agonists and antagonists at this site have separate but overlapping points of attachment (Fagg *et al.*, 1988), which might account for the observed differences in potencies.

From autoradiographic studies using [^{3}H]glutamate and [^{3}H]CPP it appears that the agonist- and antagonist-preferring states of the NMDA receptor are differentially distributed in rat brain, with high levels of antagonist binding in the cortex and relatively lower levels in the striatum. Interestingly, glycine appears to convert the receptor from being agonist preferring to antagonist preferring. Thus, glycine increased [^{3}H]glutamate binding to slices and decreased [^{3}H]D-AP5 and [^{3}H]CPP binding (Monaghan *et al.*, 1988). Biochemically, therefore, it is possible to describe the effects of glycine on the NMDA site as facilitating the effects of the agonist. The implications from the studies of Monaghan and co-workers are that glycine should increase the affinity of glutamate for its site. As a more tightly bound ligand should dissociate more slowly, the actions of glycine may be manifested as prolonged channel opening, which has been observed in single channel recordings (Ascher and Nowak, 1987).

The previous section described the profound effects of agonists and antagonists at the NMDA site on the binding of ligands to the phencyclidine site. Several studies have demonstrated, however, that phencyclidine site ligands to not alter the binding of agonists or antagonists at the NMDA site (Murphy *et al.*, 1987; Foster and Wong, 1987). These results demonstrate that there is unlikely to be direct allosteric coupling between the site for phencyclidine in the ion channel and the neurotransmitter recognition site. The effects of NMDA-like agonists are mediated by changing the access of ligands to their binding site. Such an interpretation is supported by the suggestion that the true affinity of ligands for the phencyclidine site (as opposed to the apparent affinity measured under non-equilibrium conditions) is not altered by the inclusion of glutamate in the assay (Bonhaus and McNamara, 1988).

C. The Glycine Site

The precise physiological role of glycine in the functioning of the NMDA receptor remains unclear. Early studies suggested that glycine alone could not actually activate the channel, but was capable of enhancing channel activation by NMDA or glutamate (Johnson and Ascher, 1987; Reynolds *et al.*, 1987). The ability of glycine to activate the channel as measured electrophysiologically is paralleled by its ability to increase the binding of [^{3}H]MK801 and [^{3}H]TCP at the phencyclidine site in the ion channel (Reynolds *et al.*, 1987; Wong *et al.*, 1987; Snell *et al.*, 1987; Bonhaus *et al.*, 1987; Thomas *et al.*, 1988). This is entirely consistent with the previously described model for the NMDA receptor. The activating effects of glycine are mimicked by D-serine and D-alanine, and also, less potently, by L-serine and L-alanine.

The effects of glycine and glycine mimics were not readily observed in preparations other than well-washed membranes or well-washed monolayer cultures of neurons, although two recent studies have found direct effects of glycine in brain-slice preparations (Thomson *et al.*, 1989; Jansen *et al.*, 1989). This implies that the combination of relatively high ambient glycine concentrations in these preparations with a high affinity of glycine for its site on the NMDA receptor may mask the effect of exogenously added compounds. The demonstration of positive modulatory effects of glycine on spinal cord NMDA responses (Fletcher and Lodge, 1988) and striatal slices (Ransom and Deschenes, 1989) required the use of glycine antagonists to compete against the endogenous amino acid. Early studies suggested that kynurenic acid could antagonize NMDA responses in a manner partially reversible by the addition of excess glycine (Kessler *et al.*, 1987). However, the selectivity of kynurenic acid for the glycine site compared to the NMDA site and was limited (Mayer *et al.*, 1988; Reynolds *et al.*, 1989), and kynurenic acid is also known to block the other amino acid receptor subtypes with similar potency. Cycloleucine also appears to have glycine antagonist properties, but is a very weak antagonist (Snell and Johnson, 1988). More selective antagonism was achieved with the use of HA-966 by Fletcher and Lodge (1988). This drug reduced spinal cord responses to NMDA that could be reversed by the addition of glycine but not NMDA itself. Subsequent studies have demonstrated that HA-966 can reduce [^{3}H]MK801 binding, NMDA-induced increases in intracellular Ca^{2+}, and NMDA-induced [^{3}H]GABA release from rat forebrain neurons in culture (Reynolds *et al.*, 1989). In each of these cases, HA-966 only partially reduced the response to NMDA, and the inhibition could be reversed by the addition of excess glycine. Moreover, HA-966 appears to be about 100-fold more selective for the glycine site over the NMDA site (Reynolds *et al.*, 1989).

A more recent addition to the list of glycine antagonists is 7-chlorokynurenate (7CK). 7CK inhibits [^{3}H]glycine binding to the NMDA receptor with an affinity of 0.5 μM (Kemp *et al.*, 1988). 7CK also greatly reduces NMDA-induced currents measured using patch-clamp techniques. It also appears that 7CK reduces [^{3}H]MK801 binding to a significantly greater extent than HA-966 (I. J. Reynolds, unpublished observations). Although the parent compound kynurenic acid lacks specificity, 7CK appears to be much more specific with respect to effects at other excitatoryamino acid receptors, and relatively selective for the glycine compared to the NMDA site on the NMDA receptor (Kemp *et al.*, 1988). Glycine antagonist effects of several indole carboxylic acids (Huettner, 1989) and 1-aminocyclobutane-1-carboxylate (Hood *et al.*, 1989b) have also been described. These drugs show a similar spectrum of activity as 7CK but are somewhat less potent. Their specificity remains to be determined.

There is apparently some reciprocity in the interactions between the glycine and NMDA recognition sites. Thus, where glycine increases agonist binding to the NMDA site, NMDA-like agonists increase [^{3}H]glycine binding to its recognition site (Kessler *et al.*, 1989). However, in this preparation, the effects of competitive antagonists at the NMDA site were inconsistent.

A central question regarding the role of glycine in NMDA receptor function is whether glycine is absolutely required for NMDA receptor activity, or whether it simply serves as a positive modulator of the effects of glutamate. As described above, the studies of Kleckner and Dingledine (1988) suggested that, if great care is taken to lower ambient glycine concentrations, the responses to NMDA extrapolate through zero, suggesting that glycine may be a cotransmitter rather than a positive modulator. However, a recent study by Mayer and colleagues suggested that glycine may serve to minimize desensitization of NMDA responses (Mayer *et al.*, 1989a). In the presence of very low concentrations of glycine these workers observed very transient peak responses to NMDA that decayed to plateau levels barely above baseline. The addition of glycine had little effect on the magnitude of the transient peak but greatly increased the level of the plateau. It is possible that the slower recordings made by Kleckner and Dingledine (1988) produced responses characteristic of the desensitized NMDA receptor, and thereby related the plateau level to the glycine concentration with the aforementioned conclusion.

Clearly, most of the experimental paradigms currently employed do not allow the same level of control over the ambient glycine concentrations as is possible in the oocyte system. As an alternative, the use of antagonists acting at the glycine site should, in principle, allow similar determinations to be made. However, this has proved difficult to do in practice due to the uncertain intrinsic efficacy of the putative glycine antagonists currently being used. A range of compounds has been used, as mentioned above. Glycine and D-serine represent full agonists (Reynolds *et al.*, 1987; Wong *et al.*, 1987; Snell *et al.*, 1987; Bonhaus *et al.*, 1987), while D-cycloserine has recently been demonstrated to be a partial agonist (Hood *et al.*, 1989a). HA-966 rarely, if ever, demonstrates glycine-mimetic actions, but clearly reduces the effects of added glycine (Fletcher and Lodge, 1988; Reynolds *et al.*, 1989). 7CK can apparently reduce NMDA responses to a lower level than HA-966 (Kemp *et al.*, 1988). However, glutamate-enhanced [^{3}H]MK801 binding is reduced by 90%, and is thus not completely abolished at concentrations at which 7CK is selective for the glycine site (I. J. Reynolds, unpublished observations), suggesting some residual channel activity in the absence of glycine. If one begins with the hypothesis that glycine is an absolute requirement for receptor activity and ligand binding at the phencyclidine site, then simple antagonists should completely eliminate NMDA responses. In this hypothesis 7CK represents the closest approximation to a full antagonist, and HA-966 and D-cycloserine are partial agonists. However, by analogy with benzodiazepine action at the $GABA_A$ receptor, one could propose that glycine is not an absolute requirement, and nonoccupation of the site by glycine, or occupation by an antagonist, would reduce but not eliminate NMDA responses. In this model, HA-966 would represent a prototypical antagonist, while 7CK would be an inverse agonist, binding to the site and producing an opposite effect (i.e., inhibition) to glycine. Unfortunately, it is presently difficult to distinguish between these hypotheses, as in each case the effects of HA-966 should reverse the effects of 7CK. Thus, unless it is possible to use a model system in which HA-966 consistently demonstrates agonist activity, the testing of the two models will await methods distinguishing HA-966 from glycine and 7CK. Interestingly, recent data suggests that HA-966 increases [^{3}H]CPP binding to the glutamate site, while both glycine *and* 7CK can reverse these stimulatory effects of HA-966 (Danysz *et al.* 1989). The simplest explanation of these findings, in view of the functional data with 7CK, seems to support the suggestion that 7CK is an inverse agonist. Clearly, confirmation and expansion of these findings will be an important step.

Many questions about the functional role of glycine in NMDA receptor-mediated synaptic events obviously remain. However, regardless of the actual physiological significance of the glycine site, this locus may represent an important therapeutic target as a novel approach to treating the various pathophysiological states described above. Indeed, it could be argued that negative modulation, rather than overt block, of the receptor will be a far more benign way of moderating receptor function, and thereby limiting possibly deleterious side effects of other antagonists.

D. Divalent Cation Interactions with the NMDA Receptor

From electrophysiological studies two quite distinct divalent cation effects on NMDA receptors have been proposed. Physiological concentrations of Mg^{2+} block NMDA responses by binding to a site that is almost certainly located within the channel (Mayer *et al.*, 1984; Nowak *et al.*, 1984; Ascher and Nowak, 1988). Conversely, Zn^{2+} blocks NMDA responses largely independently of membrane potential (Westbook and Mayer, 1987), suggesting a superficial site of action. A number of binding studies using [^{3}H]MK801 or [^{3}H]TCP have examined the effects of divalent cations, and have described essentially three types of effect. (1) At low concentrations (0.01–1 m*M*) several cations, including Mg^{2+}, Ca^{2+}, Sr^{2+}, and Ba^{2+}, increase binding of [^{3}H]MK801 and [^{3}H]TCP (Reynolds and Miller, 1988a; Johnson *et al.*, 1988; Loo *et al.*, 1987; Greenberg and Marks, 1988; Wong *et al.*, 1988). The magnitude of stimulation varies from two- to sixfold for g^{2+} and Sr^{2+}, respectively, and is not seen when the glutamate and glycine sites are saturated (Reynolds and Miller, 1988a; Wong *et al.*, 1988; Johnson *et al.*, 1988). (2) At higher concentrations the same cations decrease binding, and the apparent potency of inhibition increases in the presence of saturating concentrations of the receptor activators (Reynolds and Miller, 1988a;

Johnson *et al.*, 1988; Wong *et al.*, 1988; McKernan *et al.*, 1989; Greenberg and Marks, 1988). (3) Zn^{2+} and Cd^{2+} do not increase binding, and inhibit binding in a manner insensitive to the presence of glutamate and glycine (Reynolds and Miller, 1988a; McKernan *et al.*, 1989).

The type (3) effects seem to closely resemble those described for Zn^{2+} in electrophysiological paradigms (Reynolds and Miller, 1988a; Westbrook and Mayer, 1987). The potency of Zn^{2+} is very similar using the two approaches. Zn^{2+} appears to be a receptor antagonist that does not act as either the glutamate or the glycine site. Moreover, Zn^{2+} very effectively decreases the dissociation rate of [^{3}H]MK801, suggesting that Zn^{2+} allosterically prevents NMDA-induced channel opening (Reynolds and Miller, 1988b). The absence of changes in the apparent affinity in the presence of glutamate and glycine argues against a site of action within the ionophore. Thus, Zn^{2+} appears to occupy a unique site on the receptor. It is not entirely clear whether the Zn^{2+} site is allosterically coupled to other ligand recognition sites on the NMDA receptor. Zn^{2+} and Cd^{2+} decrease NMDA-sensitive glutamate binding (Monahan and Michel, 1987), and Zn^{2+} appears to reduce binding of the NMDA-site antagonist [^{3}H]CGS 19755 (I. J. Reynolds, unpublished observations), suggesting that the NMDA site may be linked to the Zn^{2+} site. However, a recent study found no effects of Zn^{2+} on [^{3}H]glycine binding (Kessler *et al.*, 1989), implying a lack of allosteric coupling.

It was recently suggested that a number of phenothiazines and tricyclic antidepressants exerted Zn^{2+}-like effects on the NMDA receptor based on their ability to slow the dissociation of [^{3}H]MK801 (Reynolds and Miller, 1988c). This effect is closely correlated with the ability of various tricyclic compounds to inhibit NMDA-induced lethality in mice (Leander, 1989). More thorough analysis, both using ligand binding studies (Reynolds and Miller, 1988d) and patch-clamp techniques (Mayer *et al.*, 1989b) has demonstrated effects probably mediated by the phencyclidine site within the channel as well as the separate locus mediating the effects on [^{3}H]MK801 binding kinetics (Reynolds and Miller, 1988b). This certainly complicates the use of these tools as probes for the Zn^{2+} site. Moreover, there may be a relationship between the ability of drugs to partition into membranes and their effects on the dissociation of [^{3}H]MK801 (Reynolds and Rush, 1990). This would imply that the "Zn^{2+}-like" effects originally observed may represent a more general membrane stabilization phenomenon rather than an effect mediated by a discrete ligand binding site.

It is difficult to describe a precise locus for type (1) and (2) cation effects on [^{3}H]MK801 and [^{3}H]TCP binding. The finding that channel activation increased the apparent potency of type (2) effects might imply a site of action that is less accessible when the receptor is not activated, as suggested above for phencyclidine-like ligands. This might correspond to the voltage-sensitive Mg^{2+} site previously described. The potency of cations at this site is closely tied to the membrane potential (Ascher and Nowak, 1988), such that Mg^{2+} should be relatively weak in the absence of a membrane potential, as is presumably the case with the membrane preparations used in standard binding assays. Indeed, the predicted potency of Mg^{2+} would be between 1 and 10 m*M* in such preparations. The values of potency for Mg^{2+} in the type (2) effects found in binding assays actually correspond reasonably well with this predicted potency range (Reynolds and Miller, 1988a; Johnson *et al.*, 1988; Wong *et al.*, 1988). Thus, type (2) cation effects may be mediated by the Mg^{2+} site within the ion channel.

As both the Mg^{2+} and phencyclidine sites are within the channel, it is possible that the two agents bind at the same site. Indeed, this was implied by the experiments of Huettner and Bean (1988), who found that Mg^{2+} could prevent the acquisition of use-dependent block of NMDA responses by MK801. An examination of the effects of Mg^{2+} on the dissociation of [^{3}H]MK801 showed that concentrations of Mg^{2+} sufficient to produce type (2) effects are sufficient to increase the dissociation rate significantly (Reynolds and Miller, 1988b). These effects were much greater than those produced by the addition of glutamate and glycine, and could be completely prevented by the addition of Zn^{2+} or AP5 (Reynolds and Miller, 1988b,d). The results demonstrate that type (2) cation effects are not mediated by ligand binding to the phencyclidine site. Moreover, the ability of AP5 to prevent the effects of Mg^{2+} in this paradigm supports the hypothesis that the site for these effects is located within the channel.

The nature of the type (1) cation effect is less clear. Although Mg^{2+} produces this effect, Sr^{2+}, Ca^{2+}, and Ba^{2+} also increase binding and are more efficacious (Reynolds and Miller, 1988a). As Sr^{2+} produces the largest effect, type (1) cation effects might be more appropriately termed "Sr^{2+} effects." Cation enhancement of binding is only observed when levels of glutamate and glycine are low. These effects are also found in solubilized receptors (McKernan *et al.*, 1989), suggesting that the site of action of type (1) cation effects is an integral part of the receptor. Several studies have suggested that Mg^{2+} at relatively low concentrations can increase binding of [^{3}H]glycine, presumably by increasing its affinity (Marvizon and Skolnick, 1988; Kessler *et al.*, 1989). Assuming that the affinity, and not the efficacy, of glycine is increased, this effect would not be observed when the glycine site was saturated, consistent with observations made using phencyclidine-site ligands. Thus, there may be a cation site that is separate from the site located within the ion channel that facilitates channel opening and acts by enhancing the effects of glycine. Unfortunately, testing this hypothesis using putative glycine antagonists may not be fruitful due to the uncertainties regarding the antagonist/inverse agonist nature of the currently available compounds. However, one might predict that low concentrations of several divalent cations would enhance Na^+ flux through the NMDA-operated channel. As this could be studied without significant divalent cation levels in the media, this could be used to test the hypothesis. In their original description of the effects of Mg^{2+}

on the NMDA receptor, Nowak and colleagues (1984) described two effects of Mg^{2+} on single channel currents. However, both of the actions of Mg^{2+} described were voltage dependent. For the reasons described for type (2) effects it seems unlikely that effects requiring a negative internal membrane potential would be manifested at the concentrations producing cation-induced increases in ligand binding to the phencyclidine site.

E. Other Sites for Modulation

The major and reasonably well-characterized sites for modulation of NMDA receptor activity have been described in the preceding sections. There have recently been descriptions of several compounds that do not seem to fit easily into the previously described classes of drug. It seems a little premature to assign separate binding sites for all of these compounds at this stage. This section describes some of these actions and explain why the compounds do not fit in the existing schemes.

Ransom and Stec (1988) recently demonstrated that the polyamines spermine and spermidine, but not their polycation precursor putrescine, substantially increase [^{3}H]MK801 binding to rat brain membranes. The effects are seen in the 5–50 μM concentration range, which is well within putative intracellular polyamine levels. The enhancement of [^{3}H]MK801 binding seen is equal to or greater than that produced by the combination of glutamate and glycine (Ransom and Stec, 1988; Reynolds and Miller, 1989), which implies a potentially substantial effect on NMDA receptor activation. The positive modulatory effect of spermidine can be blocked in an unsurmountable fashion by competitive antagonists at the NMDA recognition site, suggesting that polyamines are not simply "super glutamate." Additionally, spermidine does not displace either [^{3}H]CPP or [^{3}H]glycine binding (Ransom and Stec, 1988). Thus, polyamines may represent prototypical compounds for a novel modulatory site on the NMDA receptor. It is also possible that polyamines really produce Sr^{2+}-like effects with greater efficacy. This possibility has not yet been tested. It is interesting to note that many spider venoms, which have glutamate antagonistic properties in some species, have chemical structures that are based on polyamine molecules (Jackson and Usherwood, 1988). It will be interesting to determine whether such compounds will compete with the effects of spermine at the NMDA receptor. It will also be interesting to investigate the possibility that polyamines regulate the activity of NMDA receptors in more functional assays.

Recent studies have demonstrated that the neuroprotective agent ifenprodil and its structural analog SL 82.0715 (Gotti *et al.*, 1988), are effective NMDA receptor antagonists, based on [^{3}H]TCP binding studies (Carter *et al.*, 1988). We have recently evaluated the effects of ifenprodil using [^{3}H]MK801 (Reynolds and Miller, 1989). Ifenprodil inhibits [^{3}H]MK801 binding in a biphasic fashion.

High-affinity effects are seen at 10–30 n*M*, while low-affinity inhibition is apparent at 10–100 μ*M*. In order to determine the site of action of ifenprodil we manipulated the levels of the various positive modulators of binding. While high glutamate concentrations increased [^{3}H]MK801 binding, they did not affect the potency of ifenprodil nor the distribution of the phases of binding (about 50% in each state). The addition of glycine also did not change the potency of ifenprodil at the high-affinity site, but significantly altered the fraction of binding sensitive to low concentrations of ifenprodil (reduced to 20%). This clearly demonstrates a noncompetitive interaction between ifenprodil and glycine that is not apparent for glutamate. Addition of spermine to this assay completely abolished high-affinity actions of ifenprodil. Moreover, polyamines apparently do not interact with ifenprodil in a competitive fashion. Thus, ifenprodil seems to exert effects on the NMDA receptor that are quite distinct from other antagonists employed. It is difficult to explain these findings mechanistically. Empirically, one can suggest that ifenprodil could bind to the receptor in a state-dependent fashion that is relatively insensitive to the level of channel opening. Thus, as glycine promotes glutamate-induced channel opening and polyamines may promote this even more, ifenprodil could bind to a state that is inactive and less able to respond to glutamate or NMDA stimulation. The action of ifenprodil apparently is not sensitive to opening of the channel per se as glutamate does not alter its effects. It is tempting to suggest that ifenprodil preferentially binds to a desensitized state of the channel, although such speculation is hazardous based simply on binding data alone.

Thus, there are at least two types of drug interaction with NMDA receptors that do not easily fit within the currently accepted model. Given the complexity of the existing model, it seems that caution is appropriate before adding additional sites. However, such an action may ultimately be necessary.

IV. Summary and Conclusions

In this review we have attempted to describe the basis for current models of the NMDA receptor, and justify the need for the various binding sites that have been proposed. The NMDA receptor is clearly a complex molecule with a number of modulatory sites, any of which may have great functional significance. From the data presented above it is apparent that the NMDA recognition site is closely coupled with the glycine site, and can also be regulated by Zn^{2+}. The glycine site is reciprocally coupled to the NMDA site, and may also be coupled to a divalent-cation site outside the channel. However, the glycine site is insensitive to Zn^{2+}. The Zn^{2+} site is probably not inside the channel to any degree, but can profoundly affect the ability of NMDA site ligands to operate the channel. However, the determination of reciprocal effects at the Zn^{2+} site await the development of a suitably potent and selective ligand for this site.

Several lines of evidence suggest that the phencyclidine and channel-blocking Mg^{2+} site are located within the NMDA-operated ion channel. Glutamate, glycine, and Zn^{2+} alter the binding of ligands to these sites. However, this is most likely to be due to alteration of access of the ligands to their sites rather than a direct allosteric coupling. It does appear that phencyclidine site drugs and Mg^{2+} bind to separate sites within the channel, and that these separate sites are allosterically coupled.

This complex series of interactions, many of which are mediated by endogenous agents, may allow very fine control over the expression of NMDA receptor-mediated synaptic transmission. In addition to these ligand-produced modulatory effects, there may also be covalent modification of the channel by receptor phosphorylation. Furthermore, the voltage sensitivity of some of the effects allows control of NMDA receptor-mediated signaling by alteration of the membrane potential in the postsynaptic cell, which can be achieved in a wide variety of ways. The level of sophistication possible in adjusting the responsiveness of this receptor seems entirely appropriate given its central involvement in a wide variety of fundamental neurobiological events, and underscores the deleterious pathological sequelae of the system tilting out of balance. At the same time, the wide array of possible therapeutic targets raises hopes that it may soon be possible to treat effectively some severely debilitating and currently untreatable diseases.

References

Addae, J. I., and Stone, T. W. (1987). Involvement of *N*-methyl-D-aspartate receptors in the augmenting response in rat neocortex. *Neurosci. Lett.* **78,** 323–327.

Anis, N. A., Berry, S. C., Burton, N. R, and Lodge, D. (1983). The dissociative anaesthetics, ketamine and phenyclidine, selectively reduce excitation of central mammalian neurones by *N*-methyl-aspartate. *Br. J. Pharmacol.* **79,** 565–575.

Aram, J. A., Martin, D., Tomczyk, M., Zeman, S., Millar, J., Pohler, G., and Lodge, D. (1989). Neocortical epileptogenesis in vitro: Studies with *N*-methyl-D-asprtate, phencyclidine, *sigma* and dextromethorphan receptor ligands. *J. Pharmacol. Exp. Ther.* **248,** 320–328.

Artola, A., and Singer, W. (1987). Long term potentiation and NMDA receptors in rat visual cortex. *Nature (London)* **330,** 649–652.

Ascher, P., and Nowak, L. (1987). Electrophysiological studies of NMDA receptors. *Trends Neurosci.* **10,** 284–288.

Ascher, P., and Nowak, L. (1988). The role of divalent cations in the *N*-methyl-D-aspartate responses of mouse central neurones in culture. *J. Physiol. (London)* **399,** 247–266.

Bennett, D. A., Bernard, P. S., and Amrick, C. L. (1988). A comparison of PCP-like compounds for NMDA antagonism in two in vivo models. *Life Sci.* **42,** 447–454.

Benveniste, H., Drejer, J., Schousboe, A., and Diemer, N. H. (1984). Elevation of the extracellular concentrations of glutamate and aspartate in rat hippocampus during transient cerebral ischemia monitored by intracerebral microdialysis. *J. Neurochem.* **43,** 1369–1374.

Boast, C. A., Gerhardt, S. C., Pastor, G., Lehmann, J., Etienne, P. E., and Liebman, J. M. (1988). The *N*-methyl-D-aspartate antagonists CGS 19755 and CPP reduce ischemic brain damage in gerbils. *Brain Res.* **442,** 345–348.

Bonhaus, D. W., and McNamara, J. O. (1988). *N*-Methyl-D-aspartate receptor regulation of uncompetitive antagonist binding in rat brain membranes: Kinetic analysis. *Mol. Pharmacol.* **34,** 250–255.

Bonhaus, D. W., Burge, B. C., and McNamara, J. O. (1987). Biochemical evidence that glycine allosterically regulates an NMDA receptor-coupled ion channel. *Eur. J. Pharmacol.* **142,** 489–490.

Bowery, N. G., Wong, E. H. F., and Hudson, A. L. (1988). Quantitative autoradiography of [^{3}H]MK801 binding sites in mammalian brain. *Br. J. Pharmacol.* **93,** 944–954.

Brady, R. J., and Swann, J. W. (1986). Ketamine selectively suppresses synchronized afterdischarges in immature hippocampus. *Neurosci. Lett.* **69,** 143–149.

Bristow, D. R., Bowery, N. G., and Woodruff, G. N. (1986). Light microscopic autoradiographic localization of [^{3}H]glycine and [^{3}H]strychnine binding sites in rat brain. *Eur. J. Pharmacol.* **126,** 303–307.

Brown, T. H., Chapman, P. F., Kairiss, E. W., and Keenan, C. L. (1988). Long-term synaptic potentiation. *Science* **242,** 724–728.

Carter, C., Benavides, J., Legendre, P., Vincent, J. D., Noel, F., Thuret, F., Lloyd, K. G., Arbilla, S., Zivkovic, B., MacKenzie, E. T., Scatton, B., and Langer, S. Z. (1988). Ifenprodil and SL820175 as cerebral anti-ischemic agents II. Evidence for *N*-methyl-D-aspartate receptor antagonist properties. *J. Pharmacol. Exp. Ther.* **247,** 1222–1232.

Choi, D. W. (1988). Glutamate neurotoxicity and diseases of the nervous system. *Neuron* **1,** 623–624.

Choi, D. W., Maulucci-Gedde, M., and Kriegstein, A. R. (1987). Glutamate neurotoxicity in cortical cell culture. *J. Neurosci.* **7,** 357–368.

Choi, D. W., Koh, J.-Y., and Peters, S. (1988). Pharmacology of glutamate neurotoxicity in cortical cell culture: Attenuation by NMDA antagonists. *J. Neurosci.* **8,** 185–195.

Cline, H. T., Debski, E. A., and Constantine-Paton, M. (1987). *N*-Methyl-D-aspartate receptor antagonist desegregates eye-specific stripes. *Proc. Natl. Acad. Sci. U.S.A.* **84,** 4342–4345.

Clineschmidt, B. V. (1982). Effect of the benzodiazepine receptor antagonist Ro 15-1788 on the anticonvulsant and anticonflict actions of MK-801. *Eur. J. Pharmacol.* **84,** 119–121.

Collingridge, G. L., and Bliss, T. V. P. (1987). NMDA receptors—their role in long term potentiation. *Trends Neurosci.* **10,** 288–293.

Collingridge, G. L., Herron, C. E., and Lester, R. A. J. (1988a). Synaptic activation of *N*-methyl-D-aspartate receptors in the Schaffer collateral–commisural pathway of rat hippocampus. *J. Physiol. (London)* **399,** 283–300.

Collingridge, G. L., Herron, C. E., and Lester, R. A. J. (1988b). Frequency dependent *N*-methyl-D-aspartate receptor-mediated synaptic transmission in rat hippocampus. *J. Physiol. (London)* **399,** 301–312.

Cowburn, R., Hardy, J., Roberts, P., and Briggs, R. (1988). Presynaptic and postsynaptic function in Alzheimers disease. *Neurosci. Lett.* **86,** 109–113.

Crawford, I. L., and Connor, J. D. (1972). Zinc in maturing rat brain: Hippocampal concentration and localization. *J. Neurochem.* **19,** 1451–1458.

Croucher, M. J., Collins, J. F., and Meldrum, B. S. (1982). Anticonvulsant action of excitatory amino acid antagonists. *Science* **216,** 899–901.

Danysz, W., Fadda, E., Wroblewski, J. T., and Costa, E. (1989). Different modes of action of 3-amino-1-hydroxypyrrolidone (HA-966) and 7 chlorokynurenic acid in the modulation of *N*-methyl-D-asparate-sensitive glutamate receptors. *Mol. Pharmacol.* **36,** 912–916

Davies, J., and Watkins, J. C. (1973). Microiontophoretic studies on the depressant actions of HA-966 on chemically and synaptically excited neurones in the cat cerebral cortex and cuneate nucleus. *Brain Res.* **59,** 311–322.

Davies, S. N., Lester, R. A. J., Reymann, K. G., and Collingridge, G. L. (1989). Temporally distinct pre- and post-synaptic mechanisms maintain long-term potentiation. *Nature (London)* **338,** 500–503.

Deshpande, J. K., Siesjo, B. K., and Wieloch, T. (1987). Calcium accumulation and neuronal damage in the rat hippocampus following cerebral ischemia. *J. Cereb. Blood Flow Metab.* **7,** 89–95.

Ellison, D. W., Beal, M. F., Mazurek, M. F., Malloy, J. R., Bird, E. D., and Martin, J. B. (1987). Amino acid neurotransmitter abnormalities in Huntingdons disease and the quinolinic acid animal model of Huntingdons disease. *Brain* **110,** 1657–1673.

Fagg, G. E. (1987). Phencyclidine and related drugs bind to the activated *N*-methyl-D-aspartate receptor–channel complex in rat brain membranes. *Neurosci. Lett.* **76,** 221–227.

Fagg, G. E., Baud, J., Hall, R., and Dingwall, J. (1988). Do agonists and competitive antagonists bind to distinct sites on the NMDA receptor. *In* "Frontiers in Excitatory Amino Acid Research" (E. A. Cavalheiro, J. Lehmann, and L. Turski, eds.), pp. 59–66. Liss, New York.

Fletcher, E. J., and Lodge, D. (1988). Glycine reverses antagonism of *N*-methyl-D-aspartate (NMDA) by 1-hydroxy-3-aminopyrrolidone-2 (HA-966) but not by D-2-amino-5-phosphonovalerate (D-AP5) on rat cortical slices. *Eur. J. Pharmacol.* **151,** 161–162.

Fletcher, E. J., Martin, D., Aram, J. A., Lodge, D., and Honore, T. (1988). Quinoxalinediones selectively block quisqualate and kainate receptors and synaptic events in rat neocortex and hippocampus and frog spinal cord in vitro. *Br. J. Pharmacol.* **95,** 585–597.

Forsythe, I. D., Westbrook, G. L., and Mayer, M. L. (1988). Modulation of excitatory synaptic transmission by glycine and zinc in cultures of mouse hippocampal neurons. *J. Neurosci.* **8,** 3733–3741.

Foster, A. C., and Fagg, G. E. (1984). Acidic amino acid binding sites in mammalian neuronal membranes: Their characteristics and relationship to synaptic receptors. *Brain Res. Rev.* **7,** 103–164.

Foster, A. C., and Fagg, G. E. (1987). Comparison of L-[^{3}H]glutamate, D-[^{3}H]aspartate, DL-[^{3}H]AP5 and [^{3}H]NMDA as ligands for NMDA receptors in crude postsynaptic densities from rat brain. *Eur. J. Pharmacol.* **133,** 291–300.

Foster, A. C., and Wong, E. H. F. (1987). The novel anticonvulsant MK801 binds to the activated state of the *N*-methyl-D-aspartate receptor in rat brain. *Br. J. Pharmacol.* **91,** 403–409.

Foster, A. C., Gill, R., Kemp, J. A., and Woodruff, G. N. (1987). Systemic administration of MK801 prevents *N*-methyl-D-aspartate-induced neuronal degeneration in rat brain. *Neurosci. Lett.* **76,** 307–311.

Foster, A. C., Gill, R., and Woodruff, G. N. (1988). Neuroprotective effects of MK801 in vivo: Selectivity and evidence for delayed neurodegeneration mediated by NMDA receptor activation. *J. Neurosci.* **8,** 4745–4754.

Gilbert, M. E. (1988). The NMDA receptor antagonist MK801 suppresses limbic kindling and kindled seizures. *Brain Res.* **463,** 90–99.

Goldberg, M. P., Pham, P.-C., and Choi, D. W. (1987). Dextrorphan and dextromethorphan attenuate hypoxic injury in neuronal culture. *Neurosci. Lett.* **80,** 11–15.

Goldberg, M. P., Moyner, H., and Choi, D. W. (1988). Hypoxic neuronal injury in vitro depends on extracellular glutamine. *Neurosci. Lett.* **94,** 52–57.

Gotti, B., Duverger, D., Bertin, J., Carter, C., Dupont, R., Frost, J., Gaudilliere, B., MacKenzie, E. T., Rousseau, J., Scaton, B., and Wick, A. (1988). Ifenprodil and SL820715 as cerebral anti-ischemic agents. I. Evidence for efficacy in models of focal cerebral ischemia. *J. Pharmacol. Exp. Ther.* **247,** 1211–1221.

Greenberg, D. A., and Marks, S. S. (1988). Cation interactions with putative NMDA receptor-gated channels labeled by [^{3}H]MK801 in rat cerebral cortex. *Neurosci. Lett.* **95,** 236–240.

Gruel, J. M., Luhmann, H. J., and Singer, W. (1988). Pharmacological induction of use-dependent receptive field modifications in the visual cortex. *Science* **242,** 74–77.

Halliwell, R. F., Peters, J. A., and Lambert, J. J. (1989). The mechanism of action and pharmacological specificity of the anticonvulsant NMDA antagonist MK801: A voltage clamp study on neuronal cells in culture. *Br. J. Pharmacol.* **96,** 480–494.

Harris, R. J., and Symon, L. (1984). Extracellular pH, potassium and calcium activities in progressive ischemia of rat cortex. *J. Cereb. Blood Flow Metab.* **4,** 178–186.

Herron, C. E., Lester, R. A. J., Coan, E. J., and Collingridge, G. L. (1986). Frequency dependent involvement of NMDA receptors in the hippocampus: A novel synaptic mechanism. *Nature (London)* **322,** 265–268.

Honey, C. R., Miljkovic, Z., and MacDonald, J. F. (1985). Ketamine and phencyclidine cause a voltage-dependent block of responses to L-aspartic acid. *Neurosci. Lett.* **61,** 135–139.

Hood, W. F., Compton, R. P., and Monahan, J. B. (1989a). D-Cyloserine: A ligand for *N*-methyl-D-aspartate coupled glycine receptor has partial agonist characteristics. *Neurosci. Lett.* **98,** 91–95.

Hood, W. F., Sun, E. T., Compton, R. P., and Monahan, J. B. (1989b). 1-Aminocyclobutane-1-carboxylate (ACBC): A specific antagonist of the *N*-methyl-D-aspartate receptor coupled glycine receptor. *Eur. J. Pharmacol.* **161,** 281–282.

Huettner, J. E. (1989). Indole-2-carboxylic acid: A competitive antagonist of potentiation by glycine at the NMDA receptor. *Science* **243,** 1611–1613.

Huettner, J. E., and Bean, B. P. (1988). Block of NMDA-activated current by the anticonvulsant MK-801: Selective binding to open channels. *Proc. Natl. Acad. Sci. U.S.A.* **85,** 1307–1311.

Jackson, H., and Usherwood, P. N. R. (1988). Spider toxins as tools for dissecting elements of excitatory amino acid transmission. *Trends Neurosci.* **11,** 279–283.

Jansen, K. L. R., Dragunow, M., and Faull, R. L. M. (1989). [^{3}H]Glycine binding sites, NMDA and PCP receptors have similar distributions in the human hippocampus: An autoradiographic study. *Brain Res.* **482,** 174–178.

Jarvis, M. F., Murphy, D. E., and Williams, M. (1987). Quantitative autoradiographic localization of NMDA receptors in rat brain using [^{3}H]CPP: Comparison with [^{3}H]TCP binding sites. *Eur. J. Pharmacol.* **141,** 149–152.

Javitt, D. C., and Zukin, S. R. (1989). Interaction of [^{3}H]MK801 with multiple states of the *N*-methyl-D-aspartate receptor complex of rat brain. *Proc. Natl. Acad. Sci. U.S.A.* **86,** 740–744.

Javitt, D. C., Jotkowitz, A., Sircar, R., and Zukin, S. R. (1987). Non-competitive regulation of phencyclidine/*sigma*-receptors by the *N*-methyl-D-aspartate receptor antagonist D-(−)-2-amino-5-phosphonovaleric acid. *Neurosci. Lett.* **78,** 193–198.

Johnson, J. W, and Ascher, P. (1987). Glycine potentiates the NMDA response in cultured mouse brain neurons. *Nature (London)* **325,** 529–531.

Johnson, K. M., Snell, L. D., and Morter, R. S. (1988). *N*-Methyl-D-aspartate enhanced ^{3}H-TCP binding to rat cortical membranes: Effects of divalent cations and glycine. *In* "*Sigma* and Phencyclidine-Like Compounds as Molecular Probes in Biology" (E. F. Domino and J. M. Kamenka, eds.), pp. 259–268. NPP Books, Ann Arbor, Michigan.

Kemp, J. A., Foster, A. C., Leeson, P. D., Priestly, T., Tridgett, R., Iversen, L. L., and Woodruff, G. N. (1988). 7-Chlorokynurenic acid is a selective antagonist at the glycine modulatory site of the *N*-methyl-D-aspartate receptor complex. *Proc. Natl. Acad. Sci. U.S.A.* **85,** 6547–6550.

Kessler, M., Baudry, M., and Lynch, G. (1987). Complex interactions between a glycine binding site and NMDA receptors. *Soc. Neurosci. Abstr.* **13,** 760.

Kessler, M., Terramani, T., Lynch, G., and Baudry, M. (1989). Glycine site associated with *N*-methyl-D-aspartic acid receptors: Characterization and identification of a new class of antagonists. *J. Neurochem.* **52,** 1319–1328.

Kim, J. P., Koh, J.-Y., and Choi, D. W. (1987). L-Homocysteate is a potent neurotoxin on cultured cortical neurons. *Brain Res.* **437,** 103–110.

Kishimoto, H., Simon, J. R., and Aprison, M. H. (1981). Determination of the equilibrium dissociation constants and number of glycine binding sites in several areas of the rat central nervous system using a sodium independent system. *J. Neurochem.* **37,** 1015–1024.

Kleckner, N. W., and Dingledine, R. (1988). Requirement for glycine in activation of NMDA receptors expressed in *Xenopus* oocytes. *Science* **241,** 835–837.

Kloog, Y., Nadler, V., and Sokolovsky, M. (1988a). Mode of binding of [^{3}H]dibenzocycloalkenimine (MK-801) to the *N*-methyl-D-aspartate (NMDA) receptor and its therapeutic implication. *FEBS Lett.* **230,** 167–170.

Kloog, Y., Haring, R., and Sokolovsky, M. (1988b). Kinetic characterization of the phencyclidine *N*-methyl-D-aspartate receptor interaction: Evidence for a steric blockade of the channel. *Biochemistry* **27,** 843–848.

Kushner, L., Lerma, J., Zukin, R. S., and Bennett, M. V. L. (1988). Coexpression of *N*-methyl-D-aspartate and phencyclidine receptors in *Xenopus* oocytes injected with rat brain mRNA. *Proc. Natl. Acad. Sci. U.S.A.* **85,** 3250–3254.

Largent, B. L., Gundlach, A. G., and Snyder, S. H. (1986). Pharmacological and autoradiographic discrimination of *sigma* and phencyclidine receptor binding sites in brain with (+)-SKF 10, 047, (+)-3-[3-hydroxyphenyl]-*N*-(1-propyl)piperidine and [^{3}H]-1-[1-(2-thienyl)cyclohexyl]piperidine. *J. Pharmacol. Exp. Ther.* **238,** 739–748.

Larson, A. A., and Beitz, A. J. (1988). Glycine potentiates strychnine induced convulsions: Role of NMDA receptors. *J. Neurosci.* **8,** 3822–3826.

Leander, J. D. (1989). Tricyclic antidepressants block *N*-methyl-D-aspartic acid-induced lethality in mice. *Br. J. Pharmacol.* **96,** 256–258.

Lodge, D., Davies, S. N., Jones, M. G., Millar, J., Mallanack, D. T., Ornstein, P. L., Verberne, A. J. M., Young, N., and Beart, P. M. (1988). A comparison between the *in vivo* and *in vitro* activity of five potent and competitive NMDA antagonists. *Br. J. Pharmacol.* **95,** 957–965.

Loo, P. S., Braunwalder, A. F., Lehmann, J., and Williams, M. (1986). Radioligand binding to central phencyclidine recognition sites is dependent on excitatory amino acid receptor agonists. *Eur. J. Pharmacol.* **123,** 467–468.

Loo, P. S., Braunwalder, A. F., Lehman, J., Williams, M., and Sills, M. A. (1987). Interaction of L-glutamate and magnesium with phencyclidine recognition sites in rat brain: Evidence for multiple affinity states of the phencyclidine/*N*-methyl-D-aspartate receptor complex. *Mol. Pharmacol.* **32,** 820–830.

MacDonald, J. F., Miljkovic, Z., and Pennefather, P. (1987). Use-dependent block of excitatory amino acid currents in cultured neurons by ketamine. *J. Neurophysiol.* **58,** 251–266.

Malenka, R. C., Kauer, J. A., Zucker, R. S., and Nicholl, R. A. (1988). Postsynaptic calcium is sufficient for potentiation of hippocampal synaptic transmission. *Science* **242,** 81–84.

Maragos, W. F., Penney, J. B., and Young, A. B. (1988). Anatomic correlation of NMDA and ^{3}H-TCP-labeled receptors in rat brain. *J. Neurosci.* **8,** 493–501.

Marcoux, F. W., Probert, A. W., Goodrich, J. E., and Dominick, M. A. (1988). The NMDA antagonist ketamine blocks hypoxia-induced calcium accumulation in cultured cortical neurons and prevents ischemic hippocampal cell injury. *In* "Frontiers in Excitatory Amino Acid Research" (E. A. Cavalheiro, J. Lehmann, and L. Turski, eds.), pp. 683–686. Liss, New York.

Marvizon, J. C., and Skolnick, P. (1988). [^{3}H]Glycine binding is modulated by Mg^{2+} and other ligands of the NMDA receptor-cation channel complex. *Eur. J. Pharmacol.* **151,** 157–158.

Mayer, M. L., and Westbrook, G. L. (1987). Cellular mechanisms underlying excitotoxicity. *Trends Neurosci.* **10,** 59–61.

Mayer, M. L., Westbrook, G. L., and Guthrie, P. B. (1984). Voltage-dependent block by Mg^{2+} of NMDA responses in spinal cord neurones. *Nature (London)* **309,** 261–263.

Mayer, M. L., Westbrook, G. L., and Vyklicky, L. (1988). Sites of antagonist action on *N*-methyl-D-aspartic acid receptors studied using fluctuation analysis and a rapid perfusion technique. *J. Neurophysiol.* **60,** 645–663.

Mayer, M. L., Vyklicky, L., and Clements, J. (1989a). Regulation of NMDA receptor desensitization in mouse hippocampal neurons by glycine. *Nature (London)* **338,** 425p–427p.

Mayer, M. L., Vyklicky, L., and Sernagor, E. (1989b). A physiologist's view of the NMDA receptor: An allosteric ion channel with multiple regulatory sites. *Drug Dev. Res.* (in press).

McKernan, R. M., Castro, S., Poat, J. A., and Wong, E. H. F. (1989). Solubilization of the *N*-methyl-D-aspartate receptor channel complex from porcine brain. *J. Neurochem.* **52,** 777–785.

Millan, M. H., Patel, S., and Meldrum, B. S. (1988). The involvement of excitatory amino acid receptors within the prepiriform cortex in pilocarpine induced limbic seizures in rats. *Exp. Brain Res.* **72,** 517–522.

Monaghan, D. T., Olverman, H. J., Nguyen, L., Watkins, J. C., and Cotman, C. W. (1988). Two classes of *N*-methyl-D-aspartate recognition sites: Differential distribution and differential regulation by glycine. *Proc. Natl. Acad. Sci. U.S.A.* **85,** 9836–9840.

Monahan, J. B., and Michel, J. (1987). Identification and characterization of an *N*-methyl-D-aspartate-specific L-[^{3}H]glutamate recognition site in synaptic plasma membranes. *J. Neurochem.* **48,** 1699–1708.

Mulkeen, D., Anwyl, R., and Rowan, M. J. (1987). Enhancement of long-term potentiation by the calcium channel agonist Bayer K 8644 in CA1 of the rat hippocampus in vitro. *Neurosci. Lett.* **80,** 351–355.

Mulkeen, D., Anwyl, R., and Rowan, M. (1988). The effects of external calcium on long term potentiation in the rat hippocampal slice. *Brain Res.* **447,** 234–238.

Muller, D., and Lynch, G. (1988). Long term potentiation differentially affects two components of synaptic responses in hippocampus. *Proc. Natl. Acad. Sci. U.S.A.* **85,** 9346–9350.

Muller, D., Joly, M., and Lynch, G. (1988). Contributions of quisqualate and NMDA receptors to the induction and expression of LTP. *Science* **242,** 1694–1697.

Murphy, D. E., Schneider, J., Boehm, C., Lehmann, J., and Williams, M. (1987). Binding of [^{3}H]3-(2-carboxypiperazin-4-yl)propyl-phosphonic acid to rat brain membranes: A selective, high affinity ligand for *N*-methyl-D-aspartate receptors. *J. Pharmacol. Exp. Ther.* **240,** 778–784.

Murphy, S. N., and Miller, R. J. (1988). A glutamate receptor regulates Ca^{2+}-mobilization in hippocampal neurons. *Proc. Natl. Acad. Sci. U.S.A.* **85,** 8737–8741.

Neuman, R. S., Ben-Ari, Y., Gho, M., and Cherubini, E. (1988). Blockade of excitatory synaptic transmission by 6-cyano-7-nitroquinoxaline-2,3-dione (CNQX) in the hippocampus in vitro. *Neurosci. Lett.* **92,** 64–68.

Nicoletti, F., Wroblewski, J. T., and Costa, E. (1987). Magnesium ions inhibit the stimulation of inositol phospholipid hydrolysis by endogenous excitatory amino acids in primary cultures of cerebellar granule cells. *J. Neurochem.* **48,** 967–973.

Nicoll, R. A., Kauer, J. A., and Malenka, R. C. (1988). The current excitement in long term potentiation. *Neuron* **1,** 97–101.

Nowak, L., Bregestovski, P., Ascher, P., Herbet, A., and Prochiantz, A. (1984). Magnesium gates glutamate-activated channels in mouse central neurones. *Nature (London)* **307,** 462–465.

Olverman, H. J., Monaghan, D. T., Cotman, C. W., and Watkins, J. C. (1986). [^{3}H]CPP, a new competitive ligand for NMDA receptors. *Eur. J. Pharmacol.* **131,** 161–162.

Olverman, H. J., Jones, A. W., and Watkins, J. C. (1988). [^{3}H]D-2-Amino-5-phosphonopentanoate as a ligand for *N*-methyl-D-aspartate receptors in the mammalian central nervous system. *Neuroscience* **26,** 1–15.

Palmer, E., Monaghan, D. T., and Cotman, C. W. (1988). Glutamate receptors and phosphoinositide metabolism: Stimulation by quisqualate receptors is inhibited by *N*-methyl-D-aspartate receptor activation. *Mol. Brain Res.* **4,** 161–165.

Perez Clausell, J., and Danscher, G. (1985). Intravesicular localization of zinc in rat telencephalic boutons. A histochemical study. *Brain Res.* **337,** 91–98.

Peters, S., Koh, J., and Choi, D. W. (1987). Zinc selectively blocks the action of *N*-methyl-D-aspartate on cortical neurons. *Science* **236,** 589–593.

Prince, D. A., and Feeser, H. (1988). Dextromethorphan protects against cerebral infarction in a rat model of hypoxia ischemia. *Neurosci. Lett.* **85,** 291–296.

Ransom, R. W., and Deschenes, N. L. (1989). Glycine modulation of NMDA evoked release of [^{3}H]acetylcholine and [^{3}H]dopamine from rat striatal slices. *Neurosci. Lett.* **96,** 323–328.

Ransom, R. W., and Stec, N. L. (1988). Cooperative modulation of [^{3}H]MK-801 binding to the *N*-methyl-D-aspartate receptor-ion channel complex by L-glutamate, glycine and polyamines. *J. Neurochem.* **51,** 830–836.

Rappaport, Z. H., Young, W., and Flamm, E. S. (1987). Regional brain calcium changes in the rat middle cerebral artery occlusion model of ischemia. *Stroke* **18,** 760–764.

Reymann, K. G., Matthies, H. K., Schulzeck, K., and Matthies, H. (1989). *N*-Methyl-D-aspartate receptor activation is required for the induction of both early and late phases of long term potentiation in rat hippocampal slices. *Neurosci. Lett.* **96,** 96–101.

Reynolds, I. J., and Rush, E. A. (1990). Role of lipid solubility in the interaction of drugs with the *N*-methyl-D-asparate receptor. *Synapse* **5,** 71–76.

Reynolds, I. J., and Miller, R. J. (1988a). [^{3}H]MK801 binding to the NMDA receptor/ionophore complex is regulated by divalent cations: Evidence for multiple regulatory sites. *Eur. J. Pharmacol.* **151,** 103–112.

Reynolds, I. J., and Miller, R. J. (1988b). Multiple sites for the regulation of the *N*-methyl-D-aspartate receptor. *Mol. Pharmacol.* **33,** 581–584.

Reynolds, I. J., and Miller, R. J. (1988c). Tricyclic antidepressants block *N*-methyl-D-aspartate receptors: Similarities to the actions of zinc. *Br. J. Pharmacol.* **95,** 95–102.

Reynolds, I. J., and Miller, R. J. (1988d). [^{3}H]MK801 binding to the *N*-methyl-D-aspartate receptor reveals drug interactions with the zinc and magnesium sites. *J. Pharmacol. Exp. Ther.* **247,** 1025–1031.

Reynolds, I. J., and Miller, R. J. (1989). Ifenprodil is a novel type of NMDA receptor antagonist: Interaction with polyamines. *Mol. Pharmacol.* **36,** 758–765.

Reynolds, I. J., Murphy, S. N., and Miller, R. J. (1987). ^{3}H-Labelled MK-801 binding to the excitatory amino acid receptor complex from rat brain is enhanced by glycine. *Proc. Natl. Acad. Sci. U.S.A.* **84,** 7744–7748.

Reynolds, I. J., Harris, K. M., and Miller, R. J. (1989). NMDA receptor antagonists that bind to the strychnine-insensitive glycine binding site and inhibit NMDA-induced Ca^{2+} fluxes and [^{3}H]GABA release. *Eur. J. Pharmacol.* **172,** 9–17.

Rothman, S. M. (1984). Synaptic release of excitatory amino acid neurotransmitter mediates anoxic neuronal death. *J. Neurosci.* **4,** 1884–1891.

Rothman, S. M., Thurston, J. H., Hauhart, R. E., Clark, G. D., and Solomon, J. S. (1987). Ketamine protects hippocampal neurons from cell death. *Neuroscience* **21,** 673–678.

Salt, T. E. (1989). Modulation of NMDA receptor mediated responses by glycine and D-serine in the rat thalamus in vivo. *Brain Res.* **481,** 403–406.

Sato, K., Morimoto, K., and Okamoto, M. (1988). Anticonvulsant action of a non-competitive antagonist of NMDA receptors (MK801) in the kindling model of epilepsy. *Brain Res.* **463,** 12–20.

Simon, R. P., Griffiths, T., Evans, M. C., Swan, J. H., and Meldrum, B. S. (1984). Calcium overload in selectively vulnerable neurones of the hippocampus during and after ischemia: An electron microscopy study in the rat. *J. Cereb. Blood Flow Metab.* **4,** 350–361.

Snell, L. D., and Johnson, K. M. (1988). Cycloleucine competitively antagonizes the strychnine insensitive glycine receptor. *Eur. J. Pharmacol.* **151,** 165–166.

Snell, L. D., Morter, R. S., and Johnson, K. M. (1987). Glycine potentiates *N*-methyl-D-aspartate-induced [^{3}H]TCP binding to rat cortical membranes. *Neurosci. Lett.* **83,** 313–317.

Starmer, C. F., Packer, D. L., and Grant, A. O. (1987). Ligand binding to transiently accessible sites: Mechanisms for varying apparent binding rates. *J. Theor. Biol.* **124,** 335–341.

Sugiyama, H., Ito, I., and Hirono, C. (1987). A new type of glutamate receptor linked to inositol phospholipid metabolism. *Nature (London)* **325,** 531–533.

Thomas, J. W., Hood, W. F., Monahan, J. B., Contreras, P. C., and O'Donohue, T. L. (1988). Glycine modulation of the phencyclidine binding site in mammalian brain. *Brain Res.* **442,** 396–398.

Thomson, A. M., West, D. C., and Lodge, D. (1985). An *N*-methylaspartate receptor-mediated synapse in rat cerebral cortex: A site of action of ketamine. *Nature (London)* **313,** 479–481.

Thomson, A. M., Walker, V. E., and Flynn, D. M. (1989). Glycine enhances NMDA receptor mediated synaptic potentials in neocortical slices. *Nature (London)* **338,** 422–424.

Verdoorn, T. A., and Dingledine, R. (1988). Excitatory amino acid receptors expressed in Xenopus oocytes: Agonist pharmacology. *Mol. Pharmacol.* **34,** 298–307.

Vignon, J., Vincent, J. P., Bidard, J. N., Kamenka, J. M., Geneste, P., Monier, P., and Lazdunski, M. (1982). Biochemical properties of the brain phencyclidine receptor. *Eur. J. Pharmacol.* **81,** 531–542.

Vincent, J. P., Kartalovski, B., Geneste, P., Kamenka, J. M., and Lazdunski, M. (1979). Interaction of phencyclidine ("angel dust") with a specific receptor in rat brain membranes. *Proc. Natl. Acad. Sci. U.S.A.* **76,** 4678–4682.

Watkins, J. C. (1984). Excitatory amino acids and central synaptic transmission. *Trends Pharmacol. Sci.* **5,** 373–376.

Watkins, J. C., and Olverman, H. J. (1987). Agonists and antagonists for excitatory amino acid receptors. *Trends Neurosci.* **7,** 265–272.

Wensink, J., Molenaar, A. J., Woroniecka, U. D., and van den Hamer, J. A. (1988). Zinc uptake into synaptosomes. *J. Neurochem.* **50,** 782–789.

Westbrook, G. L., and Mayer, M. L. (1987). Micromolar concentrations of Zn^{2+} antagonize NMDA and GABA responses of hippocampal neurons. *Nature (London)* **328,** 640–643.

Whetsell, W. O., and Schwarcz, R. (1989). Prolonged exposure to submicromolar concentrations of quinolinic acid causes excitotoxic damage in organotypic cultures of rat corticostriatal system. *Neurosci. Lett.* **97,** 271–275.

Wong, E. H. F., Kemp, J. A., Priestly, T., Knight, A. R., Woodruff, G. N., and Iversen, L. L. (1986). The anticonvulsant MK 801 is a potent *N*-methyl-D-aspartate antagonist. *Proc. Natl. Acad. Sci. U.S.A.* **83,** 7104–7108.

Wong, E. H. F., Knight, A. R., and Ransom, R. (1987). Glycine modulates [^{3}H]MK-801 binding to the NMDA receptor in rat brain. *Eur. J. Pharmacol.* **142,** 487–488.

Wong, E. H. F., Knight, A. R., and Woodruff, G. N. (1988). [^{3}H]MK-801 labels a site on the *N*-methyl-D-aspartate receptor channel complex in rat brain membranes. *J. Neurochem.* **50,** 274–281.

Zukin, S. R., and Zukin, R. S. (1979). Specific [^{3}H]phencyclidine binding in rat central nervous system. *Proc. Natl. Acad. Sci. U.S.A.* **76,** 5372–5376.

Erythropoietin: Regulation of Erythropoiesis and Clinical Use

Emmanuel N. Dessypris and Sanford B. Krantz

Department of Medicine
Division of Hematology
Vanderbilt University and VA Medical Center
Nashville, Tennessee 37212

I. Introduction

During the last 30 years the role of erythropoietin (EPO) as the major, if not the single, humoral regulator of red cell production has been well established (Krantz and Jacobson, 1970; Graber and Krantz, 1978). Experimental work from various laboratories has demonstrated that there is an inverse correlation between the red cell mass and serum EPO levels. In addition, EPO has been shown to stimulate erythropoiesis *in vitro* as well as *in vivo*. In semisolid media capable of supporting clonal growth of marrow erythroid progenitor cells, EPO has been shown to be an absolute requirement for the terminal differentiation of these cells *in vitro*. EPO was initially purified from the urine of patients with aplastic anemia, and subsequently the gene encoding human EPO was isolated, cloned, and introduced into mammalian cells which became the source of unlimited amounts of recombinant protein. The availability of purified recombinant EPO has allowed studies of its action on purified erythroid cells, the identification of EPO receptors on erythroid progenitor cells and the successful administration of this recombinant hormone to patients suffering from anemia due to low EPO levels. This review summarizes the recent advances on the biology of EPO and the recent experience from its therapeutic use in humans.

II. Structure of Erythropoietin

EPO is a glycoprotein that was purified from the urine of patients with aplastic anemia. It has a molecular weight of 34,000 as determined by SDS–polyacrylamide gel electrophoresis (Miyake *et al.*, 1977) and contains about 30% carbohydrate of which 11% consists of sialic acid, 11% total hexose, and 8% *N*-acetylglucosamine (Dordal *et al.*, 1985).

The gene encoding for human EPO is contained in a 5.4-kilobase fragment of the genomic DNA in which it exists as a single copy (Lin *et al.*, 1985; Jacobs *et al.*, 1985). It contains four introns and five exons for a 193-amino acid peptide. The product of the gene includes a 27-amino acid signal peptide (leader sequence at the N terminus) which is cleaved during secretion of the hormone, and the 166-amino acid hormonal peptide with a molecular weight of 18,398 (Lin *et al.*, 1985). The C-terminal arginine predicted from the gene sequence is absent from both the urinary and the recombinant EPO, presumably because of a posttranslational processing of the genomic product by an intracellular carboxypeptidase (Recny *et al.*, 1987). The molecular weight of recombinant EPO has been determined by velocity sedimentation to be 29,000–30,000 (Browne *et al.*, 1986; Davis *et al.*, 1987), which indicates that carbohydrate makes up almost 39% of the mass of the hormone. The discrepancy between the molecular weight of the natural urinary EPO and the recombinant EPO can be attributed to the aberrant mobility of the glycoproteins on SDS–polyacrylamide gel electrophoresis.

Glycosylation of the hormonal peptide seems to be absolutely necessary for its *in vivo* activity. Asialated EPO, as well as nonglycosylated recombinant EPO produced in bacteria, have no activity *in vivo,* which can be at least partially attributed to the rapid clearance of the hormone by the liver (Goldwasser, 1975; Browne *et al.*, 1986). Nonglycosylated hormone maintains only a part of its *in vitro* activity, probably because of the instability and low solubility of the carbohydrate-lacking peptide. Recombinant EPO produced in mammalian cells is highly glycosylated, and the carbohydrate structure of the molecule is almost indistinguishable from that of the natural hormone (Sasaki *et al.*, 1987; Recny *et al.*, 1987).

The potency of EPO is expressed in units, with one unit defined as the amount of EPO present in one-tenth of one ampule of the International Reference Preparation (Cotes and Bangham, 1966). This unit had been originally defined as the amount of EPO that produced the same EPO response in the starved rat as 5 μmol of cobalt (Krantz and Jacobson, 1970). The potency of the purified recombinant EPO has been estimated to be 129,000 U/mg of total weight or 210,000 U/mg of protein (Browne *et al.*, 1986).

III. Site and Regulation of Erythropoietin Production

Almost 30 years ago, it was established that the kidney is the major organ of EPO production in adult rats (Jacobson *et al.*, 1957). In addition, in humans with end-stage renal failure, the serum EPO concentration was also found to be low and the serum level of EPO was restored to normal following successful renal transplantation (Denny *et al.*, 1966). However, failure to extract from or detect in renal tissue significant amounts of EPO has led to erroneous theories that EPO was either produced by the kidney as an inactive precursor that was enzymatically converted in the circulation into its active form (Peschle and Condorelli, 1975), or that the kidney produced an erythrogenin which activated a circulating form of inactive EPO (Zanjani *et al.*, 1971). The recent cloning of the murine EPO gene (McDonald *et al.*, 1986; Shoemaker and Mitsock, 1986) has allowed studies on the production of mRNA in renal and other tissues of the anemic animals. Bleeding or administration of cobalt has been shown to lead within an hour to the appearance of EPO-encoding mRNA in the kidney and liver of anemic mice and the kidney of anemic rats (Bondurant and Koury, 1986; Beru *et al.*, 1986; Schuster *et al.*, 1989). After severe bleeding, the EPO mRNA increases 500–1000 times compared to normal kidney EPO mRNA, whereas the liver produces only 7% of the total EPO mRNA and no EPO-encoding mRNA was detectable in normal liver even by the RNA protection assay. Even in severely hypoxic animals, no other tissue contained EPO mRNA (Bondurant and Koury, 1986). More recent evidence indicates that the increase in EPO mRNA can be partially attributed to an increased rate of transcription of the EPO gene (Schuster *et al.*, 1989). These data, along with the fact that mammalian cells transfected with the EPO gene produce intact active hormone, indicate that EPO is produced primarily by the kidney and secreted in its active form. The liver seems to be the only other organ capable of producing EPO, but its contribution to the serum EPO levels under the stress of anemia seems to be very limited in adult rodents. In sheep the liver seems to be the primary site of EPO production during fetal life (Zanjani *et al.*, 1977). EPO-encoding mRNA has also been detected in human fetal liver (Jacobs *et al.*, 1985) and in murine fetal liver in midgestation, but not in late gestation (M. J. Koury *et al.*, 1988). Thus, hepatic production of EPO may be contributing to the EPO levels in the fetal circulation, but the significance of such a contribution is not yet clear since EPO has been shown to be capable of crossing the placenta and EPO receptors have been detected in mouse and rat placenta (M. J. Koury *et al.*, 1988), but in sheep infusion of large amounts of EPO followed by biological assay of EPO in the fetal circulation failed to show any crossover to the fetus (Zanjani *et al.*, 1977).

Specialized cells capable of producing EPO have been identified in renal and hepatic tissue by the technique of *in situ* hybridization (S. T. Koury *et al.*, 1988; Lacombe *et al.*, 1988). These cells are rare in the renal tissue and even more so in the liver. They are located in the inner cortex of the renal parenchyma in the interstitium between renal tubules. Although it has been proposed that they may be of endothelial origin, their exact nature remains undetermined at the present time. Previous reports that macrophages produce EPO (Rich *et al.*, 1982) await further confirmation. Increasing demand for EPO after induction of anemia leads to the appearance of an increased number of EPO mRNA-containing cells, indicating that at the cellular level these demands are met by an increase in the number of EPO-producing cells and not by an increased production of EPO per cell (S. T. Koury *et al.*, 1989). Thus it appears that EPO is released once it is produced and there is no detectable storage pool that could be released in the event of acute hypoxia. In addition, the serum level of EPO does not seem to exert any negative feedback on the synthesis of the hormone (Cotes *et al.*, 1989).

The mechanism through which hypoxia induces synthesis of EPO by these specialized renal interstitial cells remains poorly understood. A hypothesis has been raised that hypoxia leads to release of prostaglandin E, which results in increased renal cyclic AMP (cAMP) levels, decreased intracellular calcium concentration, and eventual release of EPO. This hypothesis was based on experimental evidence from *in vivo* experiments and from experiments in tissue culture where cAMP, GMP, prostaglandin E_2, or calcium channel blockers, all at high concentrations, were found to increase EPO production (Rodgers *et al.*, 1975a,b 1976; Gross *et al.*, 1976; McGonigle *et al.*, 1987). In humans, however, neither agents inhibiting prostaglandin synthesis nor calcium channel blockers have ever been associated with alterations of the red cell mass. Recently, it has been proposed that a heme-containing protein which changes from its oxy to its deoxy form may be the sensor of hypoxia and the regulator of the transcription of EPO-encoding mRNA (Goldberg *et al.*, 1987, 1989).

IV. Erythropoietin Receptors

The availability of purified recombinant erythropoietin and the development of techniques for obtaining almost pure populations of either murine (Koury *et al.*, 1984; Sawyer *et al.*, 1987a) or human (Sawada *et al.*, 1987) EPO-responsive cells allowed studies on the mechanism of attachment of EPO to specific membrane molecules, the EPO receptors (reviewed by Sawyer, 1989b). EPO receptors were initially detected on murine erythroid cells infected by the anemic strain of Friend virus (FVA) (Krantz and Goldwasser, 1984). FVA-infected splenic erythroid cells were found to have approximately 1000 receptors per cell, of which 300–400 had a high affinity for EPO (K_d 0.08–0.10 n*M*) and the remaining a lower affinity (K_d 0.6–1.0 n*M*) (Sawyer *et al.*, 1987b,c; Fukamachi *et al.*, 1987). Purified human erythroid cells that were generated *in vitro* from circulating immature erythroid progenitors were also found to express on their membranes two classes of high- and low-affinity EPO receptors with an overall density of 1050 receptors per cell (Krantz *et al.*, 1987; Sawada *et al.*, 1988; Fukamachi *et al.*, 1987). EPO receptors have thus far been detected only on erythroid cells, erythroleukemic cell lines, fetal liver tissue rich in erythroid elements and in mouse and rat placenta (Krantz and Goldwasser, 1984; Sawyer, 1989b; M. J. Koury *et al.*, 1988; Fukamachi *et al.*, 1987).

Following binding of EPO to its receptor, the hormone is rapidly (within 1 minute) endocytosed and degraded (Sawyer *et al.*, 1987c; Sawada *et al.*, 1988; Mufson and Gesner 1987). Whether the EPO receptor is degraded along with the endocytosed hormone or recycles to the surface of the cell is not yet known; however, in the HCD33 erythroleukemic cell line that expresses only low-affinity EPO receptors, experimental evidence favors degradation over recycling (Sawyer and Hankins, 1988). The physiological significance of high- versus low-affinity EPO receptors is not fully understood at the present time, but the fact that EPO-dependent erythroleukemic cell lines have only low-affinity receptors indicates that these receptors can transmit to the cell the signal for proliferation (Sawyer and Hankins, 1988).

The density of EPO receptors on normal human erythroid progenitor cells appears to correlate with their responsiveness to and dependence on this hormone. Erythroid cells at the stage of the erythroid colony-forming unit (CFU-E) to the proerythroblast seem to have the highest density of receptors on their membrane. As the cell matures, the number of EPO receptors decreases, and eventually they disappear at the stage of the orthochromatic erythroblast (Sawyer and Koury, 1987; Sawada *et al.*, 1987; Landchulz and Boyer, 1988; Fraser *et al.*, 1988a,b). In erythroid cells earlier than the CFU-E such as the erthrythroid burst-forming unit (BFU-E), preliminary studies indicate that the number of EPO receptors is very small and increases to the density found at the CFU-E stage within the first 4 days of culture (Sawada *et al.*, 1989).

Studies of the structure of EPO receptors have demonstrated two bands of 100 and 85 kDa by SDS–polyacrylamide gel electrophoresis (Sawyer *et al.*, 1987b) that are not bridged by disulfide bonds and have less than 5% detectable carbohydrate (Hosoi *et al.*, 1988). Peptide mapping of proteolytic fragments of these two peptides showed a very similar, if not identical, pattern (Sawyer *et al.*, 1989; Sawyer, 1989a). The recent cloning of the EPO receptor gene from murine erythroleukemia cells demonstrated that the gene for this receptor encodes a 507-amino acid polypeptide with a single membrane-spanning domain and this single gene can generate both high- and low-affinity binding sites on transfected cells (D'Andrea *et al.*, 1989).

The biochemical events that follow binding of EPO to its receptor and internalization of the hormone are at the present time undetermined. Increase of the intracellular concentration of calcium, cAMP, cGMP, tyrosine-specific protein kinase, phosphatidylinositol, and protein kinase C have been considered as possible second messengers following EPO binding, but the available experimental data have so far failed to indicate that these messenger molecules have any major role in the action of EPO on erythroid cells (reviewed by Sawyer, 1989b).

V. Effects of Erythropoietin on Erythroid Cells *in Vitro* and *in Vivo*

Production of an adequate number of erythrocytes depends on the continuous replenishment of the bone marrow with erythroblasts. Erythroblasts are derived from the proliferation and differentiation of morphologically unrecognizable erythroid progenitor cells. These cells have been functionally defined by their ability to form colonies of erythroblasts in semisolid culture medium. Two major groups of erythroid progenitor cells have been recognized and studied by *in vitro* cloning techniques in semisolid media, the erythroid colony forming unit (CFU-E) and the erythroid burst-forming unit (BFU-E) (reviewed by Eaves and Eaves, 1985). In humans, the CFU-E is a cell very close to the proerythroblast that, within 7–8 days in culture in the presence of EPO, is capable of forming erythroblast colonies of 8–49 cells (Tepperman *et al.*, 1974). The BFU-E is a much more immature cell close to the hematopoietic multipotent stem cell that requires 14–16 days of culture in the presence of EPO, interleukin 3 (IL-3), and/or Granulocyte–Macrophage Colony Stimulating Factor (GM-CSF) to form huge colonies of erythroblasts consisting of 500 to many thousand cells (Gregory and Eaves, 1977).

The mechanism through which immature cells derived from the stem cell are committed to erythroid differentiation is poorly understood. There are two basic theories on this issue: one proposes that commitment is a random process for which the term stochastic is used, while the other proposes that commitment to one pathway of differentiation is the result of competitive action among the various hematopoietic growth factors (reviewed by Porter and Ogawa, 1985). At this early stage of erythropoiesis the role of EPO is still undefined. It is interesting, however, to note that cell lines with multipotent hematopoietic cell properties do express small numbers of EPO receptors on the cell surface (Sakaguchi *et al.*, 1987; Tsao *et al.*, 1988).

Once the cell is committed to erythroid differentiation, it becomes dependent on EPO for its survival and responds to the hormone by proliferation and differentiation. Only the very immature BFU-E is not dependent on EPO, and it can survive in culture for 48 hours in the absence of EPO and in the presence of other hematopoietic factors such as IL-3 or GM-CSF. Preliminary work indicates that only 20% of immature blood BFU-E have a small number of EPO receptors, which increases rapidly within the first 4 days in culture, when the cells become fully dependent on EPO (mature BFU-E) and, in its presence, proliferate and differentiate further to reach the stage of CFU-E (Sawada *et al.* 1990). Thus, mature erythroid progenitors seem to be the most sensitive cells to the hormone and, at the same time, totally dependent on its presence for their survival.

Earlier experiments in animals exposed to EPO through the induction of anemia or by injections of small quantities of impure EPO demonstrated that EPO primarily expands the CFU-E pool, whereas the effects of the hormone on the BFU-E were variable depending on the timing of bone marrow sampling (Iscove, 1977; Hara and Ogawa, 1977; Adamson *et al.*, 1978; Peschle *et al.*, 1979, 1980). Recent reports on the effects of recombinant EPO on the concentration and cycling status of erythroid and nonerythroid progenitors in patients treated with this hormone indicate that, in humans, the bone marrow responds to EPO not only by an increase in the concentration of the erythroid progenitors CFU-E and BFU-E, but also by an increase in the concentration of the progenitors for megakaryocytes and granulocytes–macrophages without a concomitant persistent increase of the blood platelet or neutrophil concentration. These changes in the concentration of hematopoietic progenitors in human marrow were accompanied by a significant increase in the percentage of these cells undergoing active DNA synthesis, indicating that the bone marrow responds to EPO as an organ rather than by selective and isolated expansion of its erythroid elements (Dessypris *et al.*, 1988; Ganser *et al.*, 1987; Reid *et al.*, 1988; Stockenhuber *et al.*, 1988; Geissler *et al.*, 1989). Although EPO may have a selective effect on the erythroid cell line when given in small single doses, its therapeutic administration to humans (multiple high doses) results in a global activation of the marrow progenitor cells, as indicated either by their increased concentration or cycling in the posttreatment marrow.

While the predominant measurable effects of EPO on early erythroid progenitor cells (BFU-E) are primarily proliferative (Dessypris and Krantz, 1984), as these cells mature and reach the stage of the CFU-E to proerythroblast, differentiation events become much more prominent, and at the orthochromatic erythroblast stage proliferation ceases. Studies on the effect of EPO on highly purified (>95%) erythroid cells derived from the spleens of FVA-infected mice (Koury *et al.*, 1984) or thiamphenicol- and phenylhydrazine-treated animals (Nijhof *et al.*, 1987) have demonstrated that EPO induces within 4 hours an increase in the synthesis of RNA, and this is closely followed by the induction of β-globin gene transcription (Koury *et al.*, 1984; Bondurant *et al.*, 1985). Previous experiments have shown that induction of RNA synthesis constitutes one of the earlier biochemical events following exposure of erythroid cells to EPO, and that stimulation of RNA synthesis is independent of DNA synthesis (Gross and Goldwasser, 1969, 1970). Other EPO-induced differentiation events include increased synthesis of transferring receptors, increased iron uptake, hemoglobin synthesis, and appearance of erythrocyte membrane proteins (bands 3 and 4.1) (Sawyer and Krantz, 1986; Koury *et al.*, 1982, 1986, 1987). Deprivation of EPO results in a decline in protein synthesis and an increase in DNA synthesis, with accumulation of small-size DNA representing DNA breakdown products with eventual cell death (Koury and Bondurant, 1988). Thus, EPO exerts profound effects on almost all stages of erythroid cell development and on their terminal differentiation.

Besides the erythroid cells, the only other hematopoietic cells that have been shown to respond to EPO were the megakaryocytes (MK) and their progenitors CFU-MK. In murine marrow, megakaryocyte colony formation can be induced by EPO even in a serum-free culture, and EPO promotes differentiation of murine megakaryocytes, whereas, in human marrow, EPO potentiates the megakaryocyte colony-stimulating activity present in lymphocyte-conditioned media (Clark and Dessypris, 1986; Ishibashi *et al.*, 1987; Dessypris *et al.*, 1987). Injections of EPO to rats have been associated with an increase of ^{35}S incorporation into newly formed platelets without a concomitant rise of the platelet count (McDonald *et al.*, 1987). It is not clear at this time whether this effect of EPO on megakaryocytopoiesis is direct or indirect and whether it has any physiological significance, since demonstrable activation of all marrow cells without concomitant persistent thrombocytosis and leukocytosis suggests that these effects may be due to indirect actions of EPO.

VI. Assays for Erythropoietin

The concentration of EPO in serum or other fluids can be determined by bioassay or radioimmunoassay (reviewed by Caro and Erslev, 1988). The traditional polycythemic mouse assay constitutes the standard against which other methods of EPO measurement have to be compared (Kazal and Erslev, 1975). In this assay, the sample to be tested is injected intravenously or intraperitoneally along with [^{59}Fe]transferrin into mice rendered polycythemic by hypertransfusion of red cells or exposure to a low oxygen atmosphere, so that endogenous EPO production is almost completely suppressed. Stimulation of erythropoiesis by the sample to be tested is evaluated by the concentration of ^{59}Fe in new erythrocytes that appear in the circulation of the mice. This method has a sensitivity of 50 mU/ml and cannot detect EPO levels present in normal human sera. The assay involves the use of a large number of experimental animals for a single measurement, it is time consuming, and the variability of results is quite large. The only advantage of this bioassay is its ability to detect EPO only in its biologically active form.

In order to overcome all these problems with the polycythemic mouse assay, a number of *in vitro* bioassays have been developed in which EPO concentrations are measured by assaying the test sample on EPO-responsive cells (marrow, spleen, fetal liver) in culture through stimulation of either [^{59}Fe]heme synthesis or formation of erythroid colonies by the EPO-responsive cells (Dunn *et al.*, 1975; Goldwasser *et al.*, 1975; McLeod *et al.*, 1974). In a modification of this system, populations of highly enriched erythroid cells are used, and the effect of EPO is quantified by the induced stimulation of DNA synthesis by these cells (Krystal, 1983). These assays are faster to perform and more sensitive than the *in vivo* bioassay, but they have the disadvantage that they are influenced by non-specific promoters and inhibitors of cell growth in culture present in the serum or the test sample, and they cannot differentiate between biologically active and inactive hormone.

Radioimmunoassays for EPO were initially developed using highly purified human urinary EPO as antigen and standard (Garcia, 1972; Sherwood and Goldwasser, 1979; Cotes, 1982) and, more recently, using recombinant EPO (Egrie and Lane, 1987; Egrie *et al.*, 1987). The radioimmunoassays are very quick and accurate and relatively inexpensive. They have the advantage of detecting very small levels of EPO in the test sample; thus, EPO levels in normal sera can be reliably quantified. Levels of EPO in normal sera range between 5 and 30 mU/ml. An inverse correlation can be established between EPO levels and the concentration of hemoglobin in the blood; however, the response to anemia seems to be widely variable among patients. The disadvantage of radioimmunoassays is that they detect immunologically reactive EPO, which does not distinguish between biologically active and inactive forms. Thus, in patients with renal failure, the levels of EPO measured by radioimmunoassay are much higher than those measured by the standard bioassay (Sherwood *et al.*, 1988; Sherwood and Goldwasser, 1979). Very recently, an enzyme-linked immunosorbent assay (ELISA) has become commercially available from AMGen Corporation (Thousand Oaks, CA).

The clinical utility of EPO assays has not yet been proved. Although measurement of EPO levels may be helpful in distinguishing primary from secondary polycythemia and may identify cases of anemia with poor EPO response, the reliability and interpretation of a single serum determination of EPO level need further investigation.

VII. Pharmacokinetics of Recombinant Erythropoietin

The pharmacokinetics of recombinant EPO have been studied in a number of patients with end-stage renal disease treated with hemodialysis (Egrie *et al.*, 1988; Wikström *et al.*, 1988; Cotes *et al.*, 1989). In these studies, EPO levels were measured by radioimmunoassay and, in one of them, confirmed also by *in vivo* bioassay. Patients were given EPO at doses ranging from 15 to 150 U/kg intravenously and studied after 1, 2, or multiple doses. The average volume of distribution was 5.5% of body weight corresponding to the plasma volume. The half-life was not influenced by the dose of EPO and averaged 9.3 ± 3.2 hours (mean ±5 SD) after the first dose of 6.2 ± 1.8 hours after the seventh dose. Continuous treatment with EPO for 3 months did not alter the half-life of the injected hormone. With a schedule of 2–3 doses per week no accumulation of EPO in the plasma was noted. Clearance of EPO was found to be 5.3 ± 1.2 ml/min and remained unchanged for at least 2 months of continuous therapy.

Subcutaneous administration of EPO resulted in a peak plasma concentration within 8–12 hours that was maintained for the next 15 hours. The peak plasma concentration of EPO after the first subcutaneous administration was only 10% of that achieved by the same dose given intravenously. After seven treatments, the peak levels were 40–70% of the levels after the first dose.

The pharmacokinetics of EPO have been also studied in patients on continuous ambulatory peritoneal dialysis and in predialysis patients (MacDougall *et al.*, 1989; Lim *et al.*, 1989). After an intravenous single dose of EPO, the calculated half-life was the same as previously determined in patients on hemodialysis. Within the first 24 hours, 2.3% of the intravenous dose was lost in the dialysate. The peak level after intravenous administration was 10 times higher than after intraperitoneal and 21 times higher-than after subcutaneous administration. The bioavailability of subcutaneous EPO was 7 times greater than that after intraperitoneal injection. Data collected from studies in predialysis patients were very similar to those from hemodialysis patients, indicating that renal clearance or metabolism of the hormone contributes very little to its disappearance from the circulation.

The lower peak levels of EPO that were observed after subcutaneous injection as compared to those after intravenous administration do not seem to affect the therapeutic response in any negative way (Bommer *et al.*, 1988). Considering the practicality of the subcutaneous route, it seems very likely that this is going to become the standard mode of EPO administration.

VIII. Treatment of the Anemia of Renal Failure with Recombinant Erythropoietin

The pathogenesis of the anemia of renal failure is multifactorial, but of all the factors contributing to the decrease of the red cell mass, the inappropriately low level of circulating EPO seem to be the predominant one (Eschbach and Adamson, 1985). Support for this view has been provided by experiments in uremic and anemic animals in which improvement or correction of the anemia was noted by infusion of crude EPO preparations or plasma containing high levels of EPO (Anagnostou *et al.*, 1977; Eschbach *et al.*, 1984; Van Stone and Max, 1979). Therefore, it appears logical that the first trials with human recombinant EPO (rEPO) were performed in anemic patients with end-stage renal failure who had been maintained by hemodialysis (Winearls *et al.*, 1986; Bommer *et al.*, 1987; Eschbach *et al.*, 1987; Cotes *et al.*, 1989). In these phase I–II studies, 48 anemic patients with hematocrits of less than 25% were given intravenous injections of rEPO in escalating doses ranging from 1.5 to 500 U/kg three times weekly after completion of the dialysis session. Within a week after initiation of treatment with doses in excess of 15 U/kg thrice weekly, an appreciable rise in the reticulocyte count was noted, and within 3–4 weeks an increase in the hematocrit could be detected. There was complete abolishment of red cell transfusion requirements and, in the patients receiving higher doses, the hematocrit returned to normal levels. Increasing hematocrit was associated with a decrease in the levels of serum iron and ferritin. The presence of hyperparathyroidism or aluminum overload did not seem to affect the response to EPO. In a number of patients, an increase in the blood pressure was noted, and one patient developed hypertensive encephalopathy with seizures. All patients reported an improved exercise tolerance, feeling of well being, and a number of them had increased libido. A number of patients reported diffuse aching in the limbs and pelvis, associated with sweating, that followed the injections of EPO and lasted for a maximum of 12 hours. The magnitude of the response was related to the dose of rEPO, and no patient developed antibodies to the recombinant hormone.

These initial findings have been confirmed in a large, prospective, multicenter study in which 333 patients with anemia of renal failure on chronic hemodialysis were treated initially with 150 or 300 U/kg of rEPO intravenously three times weekly until their hematocrits reached the level of 35 ± 3%, when the dose was reduced to 50–75 U/kg and adjusted to maintain their hematocrits at this level. In 97.4% of patients the target hematocrit level was reached within 12 weeks, and red cell transfusion requirements were eliminated in almost all patients within the first 8 weeks of therapy. The underlying illnesses in nonresponders included blood loss, myelofibrosis, osteitis fibrosa, or osteomyelitis. Exacerbation of preexisting hypertension or the appearance of hypertension was seen in 35% of patients, with seizures in 5.4%. Transient bone aches were reported by 5% of patients and, in 43%, iron deficiency developed during treatment. In patients with iron-overload secondary to multiple transfusions, the amount of ferritin in the serum decreased by 50% after 6 months of successful therapy. Significant increases in predialysis creatinine, potassium, and phosphate levels were seen, but these changes did not necessitate any alteration in the schedule or duration of dialysis. Thrombotic events, including clotting of the vascular access, were not more frequent than expected in this group of patients, and could not be attributed to a mild increase in the platelet count, which still remained within the normal range (Eschbach *et al.*, 1990). This study has confirmed that rEPO is a potent, effective, and safe agent for the treatment of the anemia of renal failure. Patients treated with rEPO should be closely observed for development or exacerbation of hypertension and for development of iron deficiency, which can limit significantly the response to EPO. The increase in the blood pressure in hemodialysis patients that may accompany the increase in the red cell mass is probably related to an increase in the peripheral vascular resistance as a result of improvement of tissue oxygenation (Buckner *et al.*, 1989; Nonnast *et al.*, 1987). This has not been seen in patients with normal renal function, e.g., patients with rheumatoid arthritis (Pincus *et al.*, 1989; Means *et al.*, 1989), and suggests that hypertensive reactions may be related to the underlying renal disease. Preliminary studies also indicated that correction of anemia by rEPO is associated with an improvement in the hemostatic defect associated with uremia (Moia *et al.*, 1987).

The safety and effectiveness of EPO were also studied in a multicenter, double-blind, placebo-controlled trial in anemic patients with renal failure at the predialysis stage. The results from a group of 28 patients have thus far been reported (Stone *et al.*, 1988; Lim *et al.*, 1989). EPO was found to be effective in increasing the red cell mass and hematocrit in patients with renal failure not undergoing hemodialysis, whereas no response was seen in any patient receiving placebo during the 8-week initial phase of the study. The rate of increase of the hematocrit was related to the dose of administered EPO. An increase in the blood pressure was documented in 5/28 patients and progression of renal failure that eventually necessitated dialysis was seen in 2 out of 28 patients, but may not have been related to rEPO therapy since this is known to occur in these patients.

The relation between progressive decline of renal function and treatment with rEPO is not at the present time well documented. Experiments in uremic and anemic rats indicated that an increase in the hematocrit by rEPO was associated with hypertension and worsening glomerular injury; however, it is not clear whether the latter was a consequence of untreated hypertension (Garcia *et al.*, 1988). Preliminary results from the multicenter trial do not support the experimental evidence derived from rats, but this issue needs further investigation.

The response of uremic nondialyzed patients to rEPO indicates that inhibitors of erythropoiesis previously assumed to have a major role in the suppression of erythropoiesis in renal failure (Ohno *et al.*, 1978; Wallner and Vantrin, 1981; Radtke *et al.*, 1981) contribute very little to the pathogenesis of the anemia.

IX. Treatment of the Anemia of Rheumatoid Arthritis with Recombinant Erythropoietin

The pathogenesis of the anemia of rheumatoid arthritis is not well understood. A shortened red cell survival, impaired release of iron from the reticuloendothelial system, and failure of the marrow to respond to anemia by increased erythropoiesis have been considered for a long time to be the basic mechanisms responsible for the anemia (Cartwright, 1966). More recently, it has been shown that EPO levels are lower in anemic patients with rheumatoid arthritis when compared to other anemic patients without an underlying inflammatory disease (Pavlovic-Kentera *et al.*, 1979; Baer *et al.*, 1987). Patients with rheumatoid arthritis are capable of responding to anemia with increased serum levels of EPO (Birgegard *et al.*, 1987), but their response is blunted (Baer *et al.*, 1987). Although EPO deficiency cannot be considered the primary factor responsible for the anemia of rheumatoid arthritis, experiments in animals have indicated that high levels of EPO may overcome the suppressive action on the erythroid marrow of various factors released during inflammation (Gutnisky and Van Dyke, 1963; Johnson *et al.*, 1989; Schooley *et al.*, 1987). It is well established that monokines, such as interleukin 1 (IL-1) and tumor necrosis factor (TNF), which are released during inflammation, suppress erythropoiesis *in vitro* (Schooley *et al.*, 1987; Roodman *et al.*, 1987) and that, in the case of IL-1, the suppressive effect can be abolished by higher concentrations of EPO. These observations provided the rationale for a clinical study aimed at investigating the potentially beneficial effect of rEPO on red cell production by anemic patients with rheumatoid arthritis. In a multicenter, randomized, placebo-controlled study, 17 patients with rheumatoid arthritis and anemia (baseline hematocrit of less than 31%) were given either placebo or 50, 100, or 150 U/kg of rEPO intravenously three times a week for 8 weeks. No increase in the hematocrit was noted in the placebo group, whereas in the EPO-treated group an increase in hematocrit was seen with a magnitude that was related to the dose of EPO (3.3, 4.3, and 7.0 points increase for 50, 100, and 150 U/kg, respectively) (Pincus *et al.*, 1989). The results from two of the treated patients that were studied in detail have already been reported (Means *et al.*, 1989). In both patients, treatment with rEPO resulted in an increase of the hematocrit from 32 to 43% and from 30 to 39%. This was further documented by an increase in the ^{51}Cr-labeled red cell volumes and a significant increase in the marrow erythroid progenitor cell compartment. It is noteworthy that, in both of these patients, the hematocrit returned to baseline levels after discontinuation of the EPO. The above multicenter study was extended further to an open-label 32-week study with dose adjustment in which 11 patients participated. All 11 increased their hematocrits by more than 5 points, and 7 of them achieved a normal hematocrit level (Pincus *et al.*, 1989). Patients with rheumatoid arthritis have a much slower response to EPO than patients with end-stage renal disease and probably require higher doses. This study indicated that rEPO may be a useful form of therapy for the anemia of rheumatoid arthritis, and it confirmed previous experimental evidence that EPO can overcome the suppression of erythropoiesis associated with chronic inflammation.

X. Other Potential Uses of Recombinant Erythropoietin

A number of trials are now in progress to evaluate the possible effectiveness of rEPO in treating the anemia associated with malignancies or myelodysplastic syndromes, in treating AIDS patients with anemia resulting from the use of zidovudine (AZT), and in improving the yield of autologous blood donation.

Malignant diseases are frequently associated with anemia, the pathogenesis of which is multifactorial (Doll and Weiss, 1985). Chronic inflammation, poor nutrition, microangiopathic hemolytic anemia, blood loss, and suppression of marrow by chemotherapeutic agents may contribute to the development of the anemia malignant disease. Tumor necrosis factor (TNF) has been recently detected in high levels in the sera of patients with a variety of malignant neoplasms (Balkwill *et al.*, 1987), and this factor has been shown to be a potent suppressor of erythropoiesis *in vitro* and *in vivo* (Roodman *et al.*, 1987; Blick *et al.*, 1987). It is conceivable that pharmacological doses of rEPO can overcome the effect of various inhibitory factors on erythropoiesis *in vivo* in a manner similar to that already described for the anemia of rheumatoid arthritis.

Myelodysplastic syndromes (preleukemia) are clonal disorders of hematopoietic stem cells characterized by cytopenias associated with a hypercellular marrow (Koeffler and Golde, 1980). Anemia due to underproduction of red cells is very frequent, and is commonly the first manifestation in these disorders. Since in these syndromes residual normal stem cells can be detected in the marrow, administration of pharmacological doses of rEPO may lead to their expansion, resulting in partial correction of anemia and alleviation of the need for regular red cell transfusions.

Zidovudine is a well-known myelosuppressive agent and its use in the treatment of AIDS frequently results in severe anemia necessitating red cell transfusions. The use of rEPO in these patients might alleviate the need for transfusions.

Autologous blood transfusions have become quite popular during the past 3 years, particularly after the association of transmission of AIDS virus with the transfusion of blood products, including red cells. An increasing number of patients scheduled for elective surgery prefer to have their blood collected and frozen before surgery and receive their own blood, if needed, during or after the operation. The major limiting factor in such an approach is that the amount of blood that can be collected within a relatively short period of time (2–3 months) is limited by the development of anemia after collection of the first couple of units and by the fact that a number of such patients are anemic before any blood collection. The combined use of iron supplementation and rEPO may allow rapid correction of the anemia so that patients can become eligible for blood donation and increase the amount of blood that can be safely collected during the preoperative period.

The majority of the studies presently in progress are aiming at studying potential uses of rEPO that seem logical based on the known facts about the physiology of this hormone. However, as with other hormones (e.g., corticosteroids), there may be effects from pharmacological doses of rEPO that are at the present time totally unknown. It is very likely that future studies will focus on the use of rEPO as a pharmacological agent rather than as a hormone.

References

Adamson, J. W., Torok-Storb, B., and Lin, N. (1978). Analysis of erythropoiesis by erythroid colony formation in culture. *Blood Cells* **4,** 89–103.

Anagnostou, A., Barone, J., Kedo, A., and Fried, W. (1977). Effect of erythropoietin therapy on the red cell volume of uraemic and nonuraemic rats. *Br. J. Haematol.* **37,** 85–91.

Baer, A. N., Dessypris, E. N., Goldwasser, E., and Krantz, S. B. (1987). Blunted erythropoietin response to anemia in rheumatoid arthritis. *Br. J. Haematol.* **66,** 559–564.

Balkwill, F., Osborne, R., and Burke, F. (1987). Evidence for tumor necrosis factor/cachectin production in cancer. *Lancet* **2,** 1229–1231.

Beru, N., McDonald, J., Lacombe, C., and Goldwasser, E. (1986). Expression of the erythropoietin gene. *Mol. Cell. Biol.* **6,** 2571–2575.

Birgegard, G., Hallgren, R., and Caro, T. (1987). Serum erythropoietin in rheumatoid arthritis and other inflammatory arthritis: Relationship to anemia and the effect of anti-inflammatory treatment. *Br. J. Haematol.* **65,** 479–483.

Blick, M., Sherwin, S. A., and Rosenblum, M. (1987). Phase I study of recombinant tumor necrosis factor in cancer patients. *Cancer Res.* **47,** 2986–2990.

Bommer, J., Kugel, M., Schoeppe, W., Brunkhorst, R., Saintlebel, W., Bramsiepe, P., and Scigalla, P. (1987). Dose-related effects of recombinant human erythropoietin on erythropoiesis. Results of a multicenter trial in patients with end-stage renal disease. *Contrib. Nephrol.* **66,** 85–94.

Bommer, J., Ritz, E., Weinreich, T., Bommer, G., and Ziegler, T. (1988). Subcutaneous erythropoietin. *Lancet* **2,** 406 (lett.).

Bondurant, M. C., and Koury, M. J. (1986). Anemia induces accumulation of erythropoietin mRNA in the kidney and liver. *Mol. Cell. Biol.* **6,** 2731–2732.

Bondurant, M. C., Lind, R. L., Koury, M. J., and Ferguson, M. E. (1985). Control of globin gene transcription by erythropoietin in erythroblasts from Friend virus-infected mice. *Mol. Cell. Biol.* **5,** 675–683.

Browne, J. K., Cohen, A. M., Egrie, J. C., Lai, P. H., Lin, F. K., Strickland, T., Watson, E., and Stebbins, N. (1986). Erythropoietin: Gene cloning, protein structure, and biological properties. *Cold Spring Harbor Symp. Quant. Biol.* **51,** 693–699.

Buckner, F. S., Eschbach, J. W., Haley, N. R., Davidson, R. R., and Adamson, J. W. (1989). Correction of the anemia in hemodialysis patients with recombinant human erythropoietin: Hemodynamic changes and risks. *Kidney Int.* **35,** 190 (abstr.).

Caro, J., and Erslev, A. J. (1988). Erythropoietin assays and their use in the study of anemias. *Contrib. Nephrol.* **66,** 54–60.

Cartwright, G. E. (1966). The anaemia of chronic disorders. *Semin. Hematol.* **3,** 351–375.

Clark, D. A., and Dessypris, E. N. (1986). Effects of recombinant erythropoietin on murine megakaryocytic colony formation in vitro. *J. Lab. Clin. Med.* **108,** 423.

Cotes, P. M. (1982). Immunoreactive erythropoietin in serum. I. Evidence for the validity of the assay method and the physiologic relevance of estimates. *Br. J. Haematol.* **50,** 427–438.

Cotes, M. P., and Bangham, D. R. (1966). The international reference preparation of erythropoietin. *Bull. W. H. O.* **35,** 751.

Cotes, M. P., and Bangham, D. R. (1966). The international reference preparation of erythropoietin. *Bull. W. H. O.* **35,** 751–753.

preparations of human erythropoietin r-HuEPO. An investigation of the pharmacokinetics of intravenous erythropoietin and its effects on erythrokinetics. *Q. J. Med.* **70,** 113–137.

D'Andrea, A. D., Lodish, H. F., and Wong, G. G. (1989). Expression cloning of the murine erythropoietin receptor. *Cell (Cambridge, Mass.)* **57,** 277–285.

Davis, J. M., Arakawa, T., Strickland, T. W., and Yphantis, D. A. (1987). Characterization of recombinant human erythropoietin produced in Chinese hamster ovary cells. *Biochemistry* **26,** 2633–2638.

Denny, W. F., Flanigan, and Zukosky, C. F. (1966). Serial erythropoietin studies in patients undergoing renal homotransplantation. *J. Lab. Clin. Med.* **67,** 386.

Dessypris, E. N., and Krantz, S. B. (1984). Effect of pure erythropoietin on DNA synthesis by human marrow day 15 erythroid burst forming units in short-term liquid culture. *Br. J. Haematol.* **56,** 295–306.

Dessypris, E. N., Gleaton, J. H., and Armstrong, O. L. (1987). Effect of human recombinant erythropoietin on human marrow megakaryocyte colony formation in vitro. *Br. J. Haematol.* **65,** 265.

Dessypris, E. N., Graber, S. E., Krantz, S. B., and Stone, T. W. (1988). Effects of recombinant erythropoietin on the concentration and cycling status of human marrow hematopoietic progenitor cells in vivo. *Blood* **72,** 2060–2062.

Doll, D. C., and Weiss, R. B. (1985). Neoplasia and the erythron. *J. Clin. Oncol.* **3,** 429–436.

Dordal, M. S., Wang, F. F., and Goldwasser, E. (1985). The role of carbohydrate in erythropoietin action. *Endocrinology (Baltimore)* **116,** 2293.

Dunn, C. D. R., Jarvis, J. H., and Greenman, J. M. (1975). A quantitative bioassay for erythropoietin using mouse fetal liver cells. *Exp. Hematol.* **3,** 65–78.

Eaves, C. J., and Eaves, A. C. E. (1985). Erythropoiesis. *In* "Hematopoietic Stem Cells" (D. W. Golde and F. Takaku, eds.), p. 19. Dekker, New York.

Egrie, J. C., and Lane, J. (1987). Development of a radioimmunoassay for erythropoietin using recombinant erythropoietin derived reagents. *In* "Molecular and Cellular Aspects of Erythropoietin and Erythropoiesis" (J. N. Rich, ed.), pp. 395–107. Springer-Verlag, Berlin.

Egrie, J. C., Cotes, M. P., Lane, J., Gaines, R. E., and Tam, R. C. (1987). Development of radioimmunoassays for human erythropoietin using recombinant erythropoietin as tracer and immunogen. *J. Immunol. Methods* **99,** 235–241.

Egrie, J. C., Eschbach, J. W., McGuire, T., and Harrison, J. W. (1988). Pharmacokinetics of recombinant human erythropoietin administered to hemodialysis patients. *Kidney Int.* **33,** 262 (abstr.).

Eschbach, J. W., and Adamson, J. W. (1985). Anemia of end-stage renal disease. Kidney Int. **28,** 1–5.

Eschbach, J. W., Mladenovic, T., Garcia, J. F., Wahl, P. W., and Adamson, J. W. (1984). The anemia of chronic renal failure in sheep. Response to erythropoietin rich plasma in vivo. *J. Clin. Invest.* **74,** 434–441.

Eschbach, J. W., Egrie, J. C., Downing, M. R., Browne, J. K., and Adamson, J. W. (1987). Correction of the anemia of end-stage renal disease with recombinant human erythropoietin. *N. Engl. J. Med.* **316,** 73–78.

Eschbach, J. W., and the Multicenter Study Group (1990). Recombinant human erythropoietin in anemic patients with end-stage renal disease. *Ann. Intern. Med.* **111,** 992–1000.

Fraser, J. K., Lin, F. K., and Berridge, M. V. (1988a). Expression of high affinity receptors on human bone marrow and HEL cells. *Exp. Hematol.* **16,** 836–842.

Fraser, J. K., Lin, F. K., and Berridge, M. V. (1988b). Expression and modulation of specific, high affinity binding sites for erythropoietin on the human erythroleukemia cell line, K562. *Blood* **71** 104–109.

Fukamachi, H., Saito, T., Tojo, A., Kitamura, T., Urabe, A., and Takaku, F. (1987). Binding of erythropoietin to CFU-E derived from fetal mouse liver cells. *Exp. Hematol.* **15,** 833–837.

Ganser, A., Bergmann, M., Völkers, B., Grützmacher, P., and Hoelzer, D. (1987). In vitro and in vivo effects of recombinant human erythropoietin on hemopoietic progenitor cells. *Contrib. Nephrol.* **66,** 123–130.

Garcia, D. L., Anderson, S., and Rennke, H. G. (1988). Anemia lessens and its prevention with recombinant human erythropoietin worsens glomerular injury and hypertension in rats with reduced renal mass. *Proc. Natl. Acad. Sci. U.S.A.* **85,** 6142.

Garcia, J. F. (1972). The radioimmunoassay of human plasma erythropoietin. *In* "Regulation of erythropoiesis" (A. S. Gordon, M. Condorelli, and C. Peschle, eds.), pp. 132–155. Il Ponte, Milano.

Geissler, K., Stockenhuber, F., Kabrina, E., Hinterberger, W., Baleke, P., and Leichner, K. (1989). Recombinant erythropoietin and hematopoietic progenitor cells in vivo. *Blood* **73,** 2229 (lett.).

Goldberg, M. A., Glass, G. A., Cunningham, J. M., and Bunn, H. F. (1987). The regulated expression of erythropoietin by two hepatoma cell lines. *Proc. Natl. Acad. Sci. U.S.A.* **84,** 7972–7977.

Goldberg, M. A., Dunning, S. P., and Bunn, H. F. (1989). Regulation of the erythropoietin gene: Evidence that the oxygen sensor is a heme protein. *Science* **242,** 1412–1414.

Goldwasser, E. (1975). Erythropoietin and the differentiation of red blood cells. *Fed. Proc., Fed. Am. Soc. Exp. Biol.* **34,** 2285–2292.

Goldwasser, E., Eliason, J. F., and Sikkema, D. (1975). An assay for erythropoietin in vitro at the milliunit level. *Endocrinology (Baltimore)* **97,** 315–319.

Graber, S. E., and Krantz, S. B. (1978). Erythropoietin and the control of red cell production. *Annu. Rev. Med.* **29,** 51–66.

Gregory, C. J., and Eaves, A. C. (1977). Human marrow cells capable of erythropoietic differentiation in vitro: Definition of three erythroid colony responses. *Blood* **49,** 855–864.

Gross, D. M., Brookins, J., Fink, G. D., and Fisher, J. W. (1976). Effects of prostaglandins A_2, E_2, and F_{2a} on erythropoietin production. *J. Pharmacol. Exp. Ther.* **198,** 489–496.

Gross, M., and Goldwasser, E. (1969). On the mechanism of erythropoietin-induced differentiation. V. Characterization of the ribonucleic acid formed as a result of erythropoietin action. *Biochemistry* **8,** 1795–1805.

Gross, M., and Goldwasser, E. (1970). On the mechanism of erythropoietin-induced differentiation. VII. The relationship between stimulated deoxyribonucleic acid synthesis and ribonucleic acid synthesis. *J. Biol. Chem.* **245,** 1632–1636.

Gutnisky, A., and Van Dyke, D. (1963). Normal response to erythropoietin or hypoxia in rats made anemic with turpentine abscess. *Proc. Soc. Exp. Biol. Med.* **112,** 75–78.

Hara, H., and Ogawa, H. (1977). Erythropoietic precursors in mice under erythropoietic stimulation and suppression. *Exp. Hematol.* **5,** 141–148.

Hosoi, T., Sawyer, S. T., and Krantz, S. B. (1988). The receptor for erythropoietin lacks detectable glycosylation. *Exp. Hematol.* **16,** 118 (abstr.).

Iscove, N. N. (1977). The role of erythropoietin in regulation of population size and cell cycling of early and late erythroid precursors in mouse bone marrow. *Cell Tissue Kinet.* **10,** 323–334.

Ishibashi, T., Koziol, J. A., and Burnstein, S. A. (1987). Human recombinant erythropoietin promotes differentiation of murine megakaryocytes in vitro. *J. Clin. Invest.* **79,** 286–289.

Jacobs, K., Shoemaker, C., Rudersdorf, R., Neill, S. D., Kaufman, R. J., Mufson, A., Seehra, J., Jones, S. S., Hewick, R., Fritsch, E. F., Kawakita, M., Shimizu, T., and Miyake, T. (1985). Isolation and characterization of genomic and cDNA clones of human erythropoietin. *Nature (London)* **313,** 806–810.

Jacobson, L. O., Goldwasser, E., Fried, W., and Plzak, L. (1957). Role of the kidney in erythropoiesis. *Nature (London)* **179,** 633–634.

Johnson, C. S., Keckler, D. J., Topper, M. I., Braunschweiger, P. G., and Furmanski, P. (1989). In vivo hematopoietic effects of recombinant interleukin-1a in mice: Stimulation of granulocytic, monocytic, and early erythroid progenitors, suppression of late-stage erythropoiesis and reversal of erythroid suppression with erythropoietin. *Blood* **73,** 678–683.

Kazal, L. A., and Erslev, A. J. (1975). The measurement of erythropoietin. *Ann. Clin. Lab. Sci.* **5,** 91–97.

Koeffler, H. P., and Golde, D. W. (1980). Human preleukemia. *Ann. Intern. Med.* **93,** 347–353.

Koury, M. J., and Bondurant, M. C. (1988). Maintenance by erythropoietin on viability and maturation of murine erythroid precursor cells. *J. Cell Biol.* **137,** 65–74.

Koury, M. J., Bondurant, M. C., Duncan, D. T., Krantz, S. B., and Hankins, W. D. (1982). Specific differentiation events induced by erythropoietin in cells infected in vitro with the anemia strain of Friend virus. *Proc. Natl. Acad. Sci. U.S.A.* **71,** 635–639.

Koury, M. J., Sawyer, S. T., and Bondurant, M. C. (1984). Splenic erythroblasts in anemia-inducing Friend disease: A source of cells for studies of erythropoietin-mediated differentiation. *J. Cell. Physiol.* **121,** 526–532.

Koury, M. J., Bondurant, M. C., and Mueller, T. J. (1986). The role of erythropoietin in the production of principal erythrocyte proteins other than hemoglobin during terminal erythroid differentiation. *J. Cell. Physiol.* **126,** 259–265.

Koury, M. J., Bondurant, M. C., and Rana, S. S. (1987). Changes in erythroid membrane proteins during erythropoietin-mediated terminal differentiation. *J. Cell. Physiol.* **133,** 438–448.

Koury, M. J., Bondurant, M. C., Graber, S. E., and Sawyer, S. T. (1988). Erythropoietin messenger RNA levels in developing mice and transfer of ^{125}I-erythropoietin by the placenta. *J. Clin. Invest.* **82,** 154–159.

Koury, S. T., Bondurant, M. C., and Koury, M. J. (1988). Localization of erythropoietin synthesizing cells in murine kidneys by *in-situ* hybridization. *Blood* **71,** 524–528.

Koury, S. T., Koury, M. J., Bondurant, M. C., Caro, J., and Graber, S. E. (1989). Quantitation of erythropoietin-producing cells in kidneys of mice by *in situ* hybridization: Correlation with hematocrit, renal erythropoietin mRNA, and serum erythropoietin concentration. *Blood* **74,** 645–651.

Krantz, S. B., and Goldwasser, E. (1984). Specific binding of erythropoietin to spleen cells infected with the anemia strain of Friend virus. *Proc. Natl. Acad. Sci. U.S.A.* **81,** 7574–7578.

Krantz, S. B., and Jacobson, L. O. (1970). Erythropoietin and the regulation of erythropoiesis. Univ. of Chicago Press, Chicago, Illinois.

Krantz, S. B., Sawada, K., Sawyer, S. T., and Civin, C. I., (1987). Specific binding of erythropoietin to human erythroid colony-forming cells. *Trans. Assoc. Am. Physicians* **100C,** 166–172.

Krystal, G. (1983). A simple microassay for erythropoietin based on ^{3}H-thymidine incorporation into spleen cells from phenylhydrazine treated mice. *Exp. Hematol.* **11,** 649–660.

Lacombe, C., DaSilva, J. L., Bruneval, P., Fournier, J. G., Wendling, F., Casadevall, N., Camilleri, J. P., Bariety, J., Varet, B., and Tambourin, P. (1988). Peritubular cells are the site of erythropoietin synthesis in the murine hypoxic kidney. *J. Clin. Invest.* **81,** 620–623.

Landschulz, K., and Boyer, S. (1988). Natural history of erythropoietin (EPO) binding during erythropoiesis. *Blood* **72** 92a.

Lim, V. S., DeGowin, R. L., Zavala, D., Kirchner, P. T., Abels, R., Perry, P., and Fangman, T. (1989). Recombinant human erythropoietin in predialysis patients. *Ann. Intern. Med.* **110,** 108–114.

Lin, F.-K., Suggs, S., Lin, C.-H., Browne, J. K., Smalling, R., Egrie, J. C., Chen, K. K., Fox, G. M., Martin, F., Stabinsky, Z., Badrawi, S. M., Lai, P. H., and Goldwasser, E. (1985). Cloning and expression of the human erythropoietin gene. *Proc. Natl. Acad. Sci. U.S.A.* **82,** 7580–7584.

MacDougall, I. C., Roberts, D. E., Neubert, P., Dharuasema, A. D., Coles, G. A., and Williams, J. D. (1989). Pharmacokinetics of recombinant human erythropoietin in patients on continuous ambulatory peritoneal dialysis. *Lancet* **1,** 425–427.

McDonald, J. D., Lin, F.-K., and Goldwasser, E. (1986). Cloning sequencing and evolutionary analysis of the mouse erythropoietin gene. *Mol. Cell. Biol.* **6,** 842–848.

McDonald, T. P., Cottrell, M. B., Clift, R. E., Culen, C. W., and Lin, F. K. (1987). High doses of recombinant erythropoietin stimulate platelet production in mice. *Exp. Hematol.* **15,** 719–724.

McGonigle, R. J. S., Brookins, J., Pegram, B. L., *et al.* (1987). Enhanced erythropoietin production by calcium entry blockers in rats exposed to hypoxia. *J. Pharmacol. Exp. Ther.* **241,** 428.

McLeod, D. L., Shreeve, M. M., and Axelrad, A. A. (1974). Improved plasma culture system for production of erythrocytic colonies in vitro: Quantitative assay method for CFU-E. *Blood* **44,** 517–523.

Means, R. T., Olsen, N. J., Krantz, S. B., Dessypris, E. N., Graber, S. E., Stone, W. J., O'Neil, V. L., and Pincus, T. (1989). Treatment of the anemia of rheumatoid arthritis with recombinant human erythropoietin: Clinical and in vitro studies. *Arthritis Rheum.* **32,** 638–642.

Miyake, T., King, C. K. H., and Goldwasser, E. (1977). Purification of human erythropoietin. *J. Biol. Chem.* **252,** 5558–5564.

Moia, M., Mannuci, M. P., Vizzotto, L., Casati, S., Cattaneo, M., and Ponticelli, C. (1987). Improvement in the hemostatic defect of uraemia after treatment with recombinant human erythropoietin. *Lancet* **2,** 1227–1229.

Mufson, R. A., and Gesner, T. G. (1987). Binding and internalization of recombinant human erythropoietin in murine erythroid precursor cells. *Blood* **69,** 1485–1490.

Nijhof, W., Wierenga, P. K., Sahr, K., Beru, N. and Goldwasser, E. (1987). Induction of globin mRNA transcription by erythropoietin in differentiating erythroid precursor cells. *Exp. Hematol.* **15,** 779.

Nonnast, D. B., Crentzig, A., Kuhn, K., Bahlmann, T., Reimers, E., Brunkhorst, R., Caspary, R., and Koch, K. M. (1987). Effect of treatment with recombinant human erythropoietin on peripheral hemodynamics and oxygenation. *Contrib. Nephrol.* **66,** 185–193.

Ohno, Y., Rege, A. B., Fisher, J. W., and Barone, J. (1978). Inhibitors of erythroid colony-forming cells in sera of azotenine patients with anemia of renal disease. *J. Lab. Clin. Med.* **92,** 916–923.

Pavlovic-Kentera, V., Ruvidic, R., Milenkovic, P., and Marinkovic, D. (1979). Erythropoietin in patients with anemia of rheumatoid arthritis. *Scand. J. Haematol.* **23,** 141–145.

Peschle, C., and Condorelli, M. (1975). Biogenesis of erythropoietin: Evidence for pro-erythropoietin in a subcellular fraction of kidney. *Science* **190,** 910–912.

Peschle, C., Cillo, C., Rappaport, I. A., Magli, M. C., Migliaccio, G., Pizzella, F., and Mastrobernandino, G. (1979). Early fluctuations of BFU-E pool size after transfusion of erythropoietin treatment. *Exp. Hematol.* **7,** 87–93.

Peschle, C., Cillo, C., Migliaccio, G., and Lettieri, F. (1980). Fluctuations of BFU-E and CFU-E cycling after erythroid perturbations: Correlation with varions of pool size. *Exp. Hematol.* **8,** 96–102.

Pincus, T., Olsen, N. J., Russell, I. J., Wolfe, F., Harris, R., Schwitzer, T., Abels, R., Bocagno, J., and Krantz, S. B. (1989). Anemia in rheumatoid arthritis: Correction using recombinant erythropoietin. *Arthritis Rheum.* **32,** Suppl. 4, S43 (abstr.).

Porter, P. P., and Ogawa, M. (1985). Pluripotent stem cells. *In* "Hematopoietic Stem Cells" (D. W. Colde and F. Takaku, eds.), pp. 3–18. Dekker, New York.

Radtke, H. W., Rege, A. B., La Marche, M. B., Bartos, D., Bartos, F., Campbell, R. A., and Fisher, J. W. (1981). Identification of spermine as an inhibitor of erythropoiesis in patients with chronic renal failure. *J. Clin. Invest.* **67,** 1623–1629.

Recny, M. A., Scoble, H. A., and Kim, Y. (1987). Structural characterization of natural human urinary and recombinant DNA-derived erythropoietin. *J. Biol. Chem.* **262,** 17156–17161.

Reid, C. D., Fidler, T., Oliver, D. O., Cotes, M. P., Pippard, M. J., and Winearls, C. G. (1988). Erythroid progenitor cell kinetics in chronic haemodialysis patients responding to treatment with recombinant human erythropoietin. *Br. J. Haematol.* **70,** 375–380.

Rich, I. N., Heit, W., and Kubanek, B. (1982). Extrarenal erythropoietin production by macrophages. *Blood* **60,** 1007–1018.

Rodgers, G. M., Fisher, J. W., and George, W. J. (1975a). The role of renal adenosine 3′,5′-monophosphate in the control of erythropoietin production. *Am. J. Med.* **58,** 31–38.

Rodgers, G. M., Fisher, J. W., and George, W. J. (1975b). Increase in hematocrit, hemoglobin and red cell mass in normal mice after treatment with cyclic AMP. *Proc. Soc. Exp. Biol. Med.* **148,** 380–382.

Rodgers, G. M., Fisher, J. W., and George, W. J. (1976). Elevated cyclic GMP concentration in rabbit bone marrow culture and mouse spleen following erythropoietin stimulation. *Biochem. Biophys. Res. Commun.* **70,** 287–294.

Roodman, G. D., Bird, A., Hutzler, D., and Montgomery, W. (1987). Tumor necrosis factor-alpha and hematopoietic progenitors: Effects of tumor necrosis factor on the growth of erythroid progenitors CFU-E and BFU-E and the hematopoietic cell lines K562, HL60, and HEL cells. *Exp. Hematol.* **15,** 928–935.

Sakaguchi, M., Koishihara, Y., Tsuda, H., Fujimoto, K., Shibuya, K., Kawakita, M., and Takatsuki, K. (1987). The expression of functional erythropoietin receptors on an interleukin-3 dependent cell line. *Biochem. Biophys. Res. Commun.* **146,** 7–12.

Sasaki, H., Bothner, B., and Dell, A. (1987). Carbohydrate structure of erythropoietin expressed in Chinese hamster ovary cells by a human erythropoietin cDNA. *J. Biol. Chem.* **262,** 12059–12064.

Sawada, K., Krantz, S. B., Kans, J. S., Dessypris, E. N., Sawyer, S. T., Glick, A. D., and Civin, C. I. (1987). Purification of human erythroid colony-forming units and demonstration of specific binding of erythropoietin. *J. Clin. Invest.* **80,** 357–366.

Sawada, K., Krantz, S. B., Sawyer, S. T., and Civin, C. I. (1988). Quantitation of specific binding of erythropoietin to human erythroid colony-forming cells. *J. Cell. Physiol.* **137,** 337–345.

Sawada, K., Krantz, S. B., Dai, C.-H., Koury, S. T., Horn, S. T., Glick, A. D., and Civin, C. I. (1990). Purification of human blood burst-forming units-erythroid and demonstration of the evolution of erythropoietin receptors. *J. Cell Biol.* **142,** 219–230.

Sawyer, S. T. (1989a). The two protein receptors are structurally similar. *J. Biol. Chem.* **264,** 13343–13347.

Sawyer, S. T. (1989b). Receptors for erythropoietin. Distribution, structure and role in receptor-mediated endocytosis in erythroid cells. *Blood Cell Biochem.* **1,** 365–402.

Sawyer, S. T., and Hankins, W. D. (1988). Metabolism of erythropoietin in erythropoietin-dependent cell lines. *Blood* **72,** 440.

Sawyer, S. T., and Koury, M. J. (1987). Erythropoietin requirements during terminal erythroid differentiation: The role of surface receptors for erythropoietin. *J. Cell Biol.* **105,** 1077.

Sawyer, S. T., and Krantz, S. B. (1986). Transferring receptor number, synthesis, and endocytosis during erythropoietin-induced maturation of Friend virus-infected erythroid cells. *J. Biol. Chem.* **261,** 9187–9195.

Sawyer, S. T., Koury, M. J., and Bondurant, M. C. (1987a). Large-scale procurement of erythropoietin-responsive erythroid cells: Assay for biological activity of erythropoietin. *In* "Methods in Enzymology" 147, pp. 340–352. Orlando, Florida.

Sawyer, S. T., Sawada, K.-I., and Krantz, S. B. (1987b). Structure of the receptor for erythropoietin in murine and human erythroid cells and murine placenta. *Blood* **70,** 590.

Sawyer, S. T., Krantz, S. B., and Goldwasser, E. (1987c). Binding and receptor-mediated endocytosis of erythropoietin in Friend virus infected erythroid cells. *J. Biol. Chem.* **262,** 5554–5562.

Sawyer, S. T., Krantz, S. B., and Sawada, K.-I. (1989). Receptors for erythropoietin in mouse and human erythroid cells and placenta. *Blood* **74,** 103–109.

Schooley, J. C., Kullgren, B., and Allison, A. C. (1987). Inhibition by interleukin-1 of the action of erythropoietin on erythroid precursors and its possible role in the pathogenesis of hypoplastic anemias. *Br. J. Haematol.* **67,** 11–17.

Schuster, S. J., Badiavas, E. V., Costa-Giomi, P., Weinmann, R., Erslev, A. J., and Caro, J. (1989). Stimulation of erythropoietin gene transcription during hypoxia and cobalt exposure. *Blood* **73,** 13–16.

Sherwood, J. B., and Goldwasser, E. (1979). A radioimmunoassay for erythropoietin. *Blood* **54,** 885–893.

Sherwood, J. B., Carmichael, L. D., and Goldwasser, E. (1988). The heterogeneity of circulating human serum erythropoietin. *Endocrinology (Baltimore)* **122,** 1472–1475.

Shoemaker, C. B., and Mitsock, L. D. (1986). Murine erythropoietin gene: Cloning, expression, and human gene homology. *Mol. Cell. Biol.* **6,** 849–858.

Stockenhuber, F., Geissler, K., Sunder-Plassman, G., Jahn, G., Hinterberger, W., and Balcke, P. (1988). Recombinant human erythropoietin activates a broad spectrum of hematopoietic stem cells. *Nephrol., Dial., Transplant.* **3,** 502 (abstr.).

Stone, W. J., Graber, S. E., Krantz, S. B., Dessypris, E. N., O'Neil, V. L., Olsen, N. J., and Pincus, T. P. (1988). Treatment of the anemia of predialysis patients with recombinant human erythropoietin: A randomized, placebo-controlled trial. *Am. J. Med. Sci.* **296,** 171–179.

Tepperman, A. D., Curtis, J. E., and McCulloch, E. A. (1974). Erythropoietic colonies in cultures of human marrow. *Blood* **44,** 659–664.

Tsao, C. J., Tojo, A., Fukamachi, H., Kitamura, T., Saito, T., and Urabe, A. (1988). Expression of the functional erythropoietin receptors on interleukin 3-dependent murine cell lines. *J. Immunol.* **140,** 89–93.

Van Stone, J. C., and Max, P. (1979). Effect of erythropoietin on anaemia of peritoneally dialyzed anephric rats. *Kidney Int.* **15,** 370–375.

Wallner, S. F., and Vantrin, R. M. (1981). Evidence that inhibition of erythropoiesis is important in the anemia of chronic renal failure. *J. Lab. Clin. Med.* **97,** 170–178.

Wikström, B., Salmonson, T., Grahnen, A., and Danielson, B. G. (1988). Pharmacokinetics of recombinant human erythropoietin in hemodialysis patients. *Nephrol., Dial., Transplant.* **3,** 503 (abstr.).

Winearls, C., Oliver, D., Pippard, M., Reid, C., Downing, M., and Cotes, M. P. (1986). Effect of human erythropoietin derived from recombinant DNA on the anaemia of patients maintained by chronic hemodialysis. *Lancet* **2,** 1175–1178.

Zanjani, E. D., McLaurin, W. D., and Gordon, A. S. (1971). Biogenesis of erythropoietin: Role of the substrate for erythrogenin. *J. Lab. Clin. Med.* **77,** 751–756.

Zanjani, E. D., Poster, J., and Burlington, H. (1977). Liver as the primary site of erythropoietin formation in the fetus. *J. Lab. Clin. Med.* **89,** 640–644.

DNA Topoisomerases as Anticancer Drug Targets

Erasmus Schneider, Yaw-Huei Hsiang, and Leroy F. Liu

Department of Biological Chemistry
The Johns Hopkins University School of Medicine
Baltimore, Maryland 21205

I. Introduction

Many clinically useful antitumor drugs are available. Based on their mechanisms of action they can be classified into different groups. In the present review, we selectively focus on one family of antitumor agents, the DNA topoisomerase poisons, whose cellular targets and primary mechanisms of action have been well defined (Liu, 1989). This class of antitumor drugs comprises a large number of structurally diverse compounds that all share the same principal mechanism of action: they interfere with the breakage–reunion reaction of mammalian DNA topoisomerase I or II by trapping a putative covalent reaction intermediate, termed the cleavable complex (Chen *et al.*, 1984; Nelson *et al.*, 1984; Hsiang *et al.*, 1985; Hsiang and Liu, 1988). These drug-stabilized cleavable complexes can be viewed as a unique type of DNA lesion, since they can be converted to protein-linked DNA breaks by treatment with a strong protein denaturant such as

Advances in Pharmacology, Volume 21

SDS or alkali (Liu *et al.*, 1983). However, in the absence of protein denaturants, cleavable complexes are readily reversed following removal of the drug, heating to 65°C, or exposure to high salt concentrations (Tewey *et al.*, 1984a,b; Hsiang and Liu, 1989).

Little is known about how reversible DNA damage can lead to cell killing. The effective cell killing following acute exposure to these drugs and the transient nature of the cleavable complexes suggest that interaction of cleavable complexes with other cellular processes, in addition to formation of the cleavable complex per se, is necessary to trigger cell killing. In the case of the topoisomerase I poison camptothecin, its S-phase specific cytotoxicity may be explained by the collision between drug-induced cleavable complexes and moving replication forks (Hsiang *et al.*, 1989a). This collision leads to replication fork arrest and the conversion of cleavable complexes into irreversible DNA strand breaks. Cell killing by topoisomerase II poisons appears to be more complex. It seems that cellular processes other than DNA replication may also be important for converting cleavable complexes into lethal DNA damage. The interaction between mammalian DNA topoisomerase II and its poisons is in many respects analogous to the interaction between bacterial topoisomerase II (DNA gyrase) and nalidixic acid (Gellert, 1981; Drlica, 1984). In *Escherichia coli* B strains or *lon*$^-$ K strains, the induction of a cell division inhibitor as part of the cellular SOS response is responsible for the acute bactericidal action of nalidixic acid (reviewed in Liu, 1989). Whether the induction of a similar cell division inhibitor is also responsible for acute killing of mammalian cells treated with topoisomerase II poisons remains to be tested.

Drug resistance to topoisomerase poisons is another complex but challenging problem. Based on the proposed mechanism of action of topoisomerase poisons, resistance may arise due to alterations in either cleavable complex formation or in subsequent steps. Recent studies with drug-resistant mutant cells have shown that resistance can indeed be due to the alteration of drug-induced complex formation. Studies on the mechanisms of drug resistance should provide useful information not only for clinical investigation but also for a better understanding of the basic cell killing mechanisms of topoisomerase poisons.

A number of reviews on several aspects of DNA topoisomerases as anticancer drug targets have appeared in recent years (Ross, 1985; Zwelling, 1985; Chen and Liu, 1986; Spadari *et al.*, 1986; Bodley and Liu, 1987, 1988; Lock and Ross, 1987; Ralph and Schneider, 1987; Liu, 1989). The importance of DNA topoisomerases as chemotherapeutic targets is further underlined by recent reports of topoisomerase poisons as antibiotics (Epstein, 1988) and antiviral (Ferrazzi *et al.*, 1988) and antifungal (Figgitt *et al.*, 1989) agents. In this review, we focus on the antitumor activity of topoisomerase poisons.

II. Mammalian DNA Topoisomerases

A. Enzymology

DNA topoisomerases are ubiquitous enzymes and have been purified from a variety of eukaryotic species, including yeast (Goto *et al.*, 1984), plant cells (Dynan *et al.*, 1981; Fukata and Fukasawa, 1982), *Drosophila* (Hsieh, 1983), and several higher eukaryote cells of avian (Pulleyblank and Ellison, 1982; Trask and Muller, 1983; Muller *et al.*, 1988) and mammalian origin (Champoux and Conaughy, 1976; Miller *et al.*, 1981; Liu, 1983a; Schmitt *et al.*, 1984; Halligan *et al.*, 1985). Although mainly found in nuclei, topoisomerases have also been found in and partially purified from animal mitochondria (Castora and Lazarus, 1984) and chloroplasts (Siedlecki *et al.*, 1983). In this review, we concentrate mainly on mammalian DNA topoisomerases.

DNA topoisomerases are a class of enzymes which catalyze the topological isomerization of DNA via the breakage–reunion of one or both DNA strands (Wang and Liu, 1979; Cozzarelli, 1980; Gellert, 1981; Liu, 1983b; Vosberg, 1985; Wang, 1985). Two major types of topoisomerases are recognized. The type I enzymes catalyze changes in the topological state of duplex DNA by performing single-strand breakage–reunion cycles without requiring an energy cofactor. The best known reaction of this type is the relaxation of supercoiled DNA, which occurs by changes in the DNA linking number by multiples of one. In contrast, type II topoisomerases catalyze changes in the topological state of DNA by passing a DNA duplex via an enzyme-bridged double-strand break, and consequently they change the linking number in steps of two (Hsieh and Brutlag, 1980; Liu *et al.*, 1980; Miller *et al.*, 1981). Because of the strand-passing mechanism, type II enzymes can catalyze a number of topological reactions of DNA such as relaxation, knotting/unknotting, and catenation/decatenation of duplex DNA (Hsieh and Brutlag, 1980; Liu *et al.*, 1980; Miller *et al.*, 1981). The bacterial type II DNA topoisomerase DNA gyrase is the only topoisomerase known to also supercoil DNA. However, all eukaryotic type II DNA topoisomerases, like DNA gyrase, require ATP or dATP as an energy cofactor.[1]

1. DNA Topoisomerase I

Human DNA topoisomerase I (M_r 100,000 Da), a type I DNA topoisomerase, is a monomeric protein encoded by a single copy gene located on chromosome

[1]*Escherichia coli* topoisomerase II′ and a type II topoisomerase from *Trypanosoma cruzi* have been shown to be ATP-independent (Brown *et al.*, 1979; Gellert *et al.*, 1979; Douc-Rasy *et al.*, 1986).

20q12-13.2 (Liu and Miller, 1981; D'Arpa *et al.*, 1988; Juan *et al.*, 1988). The enzyme is capable of relaxing both positively and negatively supercoiled DNA without requiring an energy cofactor. A putative transient intermediate involved in the topoisomerase I reaction has been characterized. This intermediate comprises a covalent enzyme–DNA complex, termed the cleavable complex, which can be detected as protein-linked single-strand DNA breaks when the topoisomerase I reaction is aborted with a strong protein denaturant, e.g., sodium dodecyl sulfate (SDS) or alkali (Champoux, 1977; Edwards *et al.*, 1982; Halligan *et al.*, 1982). Detailed characterization of the cleaved product induced by protein denaturants has shown that a topoisomerase I polypeptide is covalently linked to the 3′-phosphoryl end of the broken DNA strand via a tyrosyl–phosphate bond. The cleavable complex, which is presumably the key covalent intermediate of the breakage–reunion reaction, is at rapid equilibrium with at least one other complex, the noncleavable complex. Unlike the cleavable complex, treatment of the noncleavable complex with protein denaturants leads to dissociation of the topoisomerase I from DNA without producing strand breaks. Although the two complexes are at equilibrium, the noncleavable complex is the predominant form and only a very small fraction of the topoisomerase I can be trapped as the cleavable complex (Hsiang *et al.*, 1985). A schematic illustration of this process is shown in Fig. 1A.

Studies using single-stranded substrates have demonstrated that topoisomerase I-mediated DNA cleavage can occur in the absence of any protein denaturant (Been and Champoux, 1981; Halligan *et al.*, 1982). Furthermore, the cleaved single-stranded DNA can be covalently transferred to acceptor DNAs with 5′-OH ends (Halligan *et al.*, 1982). The strand-transfer activity of topoisomerase I suggests that the protein–DNA contact(s) is located asymmetrically relative to the transient break; the broken strand containing the protein-linked 3′ end has the protein–DNA contact(s) and the 5′-OH end is either free of protein–DNA contact(s) or minimally protected by the enzyme (Been and Champoux, 1981; Halligan *et al.*, 1982).

2. DNA Topoisomerase II

Human DNA topoisomerase II (M_r 170,000 Da), a type II DNA topoisomerase, is a homodimeric protein encoded by a single copy gene located on chromosome 17q21-22 (Miller *et al.*, 1981; Tsai-Pflugfelder *et al.*, 1988). The enzyme catalyzes a number of ATP-dependent DNA topoisomerization reactions, including relaxation of both positively and negatively supercoiled DNA, catenation/ decatenation, and knotting/unknotting via a double-strand-passing mechanism (Liu *et al.*, 1980). Unlike bacterial topoisomerase II (DNA gyrase), human topoisomerase II, at least *in vitro,* does not promote negative supercoiling of DNA.

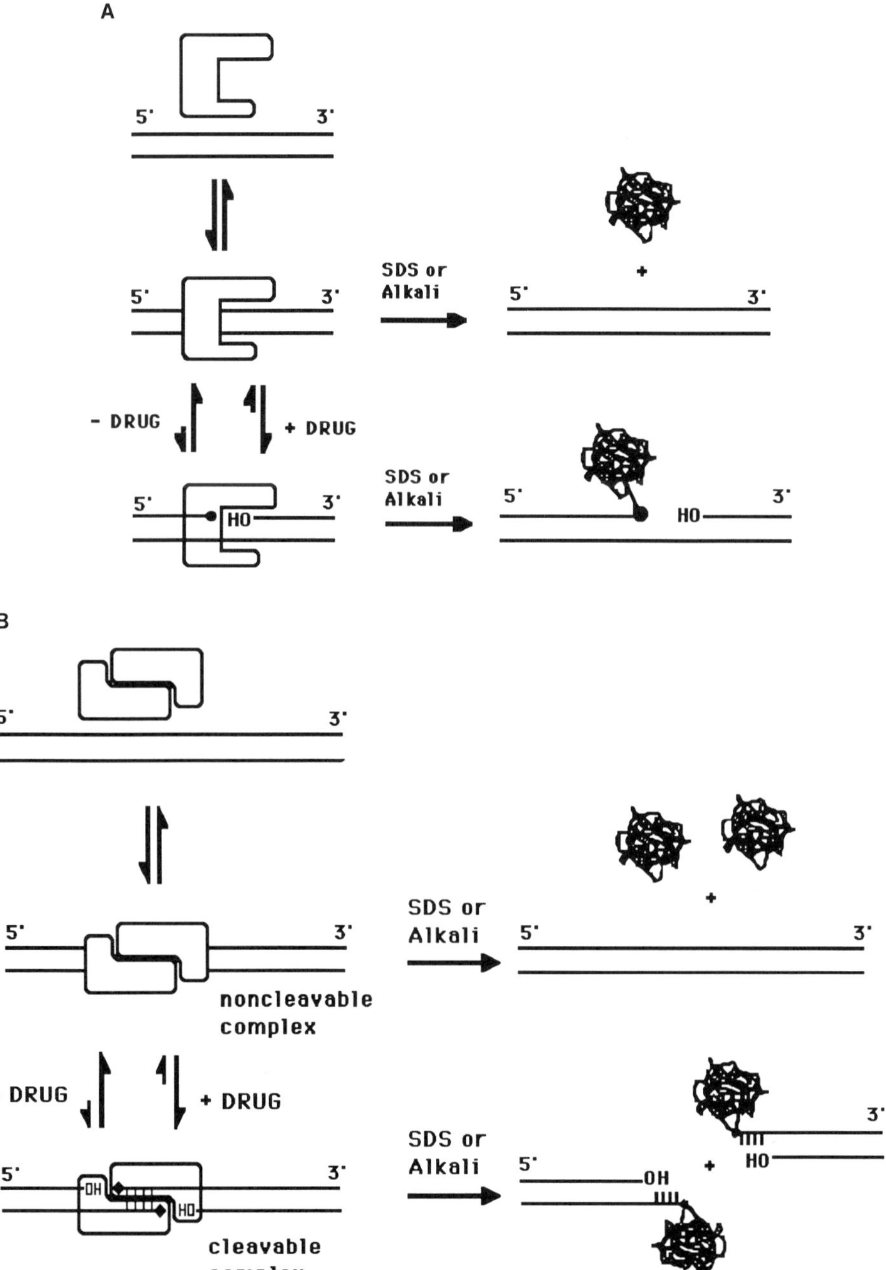

Fig. 1 (A) DNA topoisomerase I cleavable complex formation. (B) DNA topoisomerase II cleavable complex formation.

Analogous to topoisomerase I, a covalent intermediate has also been postulated and partially characterized (Liu *et al,* 1983). The topoisomerase II cleavable complex can be detected as both protein-bound single- and double-strand DNA breaks on addition of a strong protein denaturant (Liu *et al.,* 1983). Topoisomerase II-induced double-strand breaks are staggered by four base pairs and the 5′ ends of the broken strands become covalently attached to the enzyme via a phosphotyrosyl bond (Liu *et al.*, 1983; Rowe *et al.*, 1986a). The formation of the cleavable complex is proposed to be a key step in the reaction cycle. However, like with topoisomerase I, only a small fraction of all topoisomerase II–DNA complexes are in the cleavable form under normal conditions, for the reaction equilibrium clearly favors the noncleavable complex (Liu *et al.*, 1983). A simple model for this process is presented in Fig. 1B. While the formation of the cleavable complex is well documented, little is known about the actual strand-passing mechanism, although it is assumed that the intact double-stranded helix is passed through the transient enzyme-bridged break.

Recently, the existence of a second form of topoisomerase II with a molecular weight of 180 kDa has been reported in mammalian cells (Drake *et al.*, 1987). Both sequence and immunological analysis suggest that the two forms are distinct, possibly coded for by two different genes (Chung *et al.*, 1989). Both forms have been purified and identified as type II topoisomerases. However, they differ in several biochemical and pharmacological properties, like optimal salt concentration for *in vitro* catalytic activity, thermal stability and sensitivity to teniposide (Drake *et al.,* 1989). In addition, they also appear to be differentially regulated with levels of the 180 kDa form being less sensitive to the state of cell proliferation.

B. Biological Functions

Because of the double helical structure of DNA, many cellular processes involving DNA, such as replication and transcription, produce topological changes in DNA which can be resolved by topoisomerases.

1. Role of DNA Topoisomerases in DNA Replication

Studies both in yeast using mutants and in a cell-free SV40 replication system have shown that either a type I or type II topoisomerase activity is sufficient for DNA replication to proceed. However, topoisomerase II is uniquely required for the segregation of completely replicated daughter molecules during mitosis (DiNardo *et al.*, 1984; Uemura and Yanagida, 1984, 1986; Holm *et al.*, 1985, 1989b; Snapka, 1986; Brill *et al.*, 1987; Richter *et al.*, 1987; Uemura *et al.*, 1987b; Yang *et al.*, 1987; Richter and Strausfeld, 1988). Although the involvement of topoisomerases in DNA replication has been demonstrated by both *in vivo* and *in vitro* studies, the individual roles of topoisomerases in different steps of DNA replication remain to be determined.

2. Role of DNA Topoisomerases in RNA Transcription

It was generally believed until recently that negative supercoiling of DNA in bacteria is generated by DNA gyrase (the bacterial topoisomerase II) and is dynamically balanced by the opposing action of topoisomerase I (Gellert *et al.*, 1976; Gellert, 1981). However, recent studies have indicated that the translocation of the transcription machinery along the DNA duplex during RNA synthesis may also affect the supercoiling state of DNA inside the cells (Giaever and Wang, 1988; Wu *et al.*, 1988; Tsao *et al.*, 1989). According to the proposed twin-supercoiled-domain model (Liu and Wang, 1987), the rotation of the DNA duplex along its helical axis during transcription generates positive supercoils ahead of and negative supercoils behind the moving RNA polymerase. Studies in *E. coli* have suggested that DNA topoisomerase I (omega protein) is involved in the removal of negative and topoisomerase II (DNA gyrase) in the removal of positive supercoiling (torsional) waves generated by transcription (Wu *et al.*, 1988). Based on these findings, it is conceivable that the role of topoisomerases in RNA transcription could be quite complicated. Topoisomerases may affect directly the rate of RNA chain elongation and/or indirectly the rate of chain initiation depending on many parameters, such as arrangement of multiple transcription units, the sizes of the transcription units, the presence of anchorage sites on DNA, and the distribution of sites of topoisomerase activity.

The possible role of topoisomerases in transcription has been most extensively studied in yeast. It appears that transcription by both RNA polymerase I and II is affected by topoisomerases (Brill *et al.*, 1987; Uemura *et al.*, 1987a; Yamagishi and Nomura, 1988). Other studies in insects (Fleischmann *et al.*, 1984; Gilmour *et al.*, 1986; Egyhazi and Durban, 1987), *Xenopus laevis* (Glikin and Blangy, 1986), and cultured chicken cells (Muller *et al.*, 1985) have also suggested the involvement of topoisomerase I in RNA transcription. Studies using the specific topoisomerase I inhibitor camptothecin have shown that topoisomerase I-mediated DNA cleavage parallels transcription activation and that the cleavage sites are predominantly located in transcribed regions (Busk *et al,*. 1987; Gilmour and Elgin, 1987; Rowe *et al.*, 1987; Stewart and Schutz, 1987; Culotta and Sollner-Webb, 1988; Zhang *et al.*, 1988). Also, topoisomerase I appears to bind preferentially to and cleave supercoiled DNA (Camilloni *et al.*, 1988), as would be expected if it were involved in the relaxation of superhelical stress produced by the moving transcription machinery. In contrast, topoisomerase II appears to be more uniformly distributed along the chromosomes and is not enriched in actively transcribed regions (Earnshaw *et al.*, 1985; Heller *et al.*, 1986). On the other hand, mapping of topoisomerase II cleavage sites using topoisomerase II poisons revealed strong cleavage sites on both 3′ and 5′ ends of actively transcribed genes (Udvardy *et al.*, 1985, 1986; Darby *et al.*, 1986a,b; Rowe *et al.*, 1986b). However, further experiments are needed to clarify the role of topoisomerase II in transcription.

3. Other Cellular Functions

Like other topoisomerases, mammalian topoisomerases have also been proposed to participate in certain forms of illegitimate recombination (Halligan *et al.*, 1982; Ikeda, 1986; Bae *et al.*, 1988) and structural organization of chromatin (Newport, 1987; Newport and Spann, 1987; Almouzni and Mechali, 1988). In addition, topoisomerase II has been proposed to be part of the nuclear scaffold (Earnshaw *et al.*, 1985; Gasser *et al.*, 1986) and the nuclear matrix (Berrios *et al.*, 1985). The details of their roles in any of these processes, however, are largely undefined.

C. Regulation of Mammalian Topoisomerases

Accumulating lines of evidence have demonstrated that the intracellular level of mammalian DNA topoisomerase II, but not topoisomerase I, is generally sensitive to the growth state of cells. Cellular topoisomerase II levels are high in rapidly proliferating cells, but decrease when cells are arrested or induced to differentiate. In general, when cells enter a G1/G0 state, topoisomerase II levels and activities become very low. On the other hand, stimulation of quiescent cells leads to a rapid increase in topoisomerase II levels and activities (Duguet *et al.*, 1983; Miskimins *et al.*, 1983; Taudou *et al.*, 1984; Heck and Earnshaw, 1986; Bodley *et al.*, 1987; Hsiang *et al.*, 1988; Hwang *et al.*, 1989). While the level of DNA topoisomerase II is tightly regulated by growth conditions in normal cells, it is much less sensitive to these conditions in transformed cells, with levels of topoisomerase II in transformed cells maintained constantly high irrespective of growth conditions (Sullivan *et al.*, 1987; Hsiang *et al.*, 1988). Furthermore, studies using synchronized cells have shown that the cellular level of topoisomerase II remained relatively unchanged throughout the late G1, S, G2, and M phases of the cell cycle (Estey *et al.*, 1987a; Heck *et al.*, 1988; Hsiang *et al.*, 1988). Together, these results suggest that the level of topoisomerase II is primarily regulated during the entry of quiescent cells into the proliferative state or vice versa in "normal" cells. This regulation, however, is apparently altered in transformed cells (Sullivan *et al.*, 1987; Heck *et al.*, 1988; Liu, 1989).

In contrast to topoisomerase II, topoisomerase I is largely unaffected by the proliferative state of cells and appears to be present at high levels under various growth conditions (Heck *et al.*, 1988; Hsiang *et al.*, 1988; Hwang *et al.*, 1989). However, recently it was shown that treatment of density-arrested human skin fibroblasts with the tumour promotor PMA (phorbol 12-myristyl 13-acetate), epidermal growth factor, or serum induced a transient increase in topoisomerase I mRNA levels (Hwong *et al.*, 1989), similar to transient induction of c-myc mRNA after serum stimulation. In addition, analysis of clinical colon cancer tissue samples by immunoblotting showed increased levels of topoisomerase I, in parallel to increased malignancy as determined according to pathological criteria (Giovanella *et al.*, 1989). Therefore, it appears possible that topoisomerase I may also be connected to growth control, possibly in the mitogenic signal transduction process.

While there is accumulating evidence linking topoisomerase II levels to the proliferative state of cells, much less is known about the role of posttranslational modifications in the regulation of enzyme activity. Phosphorylation, which is thought to play a major role in regulating proliferation-related enzymes and proteins, has been shown to affect topoisomerases I and II activities both *in vivo* and *in vitro*. Phosphorylation of calf thymus type I topoisomerase by tyrosine protein kinases resulted in a 10-fold reduction of enzyme activity (Tse-Dinh *et al.*, 1984), but phosphorylation of topoisomerase I from Novikoff hepatoma cells by casein kinase II stimulated enzyme activity (Durban *et al.*, 1985). *In vitro* phosphorylation of the *Drosophila* type II enzyme by casein kinase II or protein kinase C led to an activation (Ackerman *et al.*, 1985, 1988; Sahyoun *et al.*, 1986), whereas a recent report showed that *in vivo* phosphorylation of topoisomerase II in HL-60 cells, probably by protein kinase C, resulted in a reduction of enzyme activity (Constantinou *et al.*, 1989). Taken together, these results indicate that phosphorylation of topoisomerases may play an important role in their regulation, but it is unclear at present what the physiological consequences are.

Modification of DNA topoisomerases by poly(ADP)ribosylation generally lead to a reduction in enzyme activity (Ferro *et al.*, 1983; Jongstra-Bilen *et al.*, 1983; Ferro and Olivera, 1984; Darby *et al.*, 1985). As with phosphorylation, the exact physiological significance of topoisomerase poly(ADP)ribosylation has not been established.

III. Mammalian DNA Topoisomerase Poisons

The identification of DNA topoisomerases as the primary targets of a number of powerful anticancer drugs has generated much interest in these enzymes. Despite their structural diversity, they all share the same specific mechanism of action, i.e., the interference with the breakage–reunion reaction of DNA topoisomerases by trapping a covalent intermediate, termed the cleavable complex. A list of topoisomerase poisons is presented in Table I and the structures of some of them are shown in Fig. 2.

Topoisomerase I poison

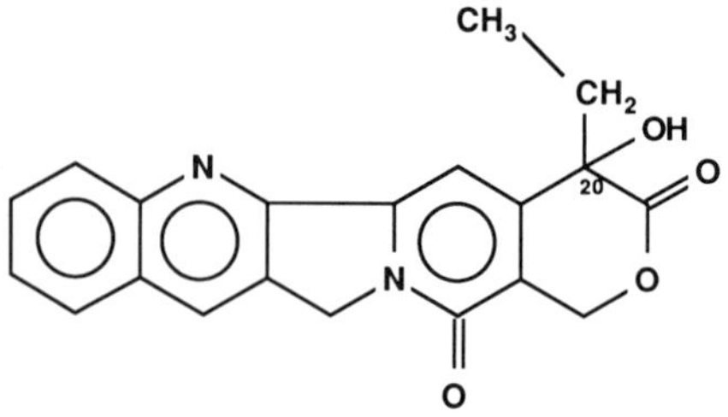

CH3
CH2
OH
N
20
O
N
O
O

Camptothecin

Topoisomerase II poisons

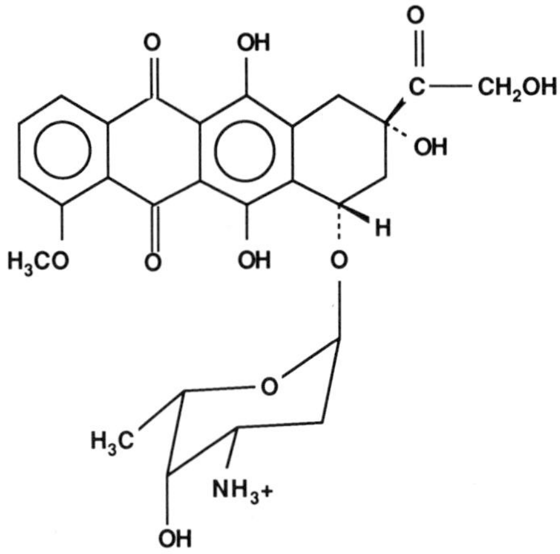

O
O
OH
C — CH2OH
OH
NHSO2CH3
H
H3CO
O
OH
O
H3CO
NH
O
H3C
NH3+
N
OH

Adriamycin

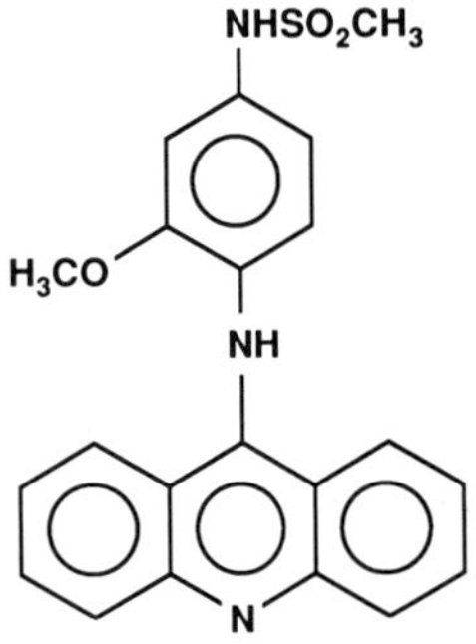

m - AMSA

O
O
H3C
C — Thr — DVal — Pro — MeGly — MeVal
O
N
O
O
H3C
C — Thr — DVal — Pro — MeGly — MeVal
O
NH2

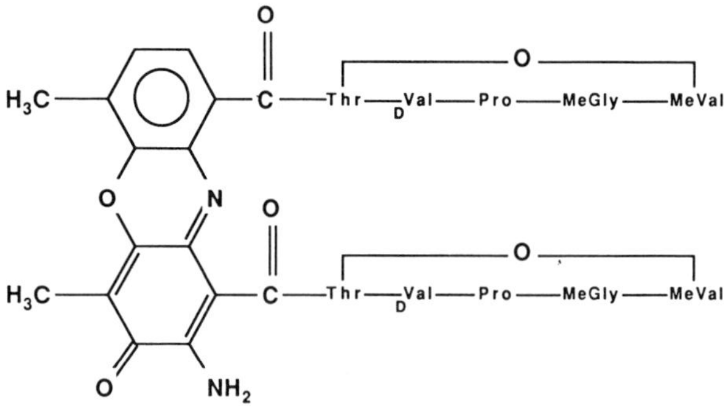

Actinomycin D

Fig. 2 Structures of DNA topoisomerase poisons.

Topoisomerase II poisons

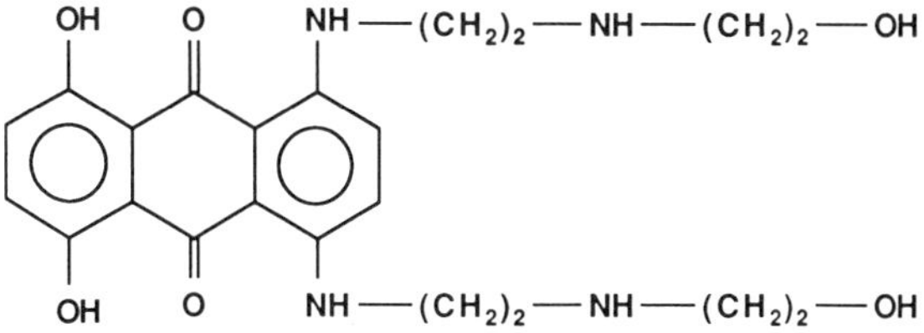

Mitoxantrone

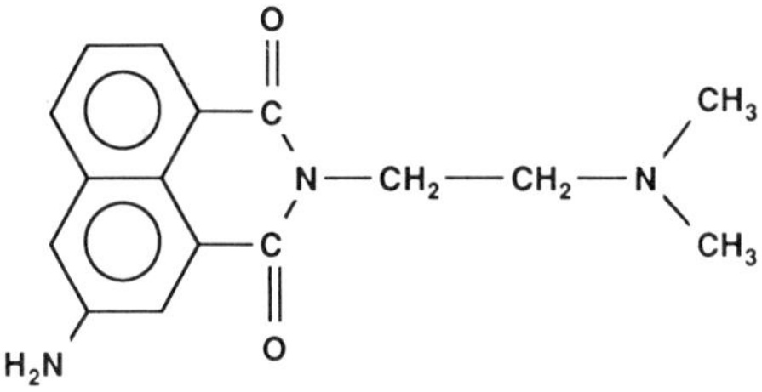

Amonafide

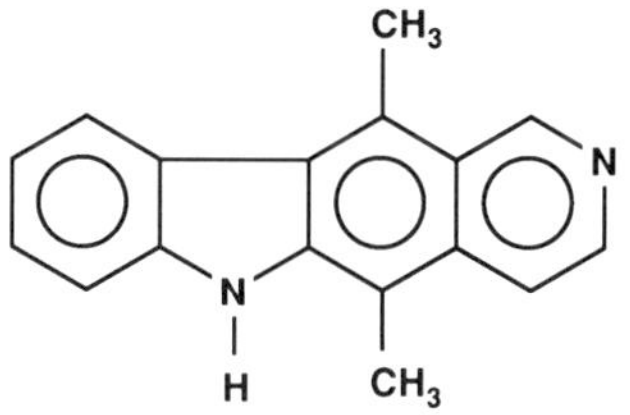

Ellipticine

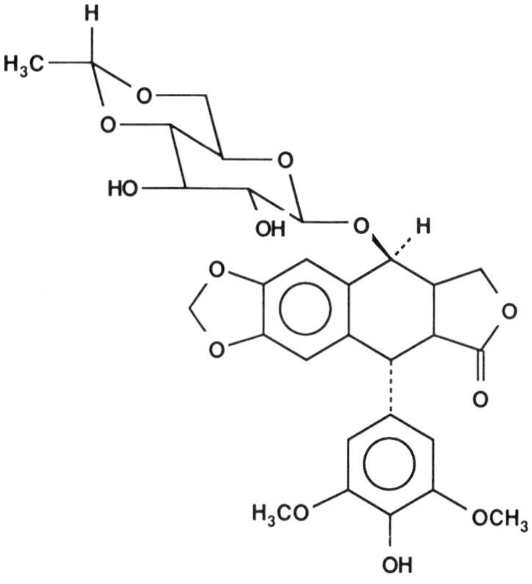

Etoposide

Fig. 2 *(continued)*

Table I
DNA Topoisomerase Inhibitors

Type of topoisomerase poison	Examples	Reference
DNA topoisomerase I poison		
Camptothecin		Hsiang *et al.* (1985)
DNA topoisomerase II poisons		
Intercalators		
Anthracyclines	Adriamycin, daunorubicin	Tewey *et al.* (1984b)
Benzisoquinolinediones	Amonafide, mitonafide	Hsiang *et al.* (1989c)
Anthracenediones	Mitoxantrone, bisantrene	Tewey *et al.* (1984b)
Acridines	*m*-AMSA	Marshall and Ralph (1985)
Actinomycins	Actinomycin D	Tewey *et al.* (1984b)
Ellipticines	2-Methyl-9-hydroxyellipticinium	Tewey *et al.* (1984a)
Nonintercalators		
Epipodophyllotoxins	Etoposide (VP-16), teniposide (VM-26)	Chen *et al.* (1984)
Isoflavones	Genistein	Markovits *et al.* (1989)

A. Mammalian DNA Topoisomerase I Poison: Camptothecin

Camptothecin, a plant alkaloid from *Camptotheca acuminata* (Horwitz, 1975), was shown to have strong antitumor activity against a wide variety of experimental tumors (Gallo *et al.*, 1971; Neil and Homan, 1973). While extracts from various parts of the tree *C. acuminata* are therapeutically used in China against certain solid tumors and leukemias, brief phase I and phase II clinical trials in the early 1970s in the United States were abandoned because of excessive nonspecific toxicity (Gottlieb and Luce, 1972; Moertel *et al.*, 1972; Muggia *et al.*, 1972). Renewed interest in camptothecin as a potential clinical antitumor drug has come from the recent identification of DNA topoisomerase I as its molecular target and the elucidation of its mechanism of action (Hsiang *et al.*, 1985; Hsiang and Liu, 1988; Covey *et al*,. 1989).

Earlier studies in cultured mammalian cells have shown that camptothecin inhibits both DNA and RNA synthesis (Bosmann, 1970; Gallo *et al.*, 1971; Horwitz *et al.*, 1971; Kessel, 1971; Kessel *et al.*, 1972; Li *et al.*, 1972; Bhuyan *et al.*, 1973). High-molecular-weight RNA synthesis is preferentially inhibited, and the inhibition is reversible on drug removal (Horwitz *et al.*, 1971; Li *et al.*, 1972). However, inhibition of DNA synthesis is only partially reversible (Horwitz *et al.*, 1971; Li *et al.*, 1972), a phenomenon which may be related to the S-phase-specific cytotoxicity of camptothecin (see below). Studies using purified DNA and RNA polymerases failed to demonstrate any inhibitory effects of camptothecin on these enzymes (Horwitz *et al.*, 1971). In addition to its inhibition of nucleic acid synthesis, camptothecin has also been found to induce reversible fragmentation of chromosomal DNA in cultured mammalian cells (Horwitz and Horwitz, 1971; Spataro and Kessel, 1972). Interestingly, camptothecin alone neither cleaves purified DNA nor binds to DNA under physiological conditions (Fukada, 1985; Hsiang *et al.*, 1985). Furthermore, like many other antitumor drugs, camptothecin induces elevated levels of sister chromatid exchanges and chromosomal aberrations (Pommier *et al.*, 1985, 1988; Lim *et al.*, 1986; Degrassi *et al.*, 1989).

While these cellular events had been well documented, DNA topoisomerase I was identified only recently as the cellular target of camptothecin (Hsiang *et al.*, 1985; Hsiang and Liu, 1988). *In vitro* studies using a purified system have shown that camptothecin induced a large number of single-strand DNA breaks in the presence, but not in the absence of, mammalian DNA topoisomerase I (Hsiang *et al.*, 1985). A topoisomerase I polypeptide was found covalently linked to the 3′-phosphoryl end of the broken strand (Hsiang *et al.*, 1985). Treatment of the reaction mixture with a strong protein denaturant such as SDS or alkali was necessary to reveal the topoisomerase I-mediated DNA cleavage (Hsiang *et al.*, 1985). If the reaction mixture was exposed to higher salt concentrations or briefly heated to 65°C prior to the addition of protein denaturants, the level of DNA strand breaks was greatly reduced (Hsiang *et al.*, 1985; Hsiang and Liu, 1988). Based on these observations, the following mechanism of action for camptothecin was proposed (Hsiang *et al.*, 1985). Camptothecin interferes with the breakage–reunion reaction of mammalian DNA topoisomerase I by trapping a key covalent intermediate, the cleavable complex. In the absence of camptothecin, the cleavable complex, which is at rapid equilibrium with the non-cleavable complex, exists at a very low concentration (see Section II,A,1 and Fig. 1A). However, in the presence of camptothecin the equilibrium is shifted toward the cleavable complex, which accumulates as a drug–enzyme–DNA ternary complex. The subsequent exposure of drug-induced cleavable complexes to a strong protein denaturant leads to topoisomerase I-linked single-strand breaks.

Essentially the same results were obtained in cultured mammalian cells (Hsiang and Liu, 1988), supporting the hypothesis that camptothecin-induced fragmentation of chromosomal DNA is due to the formation of reversible topoisomerase I-cleavable complexes in cells. Studies have shown that more than 90% of the cellular topoisomerase I molecules were trapped covalently on chromosomal DNA in L1210 cells treated with 25 μM camptothecin, but were rapidly released following a brief heat treatment of the drug-treated cells (Hsiang and Liu, 1988).

Accumulating lines of evidence have shown that camptothecin-induced topoisomerase I–DNA cleavable complexes are responsible for most if not all of its biological effects. Structure–activity–relationship studies of camptothecin and of a large number of its structural analogs have shown a quantitative correlation between the amounts of drug-induced cleavable complexes and their antitumor activities (Hertzberg *et al.*, 1989; Hsiang *et al.*, 1989b; Jaxel *et al.*, 1989). These studies also showed that the opening of the lactone ring reduced camptothecin activity 10-fold (Hertzberg *et al.*, 1989). Furthermore, it was demonstrated that the 20-hydroxy group was critical for antitumor activity and needed to be in the correct steric conformation at C-20, since only the 20(S)-camptothecin showed antitumor activity and topoisomerase I-mediated DNA cleavage (Hertzberg *et al.*, 1989). Studies with yeast mutants have shown that the cellular effects of camptothecin can be entirely attributed to its action on topoisomerase I (Nitiss and Wang, 1988; Eng *et al.*, 1989). Furthermore, camptothecin resistance in mutant mammalian cells was found to be due to drug-resistant topoisomerase I (Andoh *et al.*, 1987), which provides further evidence that topoisomerase I is the sole target for camptothecin.

B. Mammalian DNA Topoisomerase II Poisons

Many DNA intercalating drugs have been found to exhibit antitumor activity (Waring, 1981; Neidle and Waring, 1983; Ralph *et al.*, 1983; Marshall and Ralph, 1985). Since these drugs are capable of unwinding, expanding, and distorting the DNA double helix, it was conjectured that they would interfere with DNA replication and, possibly, other processes involving DNA. However, studies using a large number of analogs did not reveal any correlation between any of the known parameters of intercalative compounds (e.g., DNA-binding strength, ability to inhibit DNA synthesis, drug hydrophobicity) and cytotoxicity or antitumor activity (Cain *et al.*, 1971; Cain and Atwell, 1974, 1976; Ferguson and Denny, 1979; Baguley and Nash, 1981; Baguley *et al.*, 1981; Wilson *et al.*, 1981; Baguley and Cain, 1982). The most striking example of this observation is the pair of structural isomers *m*-AMSA [4′-(9-acridinylamino)methanesulfon-*m*-anisidide] and *o*-AMSA. Despite having equal DNA intercalation strength, only *m*-AMSA has antitumor activity (Wilson *et al.*, 1981). These studies eventually led to the suggestion that antitumor activity was dependent on (1) intercalation and (2) some interaction with a nuclear factor (Baguley and Nash, 1981; Baguley *et al.*, 1981; Wilson *et al.*, 1981). Later, they were found to act by a common mechanism, i.e., interference with the topoisomerase II reaction by stabilizing the cleavable complex, a key covalent intermediate in the DNA topoisomerase II-catalyzed reaction (see below). These intercalative antitumor drugs and the nonintercalative epipodophyllotoxins and genistein are now generally referred to as DNA topoisomerase II poisons (Liu, 1989).

1. Intercalative Topoisomerase II Poisons

Members of this group include the anthracyclines (e.g., adriamycin, daunorubicin), ellipticines (e.g., 2-methyl-9-hydroxyellipticinium), acridines (e.g., *m*-AMSA, CI-921), actinomycins (e.g., actinomycin D), anthracenediones (e.g., mitoxantrone, bisantrene), and benzisoquinolinediones (e.g., amonafide, mitonafide) (see also Table I). Originally, it was thought that the process of intercalation itself prevented cells from replicating their DNA, thus causing cell death (Neidle and Waring, 1983). However, careful examination of the DNA from drug-treated cells revealed that the DNA was rapidly broken following the addition of drugs to cells (Burr-Furlong *et al.*, 1978; Ross *et al.*, 1978; Kohn, 1979; Ralph, 1980; Zwelling *et al.*, 1982b). Since the initial studies used alkaline sucrose density gradients, it was thought that intercalating drugs mainly produced DNA single-strand breaks (Burr-Furlong *et al.*, 1978). Later experiments using neutral sucrose density gradients (Marshall and Ralph, 1982a,b), viscosity measurements (Marshall and Ralph, 1982c), or filter elution techniques (Ross *et al.*, 1978; Kohn, 1979; Ross and Bradley, 1981; Zwelling *et al.*, 1981, 1982b) showed that agents such as *m*-AMSA, adriamycin, or 2-methyl-9-hydroxyellipticinium also induced double-strand breaks in the DNA of treated cells. Furthermore, the fact that proteinase K treatment was necessary to reveal these breaks suggested that the DNA fragments were protein-bound (Ross *et al.*, 1978; Zwelling *et al.*, 1981, 1982b). It was also estimated that the ratio of DNA breaks to DNA–protein cross-links was close to unity, suggesting that the two phenomena were related and that the protein bound was at or near one end of the broken DNA (Ross *et al.*, 1979; Zwelling *et al.*, 1981, 1982b). Further analysis of the *m*-AMSA-induced DNA fragments from mouse cells with specific exonucleases revealed that the DNA had blocked 5′ ends, suggesting the presence of a bound protein (Marshall *et al.*, 1983). In addition, drug-induced DNA cleavage was rapidly reversible on dilution (Ross and Smith, 1982) and both formation and disappearance of DNA breaks were reduced at lower temperatures (Zwelling *et al.*, 1981, 1982b). These observations and the saturation behavior of DNA break formation (Zwelling *et al.*, 1981, 1982b) suggested that drug-induced DNA cleavage was an enzymatic process, and it was proposed at that time that a nuclease or DNA topoisomerase might be involved.

Using purified DNA topoisomerase II, it was shown that *m*-AMSA dramatically stimulated the formation of topoisomerase II–DNA complexes that are detected on protein–denaturant treatment (Nelson *et al.*, 1984). Both single- and double-strand DNA breaks were produced and a topoisomerase II subunit was covalently linked to each 5′ end of the broken DNA strands. The noncytotoxic isomer *o*-AMSA, which did not induce any significant amount of DNA–protein cross-links in cultured cells, was also inactive in the *in vitro* system. Similar results were also obtained with other intercalative antitumor drugs (Tewey *et al.*, 1984a,b). In addition, a protein of M_r 175,000 Da was found to be covalently attached to broken DNA from *m*-AMSA-treated cells (Ralph and Hancock, 1985). The covalent bond was eventually shown to be a phosphotyrosyl bond to the 5′ end of the broken DNA (Rowe *et al.*, 1986a) and the protein was isolated and identified as DNA topoisomerase II (Yang *et al.*, 1985; Minford *et al.*, 1986; Rowe *et al.*, 1986a).

2. Nonintercalative DNA Topoisomerase Poisons

Epipodophyllotoxins are semisynthetic derivatives of the natural product podophyllotoxin. Two members of this class, etoposide (VP-16) and teniposide (VM-26), have significant *in vivo* antitumor activity and are now widely used in clinical cancer chemotherapy. In cells treated with these agents, a high incidence of chromosomal aberrations, sister chromatid exchange (Singh and Gupta, 1983), and DNA strand breaks (Loike and Horwitz, 1976) was observed. *In vitro* studies using the purified enzyme showed that these drugs interfere with the breakage–reunion reaction of mammalian DNA topoisomerase II in a manner similar to intercalative antitumor drugs described above (Chen *et al.*, 1984; Ross *et al.*, 1984). Essentially the same conclusions were reached from *in vivo* cleavage mapping studies and the protein covalently bound to the DNA fragments was shown to be topoisomerase II by immunoprecipitation with anti-topoisomerase II antibodies (Yang *et al.*, 1985). However, no intercalation or binding of epipodophyllotoxins to DNA was detected (Chen *et al.*, 1984; Glisson *et al.*, 1986b). Protein-associated DNA breaks were produced in a dose-dependent manner both *in vivo* and *in vitro*, and this generally correlated with cytotoxicity (Wozniak and Ross, 1983; Long *et al.*, 1984, 1985, 1986). Although their interaction with topoisomerase II and the cleavable complex both in the purified *in vitro* system and in cells is now well established (Hsiang and Liu, 1989), it remains to be shown if interaction with DNA is also necessary for their activity.

Recently, the isoflavon derivative genistein, originally described as a specific inhibitor of tyrosine-specific protein kinases (Akiyama *et al.*, 1987), was shown to be cytotoxic against transformed cells (Okura *et al.*, 1988). In addition, it also inhibits topoisomerase II catalytic activity and stimulates topoisomerase II-mediated DNA strand breaks in a similar manner to the topoisomerase II poisons described (Markovits *et al.*, 1989). Since it does not intercalate, it appears to be a new member of the nonintercalative topoisomerase poison family.

3. The "Misalignment" Model for the Action of DNA Topoisomerase II Poisons

It is now well established that the primary target of both the intercalative and nonintercalative antitumor drugs described above is DNA topoisomerase II. While the exact mechanism of action has not been established, it was proposed that these drugs interfere with the breakage–reunion reaction of topoisomerase II by increasing the half-life of a covalent intermediate, termed the cleavable complex. Recently, a model for the mechanism of action of intercalative topoisomerase II poisons has been proposed (Fig. 3; D'Arpa and Liu, 1989). In this model, topoisomerase II binds to DNA in such a way that the cleavage site is

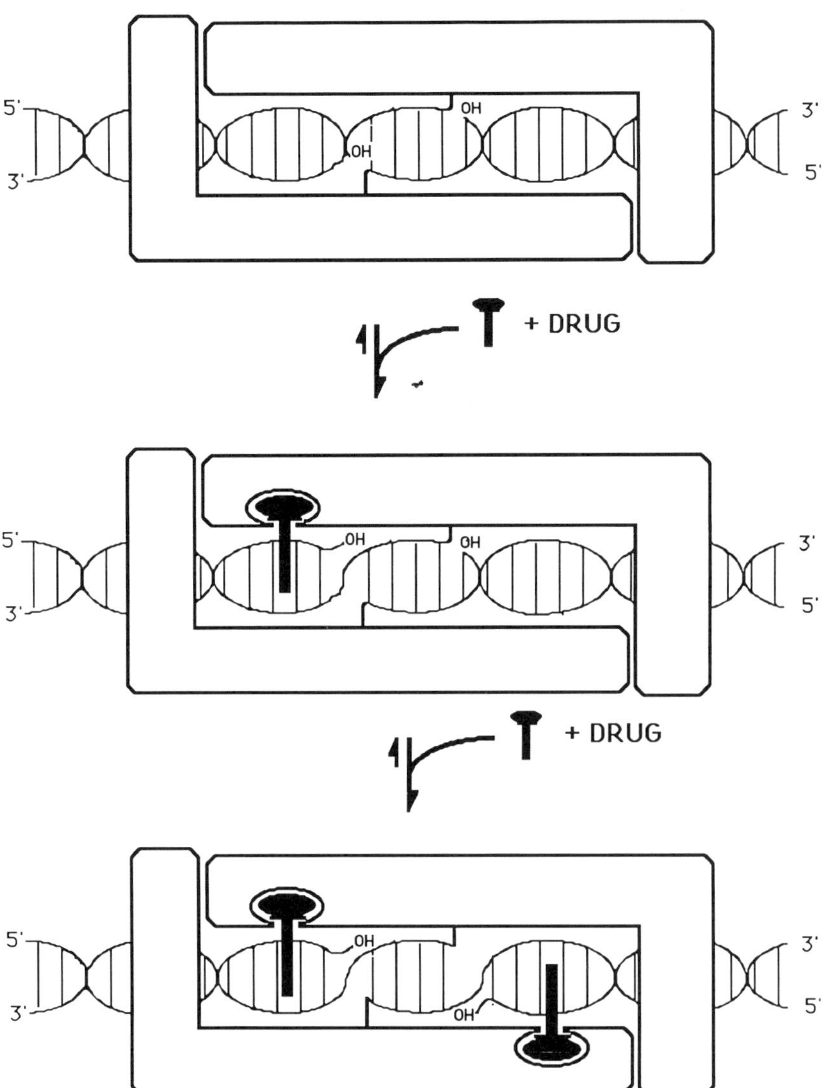

Fig. 3 The misalignment model for the action of topoisomerase II poisons.

flanked by protein–DNA contacts. It is conjectured that the protein–DNA contacts effectively separate the DNA inside the protein–DNA cleavable complex from the rest of the bulk DNA topologically. It is presumed that in the cleavable state the DNA strands are cleaved and that the enzyme subunits are covalently linked to the 5′ ends of the broken DNA strands. The corresponding 3′ and 5′ ends of each pair of the transiently broken DNA can rotate relative to each other due to thermal fluctuation. However, due to the short length of the bound DNA, only limited rotation of the order of a few degrees can occur. In contrast, when a drug molecule intercalates within this subdomain of bound DNA, a large displacement (or misalignment) of the corresponding ends relative to each other occurs, due to the relatively large unwinding angles (typically 10–30°) of the intercalative drugs. Thermal fluctuation is then ineffective to realign the two ends for religation.

Several consequences arise from this model. First, intercalation has to occur after formation of the protein–DNA complex. Second, the half-life of the cleavable complex is dependent on the residence time of the drug in the protein–DNA complex. Third, although intercalation is necessary for displacement of the broken ends, drug–enzyme interaction is probably also an important parameter in determining the residence time of the drug within the cleavable complex. However, this drug–enzyme interaction may be mostly steric and needs not to be specific and of high affinity. This could explain why effective topoisomerase II-directed antitumor drugs seem to have a common minimal structural requirement of an intercalating group and at least one bulky side chain that also has to be in the proper position with respect to the intercalating part. The bulky side chain(s) presumably provide the steric interaction with the bound enzyme molecule necessary to increase the residence time of the drug, due to a cage effect. However, the actual composition of these two structural elements appears to be less important, as long as they are compatible with intercalation and proper steric interaction with the enzyme (Cheng, 1988). This explains why many structurally diverse intercalative antitumor drugs can similarly trap topoisomerase II in the cleavable complex.

While this model can adequately explain the mechanism of action of intercalative antitumor drugs, its generalization to include the nonintercalative drugs is more difficult. However, it is possible that these drugs may intercalate into DNA weakly and are stabilized in the ternary complex because of the steric interaction with the enzyme. Indeed, it was recently proposed, based on computer molecular modeling studies, that the etoposide molecule was sterically well suited for partial intercalation and that its failure to do so may be related to a very low association constant between etoposide and DNA (Lock and Ross, 1987).

IV. Possible Mechanisms of Cell Killing

A. Apoptosis

It is now generally accepted that the formation and stabilization of the cleavable complex by DNA topoisomerase I and II poisons is responsible for cell killing. However, little is known about how the formation of these complexes actually leads to cell death. While it was proposed that cleavable complex formation is an early step in a cascade of events eventually leading to cell death (Nelson *et al.*,

1984; Rowe *et al.*, 1986a), none of the later steps has been identified. Possibilities include interaction with replication forks, helicases, RNA transcription machinery, or even nucleases or proteases. Furthermore, the level of cleavable complexes formed is often (Pommier *et al.*, 1985; Glisson *et al.*, 1986a; Rowe *et al.*, 1986a; Sullivan *et al.*, 1986, 1987; Estey *et al.*, 1987b; Markovits *et al.*, 1987; Robbie *et al.*, 1988; Schneider *et al.*, 1988a), but not always sufficient to predict cytotoxicity (Zwelling *et al.*, 1982a, 1987; Chow and Ross, 1987; Schneider *et al.*, 1988b).

Two modes of cell death are distinguished in pathology, namely necrosis and apoptosis (Duvall and Wyllie, 1986; Wyllie, 1987). While neither of these has been identified as responsible for topoisomerase-poison-mediated cell killing, several lines of evidence suggest that apoptosis may be involved. First, active protein synthesis, which is a requirement for apoptosis, and possibly RNA synthesis were shown to be necessary for *m*-AMSA- and VM-26-mediated cell killing (Chow *et al.*, 1988; Schneider *et al.*, 1989). However, no reduction in protein–DNA complex formation was observed when cells were pretreated with cycloheximide or cordycepin prior to *m*-AMSA treatment (Schneider *et al.*, 1989), suggesting that it was the downstream cleavable complex processing which was somehow affected by protein synthesis inhibition. Second, within 6 hours after VP-16 or camptothecin treatment of HL-60 cells, their DNA was degraded into small pieces (Kaufmann, 1989). A similar effect was also observed in concanavalin A-stimulated mouse splenocytes after camptothecin or VM-26 treatment (Jaxel *et al.*, 1988). This is reminiscent of the effect of a calcium–magnesium-activated neutral endonuclease in apoptosis (Wyllie, 1987).

In conclusion, it appears likely that the formation of cleavable complexes can induce a programmed sequence of events eventually leading to cell death. While some of these events may be common to all dying cells, others are possibly unique to the type of initial (DNA) damage induced by the topoisomerase poisons (Fornace *et al.*, 1988).

Recent observations that tumor necrosis factor can synergistically enhance *in vivo* antitumor efficacy and *in vitro* cytotoxicity of topoisomerase II poisons (Alexander *et al.*, 1987a,b) indicate that it may be possible to enhance topoisomerase poison-mediated tumor cell killing specifically. Furthermore, enhancement of L929 tumor cell killing by natural cell-mediated cytotoxicity was observed following treatment of the target cells with various topoisomerase poisons (Utsugi *et al.*, 1989). Together, these data provide a basis for rational selection of chemotherapeutic drugs and immunomodulators that, when used in combination therapy, would synergize for tumor destruction *in vivo*.

B. Role of Nucleic Acid Synthesis

The well-known S-phase specificity of camptothecin (Kessel *et al.*, 1972; Li *et al.*, 1972; Bhuyan *et al.*, 1973; Hsiang *et al.*, 1989a) was further confirmed by the observation that aphidicolin, a specific inhibitor of DNA polymerase α and δ, protected cells from camptothecin cytotoxicity but apparently did not prevent the formation of the cleavable complex (Holm *et al.*, 1989a; Hsiang *et al.*, 1989a). These results indicate that it is the collision of the replication fork with the drug-stabilized cleavable complex that is the major event leading to DNA synthesis inhibition and cell death (Fig. 4; Hsiang *et al.*, 1989a).

The role of DNA replication is much less clear in topoisomerase II-poison-mediated cell killing, since aphidicolin did not protect P815 mouse mastocytoma cells against *m*-AMSA cytotoxicity (Schneider *et al.*, 1989). In contrast, however, aphidicolin provided partial protection against VP-16 cytotoxicity in DC3F cells (Holm *et al.*, 1989a). It is also interesting to note that maximal cytotoxicity of *m*-AMSA was observed in S-phase HeLa cells, while maximal DNA breakage occurred in G2/M-phase cells (Estey *et al.*, 1987a). Furthermore, S-phase specificity has been observed only for low concentrations of *m*-AMSA, whereas at higher concentrations it killed cells in all phases of the cycle (Wilson and Whitmore, 1981; Drewinko *et al.*, 1982). This was further substantiated by recent results in our laboratory, when aphidicolin protected S-phase V-79 cells from the lethal effects of low doses of *m*-AMSA, but provided only partial protection at higher concentrations of the drug (P. D'Arpa, personal communication). Therefore, it appears likely that additional cellular processes are involved in cell killing mediated by topoisomerase II poisons. A possible explanation for this phenomenon may come from the well documented observation that low doses of drug produce predominantly single strand breaks (Ross *et al.*, 1979; Long *et al.*, 1985, 1986). Under these conditions, it may require the collision with the replication fork for the breaks to become irreversible and lethal. In contrast, at high concentrations, topoisomerase II-linked double-strand breaks are more abundant (Long *et al.*, 1985, 1986) and may become lethal through interaction with other cellular processes. One such process is probably RNA transcription, since a number of transcription inhibitors protected cells from high doses of *m*-AMSA (Schneider *et al.*, 1989; P. D'Arpa, personal communication).

V. Possible Mechanisms of Drug Resistance

Two different types of resistance against topoisomerase poisons are apparent: (1) dependence on the state of proliferation and (2) multidrug resistance. Both are being investigated and both seem to have clinical relevance.

A. Drug Resistance and State of Cell Proliferation

It is well known that solid tumors contain only a small fraction of cells that actively undergo proliferation. It is also known that topoisomerase II poisons have poor anticancer activity against solid tumors. While part of the reasons for

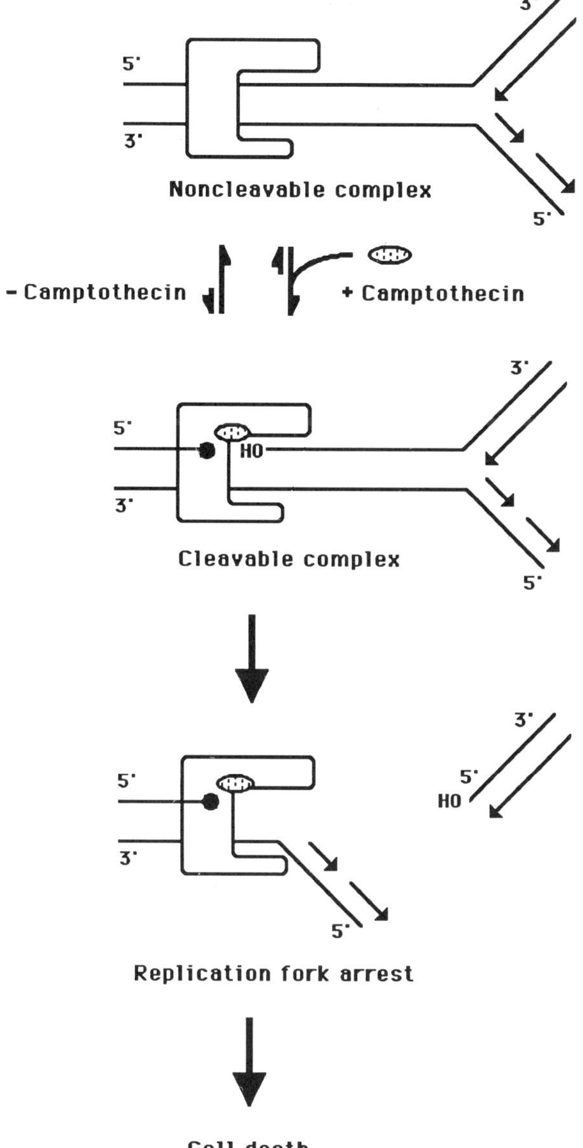

Fig. 4 Camptothecin Topoisomerase I cleavable complex mediated replication fork arrest.

this may be the poor vascularity of solid tumors and the limited accessibility of the drugs to cells in the interior of a tumor, the nonproliferative nature of these cells may be another possible cause of resistance.

As already described in Section II,C, the amount of topoisomerase II in cells is dependent on their growth state, with little or no enzyme detected in nongrowing (normal) cells. Several studies compared sensitivity to topoisomerase II poisons with topoisomerase II activity in cycling versus noncycling cultured cells. For example, it was found that when Chinese hamster ovary (CHO) cells were grown to plateau phase they gradually became less sensitive to VP-16 or *m*-AMSA, concomitant with a reduction in both topoisomerase II strand-passing activity and protein–DNA complex formation (Sullivan *et al.*, 1986; Robbie *et al.*, 1988). Similar results were also obtained in other systems (Drewinko *et al.*, 1982; Markovits *et al.*, 1987). In contrast, although *m*-AMSA sensitivity and drug-stimulated protein–DNA complex formation were significantly lower in plateau phase than in log phase CHO-AA8 cells, only a 2-fold difference in topoisomerase II unknotting activity was observed (Schneider *et al.*, 1988a). These examples demonstrate that, while the amount of drug target, i.e., topoisomerase II, may be an important factor in some cells, additional factors, e.g., the state of cell proliferation (Hwang *et al.*, 1989), may also be involved in determining drug sensitivity in others.

In a recent study, *in vitro* exposure to adriamycin resulted in no detectable DNA cleavage in lymphocytes from patients with B cell chronic lymphotic leukemia (CLL) or in either B or T lymphocytes from normal donors (Potmesil *et al.*, 1988). These cells were arrested in the G1 phase of the cell cycle and had undetectable topoisomerase II levels. This is the first report in which clinical drug resistance was directly correlated with cellular levels of topoisomerase II and indicates that topoisomerase II levels may indeed be a factor in clinical drug resistance. In contrast, adriamycin induced DNA cleavage in T cells from CLL patients, despite the absence of detectable topoisomerase II in these cells, suggesting that additional factors may also be involved in drug resistance.

B. Multidrug Resistance

One of the major obstacles to successful anticancer chemotherapy is the relatively rapid emergence of a drug-resistant subpopulation of cells in tumors. These cells usually display a multidrug-resistant phenotype (MDR), i.e., they are cross-resistant to several other unrelated drugs with different mechanisms of action, irrespective of what the original treatment was. Quite often, this is accompanied by overexpression of P-170 glycoprotein, a membrane protein which is the product of the amplified *mdr1* gene, resulting in a lower intracellular drug concentration due to increased active drug efflux (Riordan and Ling, 1986; Ueda *et al.*, 1986). The ineffectiveness of topoisomerase II poisons in treating certain solid tumors (e.g., human colon tumors) may be due to the overexpression of the *mdr1* gene. Interestingly, a recent study showed that 9-amino-camptothecin was highly effective against human colon tumor xenografts in nude mice, suggesting that camptothecin may bypass the *mdr1* related multidrug resistance in solid tumors (Giovanella *et al.*, 1989).

Recently, a type of multidrug resistance affecting only topoisomerase II poisons has been described (Danks *et al.*, 1987, 1988). These authors showed that two sublines of human leukemic CCRF-CEM cells, selected for resistance to VM-26, were highly cross-resistant to VP-16, doxorubicin, and *m*-AMSA, but not to vinblastine and vincristine, two inhibitors of mitotic spindle formation. No difference in the amount of immunoreactive topoisomerase II in nuclear extracts was found between resistant and sensitive parent cells. However, both unknotting and DNA cleavage activities were significantly altered, with the effect of VM-26 on both strand passing and DNA cleavage being inversely related to the degree of primary resistance of each cell line. Several other cell lines which are resistant to topoisomerase II poisons have also been reported (Glisson *et al.*, 1986a,b; Pommier *et al.*, 1986; Estey *et al.*, 1987b; Per *et al.*, 1987; Charcosset *et al.*, 1988). While a direct comparison of these cell lines is difficult because of the different assays that were used, they all seem to share a change in drug-induced cleavable complex formation. So far, no clear biochemical explanation has been found for these observations, although the presence of a modulating factor(s) has been proposed (Pommier *et al.*, 1986; Danks *et al.*, 1988). Indeed, an activity promoting *m*-AMSA-induced protein–DNA complex formation in isolated nuclei has recently been reported (Darkin and Ralph, 1989), and was found to be several-fold reduced in drug-resistant cells (S. Darkin, personal communication). However, its physiological significance has not yet been established.

Reduced topoisomerase II activity and levels have been implied in adriamycin resistance of a mutant P388 murine leukemia cell line (Deffie *et al.*, 1989a). The molecular basis of the reduced topoisomerase II levels has now been found to be due to the expression of a mutant allele of the topoisomerase II gene (Deffie *et al.*, 1989b). Therefore, it appears that both genetic and epigenetic modificatons can contribute to topoisomerase II drug resistance.

VI. Perspectives

Much progress has been made in recent years in understanding the mechanism of action of antitumor drugs that target topoisomerases. However, while it is now well established that these drugs interact with the cleavable complex, molecular details of the protein–DNA–drug interaction are only just starting to emerge. The large body of information available from the study of drug analogs has provided some detailed information on the structural requirements for drugs to interact successfully with the cleavable complex. Further progress in this area may be accelerated by X-ray crystallographic studies of enzyme–DNA–drug complexes.

Little is known about the actual cell killing mechanism. This question, which involves events beyond cleavable complex formation and its interaction with drugs, is becoming more and more important. Knowledge of the signals and events involved in cell killing, in particular the early signals induced by drug-mediated DNA damage, might eventually lead to the discovery and identification of new targets for antitumor drugs. Furthermore, general principles for tumor cell killing by other antitumor drugs may also emerge from these studies.

Acknowledgments

We wish to thank Drs. A. L. Bodley, P. D'Arpa, and K. Lau for critically reading the manuscript and Mrs. Janice Burgess for her help with the library work. E. S. and L. F. L. are recipients of a Swiss National Science Foundation advanced career fellowship and an American Cancer Society Faculty research award, respectively.

References

Ackerman, P., Glover, C. V. C., and Osheroff, N. (1985). Phosphorylation of DNA topoisomerase II by casein kinase II: Modulation of eukaryotic topoisomerase II activity in vitro. *Proc. Natl. Acad. Sci. U.S.A.* **82,** 3164–3168.

Ackerman, P., Glover, C. V. C., and Osheroff, N. (1988). Phosphorylation of DNA topoisomerase II in vivo and in total homogenates of *Drosophila* Kc cells. *J. Biol. Chem.* **263,** 12653–12660.

Akiyama, T., Ishida, J., Nakagawa, S., Ogawara, H., Watanabe, S., Itoh, N., Shibuya, M. and Fukami, Y. (1987). Genistein, a specific inhibitor of tyrosine-specific protein kinanses. *J. Biol. Chem.* **262,** 5592–5595.

Alexander, R. B., Isaacs, J. T., and Coffey, D. S. (1987a). Tumour necrosis factor enhances *in vitro* and *in vivo* efficacy of chemotherapeutic drugs targeted at DNA topoisomerase II in treatment of murine bladder cancer. *J. Urol.* **138,** 427–430.

Alexander, R. B., Nelson, W. G. and Coffey, D. S. (1987b). Synergistic enhancement by tumor necrosis factor of *in vitro* cytotoxicity from chemotherapeutic drugs targeted at DNA topoisomerase II *Cancer Res.* **47,** 2403–2406.

Almouzni, G., and Mechali, M. (1988). Assembly of spaced chromatin involvement of ATP and DNA topoisomerase activity. *EMBO J.* **7,** 4355–4365.

Andoh, T., Ishii, K., Suzuki, Y., Ikegami, Y., Kusunoki, Y., Takemoto, Y., and Okada, K. (1987). Characterization of a mammalian mutant with a camptothecin resistant DNA topoisomerase I. *Proc. Natl. Acad. Sci. U.S.A.* **84,** 5565–5569.

Bae, Y.-S., Kawasaki, I., Ikeda, H., and Liu, L. F. (1988). Illegitimate recombination mediated by calf thymus DNA topoisomerase II in vitro. *Proc. Natl. Acad. Sci. U.S.A.* **85,** 2076–2080.

Baguley, B. C., and Cain, B. F. (1982). Comparison of the *in vivo* and *in vitro* antileukemic activity of monosubstituted derivatives of 4′-(9-acridinylamino)methanesulfon-*m*-anisidide. *Mol. Pharmacol.* **22,** 486–492.

Baguley, B. C., and Nash, R. (1981). Antitumour activity of substituted 9-anilinoacridines: Comparison of *in vivo* and *in vitro* testing systems. *Eur. J. Cancer* **17,** 671–679.

Baguley, B. C., Denny, W. A., Atwell, G. J., and Cain, B. F. (1981). Potential antitumour agents.

35. Quantitative relationships between antitumour (L1210) potency and DNA binding for 4′-(9-acridinylamino)methanesulfon-*m*-anisidide analogues. *J. Med. Chem.* **24,** 520–525.

Been, M. D., and Champoux, J. J. (1981). DNA breakage and closure by rat liver type I topoisomerase: Separation of the half-reactions by using single-stranded DNA substrate. *Proc. Natl. Acad. Sci. U.S.A.* **78,** 2883–2887.

Berrios, M., Osheroff, N., and Fisher, P. A. (1985). In situ localization of DNA topoisomerase II, a major polypeptide component of the Drosophila nuclear matrix fraction. *Proc. Natl. Acad. Sci. U.S.A.* **82,** 4142–4146.

Bhuyan, B. K., Fraser, T. J., Gray, L. G., Kuentzel, S. L., and Neil, G. L. (1973). Cell-kill kinetics of several S-phase-specific drugs. *Cancer Res.* **33,** 888–894.

Bodley, A. L., and Liu, L. F. (1987). Roles of DNA topoisomerases in drug cytotoxicity and drug resistance. *Bristol-Myers Cancer Symp.* **9,** 277–286.

Bodley, A. L., and Liu, L. F. (1988). Topoisomerases as novel targets for cancer chemotherapy. *Bio/Technology* **6,** 1315–1319.

Bodley, A. L., Wu, H.-Y., and Liu, L. F. (1987). Regulation of DNA topoisomerases during cellular differentiation. *NCI Monogr.* **4,** 31–35.

Bosmann, H. B. (1970). Camptothecin inhibits macromolecular synthesis in mammalian cells but not in isolated mitochondria or *E. coli*. *Biochem. Biophys. Res. Commun.* **41,** 1412–1420.

Brill, S. J., DiNardo, S., Voelkel-Meiman, K., and Sternglanz, R. (1987). Need for DNA topoisomerase activity as a swivel for DNA replication for transcription of ribosomal RNA. *Nature (London)* **326,** 414–416.

Brown, P. O., Peebles, C. L., and Cozarelli, N. R. (1979). A topoisomerase from *Escherichia coli* related to DNA gyrase. *Proc. Natl. Acad. Sci. U.S.A.* **76,** 6110–6119.

Burr-Furlong, N., Sato, J., Brown, T., Chavez, F., and Hurlbert, R. B. (1978). Induction of limited DNA damage by the anti-tumour agent Cain's acridine. *Cancer Res.* **38,** 1329–1335.

Busk, H., Thomson, B., Bonven, B. J., Kjeldsen, O. F., and Westergaard, O. (1987). Preferential relaxation of supercoiled DNA containing a hexadecameric recognition sequence of topoisomerase I. *Nature (London)* **327,** 638–640.

Cain, B. F., and Atwell, G. J. (1974). The experimental antitumour properties of three congeners of the acridinylmethanesulfonanilide (AMSA) series. *Eur. J. Cancer* **10,** 539–549.

Cain, B. F., and Atwell, G. J. (1976). Potential antitumour agents, 19. Multiply substituted 4′-9-(acridinylamino)methanesulfonanilides. *J. Med. Chem.* **19,** 1124–1129.

Cain, B. F., Atwell, G. J., and Seelye, R. N. (1971). Potential antitumour agents. 11. 9-Anilinoacridines. *J. Med. Chem.* **14,** 311–315.

Camilloni, G., Martin, E. D., Caserta, M., and di Mauro, E. (1988). Eukaryotic DNA topoisomerase I reaction is topology dependent. *Nucleic Acids Res.* **16,** 7071–7085.

Castora, F. J., and Lazarus, G. M. (1984). Isolation of mitochondrial DNA topoisomerase from human leukemia cells. *Biochem. Biophys. Res. Commun.* **121,** 77–86.

Champoux, J. J. (1977). Strand breakage by the DNA untwisting enzyme results in covalent attachment of the enzyme to DNA. *Proc. Natl. Acad. Sci. U.S.A.* **74,** 3800–3804.

Champoux, J. J., and Conaughy, B. L. (1976). Purification and characterization of the DNA untwisting enzyme from rat liver. *Biochemistry* **15,** 4638–4642.

Charcosset, J.-Y., Saucier, J.-M., and Jacquemin-Sablon, A. (1988). Reduced DNA topoisomerase II activity and drug-stimulated DNA cleavage in 9-hydroxyellipticine resistant cells. *Biochem. Pharmacol.* **37,** 2145–2149.

Chen, G. L., and Liu, L. F. (1986). DNA topoisomerases as therapeutic targets in cancer chemotherapy. *Annu. Rep. Med. Chem.* **21,** 257–262.

Chen, G. L., Yang, L., Rowe, T. C., Halligan, B. D., Tewey, K. M., and Liu, L. F. (1984). Nonintercalative antitumor drugs interfere with the breakage-reunion reaction of mammalian DNA topoisomerase II. *J. Biol. Chem.* **259,** 13560–13566.

Cheng, C. C. (1988). Structural aspects of antineoplastic agents: A new approach. *Progr. Med. Chem.* **25,** 35–83.

Chow, K. C., and Ross, W. E. (1987). Topoisomerase-specific drug sensitivity in relation to cell cycle progression. *Mol. Cell. Biol.* **7,** 3119–3123.

Chow, K. C., King, C. K., and Ross, W. E. (1988). Abrogation of etoposide-mediated cytotoxicity by cycloheximide. *Biochem. Pharmacol.* **37,** 1117–1122.

Chung, T. D. Y., Drake, F. H., Tan, K. B., Per, S. R., Crooke, S. T. and Mirabelli, C. K. (1989). Characterization and immunological identification of cDNA clones encoding two human DNA topoisomerase II isozymes. *Proc. Natl. Acad. Sci. U.S.A.* **86,** 9431–9435.

Constantinou, A., Henning-Chubb, C., and Huberman, E. (1989). Novobiocin and phorbol-12 myristate-13-acetate-induced differentiation of human leukemia cells associated with a reduction in topoisomerase II activity. *Cancer Res.* **49,** 1110–1117.

Covey, J. M., Jaxel, C., Kohn, K. W., and Pommier, Y. (1989). Protein-linked DNA strand breaks induced in mammalian cells by camptothecin, an inhibitor of topoisomerase I. *Cancer Res.* **49,** 5016–5022.

Cozzarelli, N. R. (1980). DNA gyrase and the supercoiling of DNA. *Science* **207,** 953–960.

Culotta, V., and Sollner-Webb, B. (1988). Sites of topoisomerase I action on *X. laevis* ribosomal chromatin: Transcriptionally active rDNA has a +200 bp repeating structure. *Cell* **52,** 585–597.

Danks, M. K., Yalowich, J. C., and Beck, W. T. (1987). Atypical multiple drug resistance in a human leukemic cell line selected for resistance to teniposide (VM-26). *Cancer Res.* **47,** 1297–1301.

Danks, M. K., Schmidt, C. A., Cirtain, M. C., Suttle, D. P., and Beck, W. T. (1988). Altered catalytic activity of and DNA cleavage by DNA topoisomerase II from human leukemic cells selected for resistance to VM-26. *Biochemistry* **27,** 8861–8869.

Darby, M. K., Schmitt, B., Jongstra-Bilen, J., and Vosberg, H. P. (1985). Inhibition of calf thymus type II DNA topoisomerase by poly(ADP)ribosylation. *EMBO J.* **4,** 2129–2134.

Darby, M. K., Herrera, R. E., Vosberg, H. P., and Nordheim, A. (1986). DNA topoisomerase II cleaves at specific sites in the 5′-flanking region of c-fos proto-oncogenes in vitro. *EMBO J.* **5,** 2257–2265.

Darkin, S. J., and Ralph, R. K. (1989). A protein factor that enhances amsacrine-mediated formation of topoisomerase II–DNA complexes in murine mastocytoma cell nuclei. *Biochim. Biophys. Acta* **1007,** 295–300.

D'Arpa, P., and Liu, L. F. (1989). Topoisomerase-targeting antitumour drugs. *Biochem. Biophys. Acta* **989,** 163–177.

D'Arpa, P., Machlin, P. S., Ratrie, H., III, Rothfield, N. F., Cleveland, D. W., and Earnshaw, W. C. (1988). cDNA cloning of human DNA topoisomerase I: Catalytic activity of a 67.7-kDa carboxyl-terminal fragment. *Proc. Natl. Acad. Sci. U.S.A.* **85,** 2543–2547.

Deffie, A. M., Batra, J. K. and Goldenberg, G. J. (1989a). Direct correlation between DNA topoisomerase II activity and cytotoxicity in adriamycin-sensitive and -resistant P388 leukemia cell lines. *Cancer Res.* **49,** 58–62.

Deffie, A. M., Bosman, D. J. and Goldenberg, G. J. (1989b). Evidence for a mutant allele of the gene for DNA topoisomerase II in adriamycin-resistant P388 murine leukemia cells. *Cancer Res.* **49,** 6879–6882.

Degrassi, F., De Salvia, R., Tanzarella, C., and Palitti, F. (1989). Induction of chromosomal aberrations and SCE by camptothecin, an inhibitor of mammalian topoisomerase I. *Mutat. Res.* **211,** 125–130.

DiNardo, S., Voelkel, K., and Sternglanz, R. (1984). DNA topoisomerase II mutant of *Saccharomyces cerevisiae:* Topoisomerase II is required for segregation of daughter molecules at the termination of DNA replication. *Proc. Natl. Acad. Sci. U.S.A.* **81,** 2616–2620.

Douc-Rasy, S., Kayser, A., Riou, J. F., Riou, G. (1986). ATP-independent type II topoisomerase from trypanosomes. *Proc. Natl. Acad. Sci. U.S.A.* **83,** 7152–7156.

Drake, F. H., Zimmermann, J. P., McCabe, F. L., Bartus, H. F., Per, S. R., Sullivan, D. M., Ross, W. E., Mattern, M. R., Johnson, R. K., Crooke, S. T., and Mirabelli, C. K. (1987). Purification of topoisomerase II from amsacrine-resistant P388 leukemia cells. Evidence for two forms of the enzyme. *J. Biol. Chem.* **262,** 16739–16747.

Drake, F. H., Hofmann, G. A., Bartus, H. F., Mattern, M. R., Crooke, S. T. and Mirabelli, C. K. (1989). Biochemical and pharmacological properties of p170 and p180 forms of topoisomerase II. *Biochemistry* **28,** 8154–8160.

Drewinko, B., Yang, L. Y., and Barlogie, B. (1982). Lethal activity and kinetic response of cultured human cells to 4′-(9-acridinylamino)methanesulfon-*m*-anisidine. *Cancer Res.* **42,** 107–111.

Drlica, K. (1984). Biology of bacterial DNA topoisomerases. *Microbiol. Rev.* **48,** 273–289.

Duguet, M., Lavenot, C., Harper, F., Mirambeau, G., and DeRecondo, A. M. (1983). DNA topoisomerases from rat liver: Physiological variations. *Nucleic Acids Res.* **11,** 1059–1075.

Durban, E., Goodenough, M., Mills, J., and Busch, H. (1985). Topoisomerase I phosphorylation in vitro and in rapidly growing Novikoff hepatoma cells. *EMBO J.* **4,** 2921–2926.

Duvall, E., and Wyllie, A. H. (1986). Death and the cell. *Immunol. Today* **7,** 115–119.

Dynan, W. S., Jendrisak, J. J., Hager, D. A., and Burgess, R. R. (1981). Purification and characterization of wheat germ DNA topoisomerase I (nicking-closing enzyme). *J. Biol. Chem.* **256,** 5860–5865.

Earnshaw, W. C., Halligan, B., Cooke, C., Heck, M. M. S., and Liu, L. F. (1985). Topoisomerase II is a structural component of mitotic chromosome scaffolds. *J. Cell Biol.* **100,** 1706–1715.

Edwards, K. A., Halligan, B. D., Davis, J. L., Nevera, N. L., and Liu, L. F. (1982). Recognition sites of eukaryotic DNA topoisomerase I. DNA nucleotide sequencing analyses of topo I cleavage sites on SV40 DNA. *Nucleic Acids Res.* **10,** 2565–2576.

Egyhazi, E., and Durban, E. (1987). Microinjection of anti-topoisomerase I immunoglobulin G into nuclei of *Chironomus tentans* salivary gland cells leads to blockage of transcription elongation. *Mol. Cell. Biol.* **7,** 4308–4316.

Eng, W.-K., Faucette, L., Johnson, R. K., and Sternglanz, R. (1989). Evidence that DNA topoisomerase I is necessary for the cytotoxic effects of camptothecin. *Mol. Pharmacol.* **34,** 755–760.

Epstein, R. J. (1988). Topoisomerases in human disease. *Lancet.* **1,** 521–524.

Estey, E. H., Adlakha, R. C., Hittelman, W. N., and Zwelling, L. A. (1987a). Cell cycle stage dependent variations in drug induced topoisomerase II mediated DNA cleavage and cytotoxicity. *Biochemistry* **26,** 4338–4344.

Estey, E. H., Silberman, L., Beran, M., Andersson, B. S., and Zwelling, L. A. (1987b). The interaction between nuclear topoisomerase II activity from human leukemia cells, exogenous DNA, and 4′-(9-acridinylamino)methanesulfon-*m*-anisidide (*m*-AMSA) or 4-(4,6-*O*-ethylidene-β-D-glucopyranoside) (VP-16) indicates the sensitivity of the cells to the drugs. *Biochem. Biophys. Res. Commun.* **144,** 787–793.

Ferguson, L. R., and Denny, W. A. (1979). Potential antitumour agents. 30. Mutagenic activity of some 9-anilinoacridines: Relationships between structure, mutagenic potential, and antileukemic activity. *J. Med. Chem.* **22,** 251–255.

Ferrazzi, E., Peracchi, M., Biasolo, M. A., Faggionato, O., Stefanelli, S., and Palu, G. (1988). Antiviral activity of gyrase inhibitors norfloxacin, coumermycin A_1, and nalidixic acid. *Biochem. Pharmacol.* **37,** 1885–1886.

Ferro, A. M., and Olivera, B. M. (1984). Poly(ADP)ribosylation of DNA topoisomerase I from calf thymus. *J. Biol. Chem.* **259,** 547–554.

Ferro, A. M., Higgins, N. P., and Olivera, B. M. (1983). Poly (ADP)ribosylation of a DNA topoisomerase. *J. Biol. Chem.* **258,** 6000–6003.

Figgitt, D. P., Denyer, S. P., Dewick, P. M., Jackson, D. E., and Williams, P. (1989). Topoisomerase II: A potential target for novel antifungal agents. *Biochem. Biophys. Res. Commun.* **160,** 257–262.

Fleischmann, G., Pflugfelder, G., Steiner, E. K., Javaherian, K., Howard, G. C., Wang, J. C., and Elgin, S. C. R. (1984). Drosophila DNA topoisomerase I is associated with transcriptionally active regions of the genome. *Proc. Natl. Acad. Sci. U.S.A.* **81,** 6958–6962.

Fornace, A. J., Alamo, I., Jr., and Hollander, M. C. (1988). DNA damage-inducible transcripts in mammalian cells. *Proc. Natl. Acad. Sci. U.S.A.* **85,** 8800–8804.

Fukada, M. (1985). Action of camptothecin and its derivatives on deoxyribonucleic acid. *Biochem. Pharmacol.* **34,** 1225–1230.

Fukata, H., and Fukasawa, H. (1982). Isolation and partial characterization of two distinct DNA topoisomerases from cauliflower inflorescence. *J. Biochem. (Tokyo)* **91,** 1337–1342.

Gallo, R. C., Whang-Peng, J., and Adamson, R. H. (1971). Studies on the antitumor activity, mechanism of action, and cell cycle effects of camptothecin. *J. Natl. Cancer Inst. (U.S.)* **46,** 789–795.

Gasser, S. M., Laroche, T., Falquet, J., Boy de la Tour, E., and Laemmli, U. K. (1986). Metaphase chromosome structure: Involvement of topoisomerase II. *J. Mol. Biol.* **188,** 613–630.

Gellert, M. (1981). DNA topoisomerases. *Annu. Rev. Biochem.* **50,** 879–910.

Gellert, M., Mizuuchi, K., O'Dea, M. H., and Nash, H. A. (1976). DNA gyrase, an enzyme that introduces superhelical turns into DNA. *Proc. Natl. Acad. Sci. U.S.A.* **73,** 3872–3876.

Gellert, M., Fisher, L. M., and O'Dea, M. H. (1979). DNA gyrase: Purification and catalytic properties of a fragment of gyrase B protein. *Proc. Natl. Acad. Sci. U.S.A.* **76,** 6289–6293.

Giaever, G. N., and Wang, J. C. (1988). Supercoiling of intracellular DNA can occur in eukaryotic cells. *Cell (Cambridge, Mass.)* **55,** 849–856.

Gilmour, D. S., and Elgin, S. C. R. (1987). Localization of specific topoisomerase I interactions within the transcribed region of active heat shock genes by using the inhibitor camptothecin. *Mol. Cell. Biol.* **7,** 141–148.

Gilmour, D. S., Pflugfelder, G., Wang, J. C., and Lis, J. T. (1986). Topoisomerase I interacts with transcribed regions in *Drosophila* cells. *Cell (Cambridge, Mass.)* **44,** 401–407.

Giovanella, B. C., Stehlin, J. S., Wall, M. E., Wani, M. C., Nicholas, A. W., Liu, L. F., Silber, R. and Potmesil, M. (1989). DNA topoisomerase I-targeted chemotherapy of human colon cancer in xenografts. *Science* **246,** 1046–1048.

Glikin, G. C., and Blangy, D. (1986). In vitro transcription by *Xenopus* oocytes RNA polymerase III requires a DNA topoisomerase II activity. *EMBO J.* **5,** 151–156.

Glisson, B., Gupta, R., Smallwood-Kentro, S., and Ross, W. (1986a). Characterization of acquired epipodophyllotoxin resistance in a Chinese hamster ovary cell line: Loss of drug stimulated DNA cleavage activity. *Cancer Res.* **46,** 1934–1938.

Glisson, B., Gupta, R., Hodges, P., and Ross, W. (1986b). Cross-resistance to intercalating agents in an epipodophyllotoxin-resistant Chinese hamster ovary cell line: Evidence for a common intracellular target. *Cancer Res.* **46,** 1939–1942.

Goto, T., Laipsis, P., and Wang, J. C. (1984). The purification and characterization of DNA topoisomerases I and II of the yeast *Saccharomyces cerevisiae*. *J. Biol. Chem.* **259,** 10422–10429.

Gottlieb, J. A., and Luce, J. K. (1972). Treatment of malignant melanoma with camptothecin (NSC-100880). *Cancer Chemother. Rep.* **56,** 103–105.

Halligan, B. D., Davis, J. L., Edwards, K. A., and Liu, L. F. (1982). Intra- and intermolecular strand transfer by HeLa DNA topoisomerase I. *J. Biol. Chem.* **257,** 3995–4000.

Halligan, B. D., Edward, K. A., and Liu, L. F. (1985). Purification and characterization of a type II DNA topoisomerase from bovine calf thymus. *J. Biol. Chem.* **260,** 2475–2482.

Heck, M. M. S., and Earnshaw, W. C. (1986). Topoisomerase II: A specific marker for cell proliferation. *J. Cell Biol.* **103,** 2569–2581.

Heck, M. M. S., Hittelman, W. N., and Earnshaw, W. C. (1988). Differential expression of DNA topoisomerase I and II during the eukaryotic cell cycle. *Proc. Natl. Acad. Sci. U.S.A.* **85,** 1086–1090.

Heller, R. A., Shelton, E. R., Dietrich, V., Elgin, S. C. R., and Brutlag, D. L. (1986). Multiple forms and cellular localization of *Drosophila* DNA topoisomerase II. *J. Biol. Chem.* **261,** 8063–8069.

Hertzberg, R. P., Caranfa, M. J., Holdern, K. G., Jakas, D. R., Gallagher, G., Mattern, M. R., Mong, S.-M., Bartus, J. O., Johnson, R. K., and Kingsbury, W. D. (1989). Modification of the hydroxy lactone ring of camptothecin: Inhibition of mammalian topoisomerase I and biological activity. *J. Med. Chem.* **32,** 715–720.

Holm, C., Goto, T., Wang, J. C., and Botstein, D. (1985). DNA topoisomerase II is required at the time of mitosis in yeast. *Cell (Cambridge, Mass.)* **41,** 553–563.

Holm, C., Covey, J. M., Kerrigan, D. and Pommier, Y. (1989a). Differential requirement of DNA replication for the cytotoxicity of DNA topoisomerase I and II inhibitors in Chinese hamster DC3F cells. *Cancer Res.* **49,** 6365–6368.

Holm, C., Stearns, T., and Botstein, D. (1989b). DNA topoisomerase II must act at mitosis to prevent nondisjunction and chromosome breakage. *Mol. Cell. Biol.* **9,** 159–168.

Horwitz, M. S., and Horwitz, S. B. (1971). Intracellular degradation of HeLa and adenovirus type 2 DNA induced by camptothecin. *Biochem. Biophys. Res. Commun.* **45,** 723–727.

Horwitz, S. B. (1975). Camptothecin. *In* "Antibiotics" (J. W. Corcoran and F. E. Hahn, eds.), Vol. 3, pp. 48–57. Springer-Verlag, Berlin.

Horwitz, S. B., Chang, C.-K., and Grollman, A. P. (1971). Studies on camptothecin: Effects on nucleic acid and protein synthesis. *Mol. Pharmacol.* **7,** 632–644.

Hsiang, Y.-H., and Liu, L. F. (1988). Identification of mammalian DNA topoisomerase I as an intracellular target of the anticancer drug camptothecin. *Cancer Res.* **48,** 1722–1726.

Hsiang, Y.-H., and Liu, L. F. (1989). Evidence for the reversibility of cellular DNA lesion induced by mammalian topoisomerase II poisons. *J. Biol. Chem.* **264,** 9713–9715.

Hsiang, Y.-H., Hertzberg, R., Hecht, S., and Liu, L. F. (1985). Camptothecin induces protein-linked DNA breaks via mammalian DNA topoisomerase I. *J. Biol. Chem.* **260,** 14873–14878.

Hsiang, Y.-H., Wu, H. Y., and Liu, L. F. (1988). Proliferation-dependent regulation of DNA topoisomerase II in cultured human cells. *Cancer Res.* **48,** 3230–3235.

Hsiang, Y.-H., Lihou, M. G., and Liu, L. F. (1989a). Mechanism of cell killing by camptothecin: Arrest of replication forks by drug-stabilized topoisomerase I-DNA cleavable complexes. *Cancer Res.* **49,** 5077–5082.

Hsiang, Y.-H., Liu, L. F., Wall, M. E., Wani, N. C., Nicholas, A. W., Manikumar, G., Kirschenbaum, S., Silber, R., and Potmesil, M. (1989b). DNA topoisomerase I mediated DNA cleavage and cytotoxicity of camptothecin analogs. *Cancer Res.* **49,** 4385–4389.

Hsiang, Y.-H., Jiang, J., and Liu, L. F. (1989c). Topoisomerase II-mediated DNA cleavage by amonafide and its structural analogs. *Mol. Pharmacol.* **36,** 371–376.

Hsieh, T. S. (1983). Purification and properties of type II DNA topoisomerase from embryos of *Drosophila melanogaster*. *In* "Methods in Enzymology" (R. Wu, L. Grossman, and K. Moldave, eds.), Vol. 100, pp. 161–170. Academic Press, New York.

Hsieh, T. S., and Brutlag, D. (1980). ATP dependent DNA topoisomerase from *D. melanogaster* reversibly catenates duplex DNA rings. *Cell (Cambridge, Mass.)* **21,** 115–125.

Hwang, J., Shyy, S., Chen, A. Y., Juan, C.-C., and Whang-Peng, J. (1989). Studies of topoisomerase-specific antitumor drugs in human lymphocytes using rabbit antisera against recombinant human topoisomerase II polypeptide. *Cancer Res.* **49,** 958–962.

Hwong, C.-L., Chen, M.-S. and Hwang, J. (1989). Phorbol ester transiently increases topoisomerase I mRNA levels in human skin fibroblasts. *J. Biol. Chem.* **264,** 14923–14926.

Ikeda, H. (1986). Illegitimate recombination: Role of type II DNA topoisomerase. *Adv. Biophys.* **21,** 149–160.

Jaxel, C., Taudou, G., Portemer, C., Mirambeau, G., Panijel, J., and Duguet, M. (1988). Topoisomerase inhibitors induce irreversible fragmentation of replicated DNA in concanavalin A stimulated splenocytes. *Biochemistry* **27,** 95–100.

Jaxel, C., Kohn, K. W., Wani, M. C., Wall, M. E., and Pommier, Y. (1989). Structure-activity study of the actions of camptothecin derivatives on mammalian topoisomerase I: Evidence for a specific receptor site and a relation to antitumor activity. *Cancer Res.* **49,** 1465–1469.

Jongstra-Bilen, J., Ittel, M. E., Niedergang, C., Vosberg, H. P., and Mandel, P. (1983). DNA topoisomerase I from calf thymus is inhibited in vitro by poly(ADP)ribosylation. *Eur. J. Biochem.* **136,** 391–396.

Juan, C.-C., Hwang, J., Liu, A. A., Whang-Peng, J., Knutsen, T., Huebner, K., Croce, C. M., Zhang, H., Wang, J. C., and Liu, L. F. (1988). Human DNA topoisomerase I is encoded by a single-copy gene that maps to chromosome region 20q12-13.2. *Proc. Natl. Acad. Sci. U.S.A.* **85,** 8910–8913.

Kaufmann, S. H. (1989). Induction of endonucleolytic DNA cleavage in human acute myelogenous leukemia cells by etoposide, camptothecin, and other cytotoxic anticancer drugs: A cautionary note. *Cancer Res.* **49,** 5870–5878.

Kessel, D. (1971). Effects of camptothecin on RNA synthesis in leukemia cells. *Biochim. Biophys. Acta* **246,** 225–232.

Kessel, D., Bosmann, H. B, and Lohr, K. (1972). Camptothecin effects on DNA synthesis in murine leukemia cells. *Biochim. Biophys. Acta* **269,** 210–216.

Kohn, K. W. (1979). DNA as a target in cancer chemotherapy: Measurement of macromolecular DNA damage produced in mammalian cells by anticancer agents and carcinogens. *Methods Cancer Res.* **16,** 291–345.

Li, L. H., Fraser, T. J., Olin, E. J., and Bhuyan, B. K. (1972). Action of camptothecin on mammalian cells in culture. *Cancer Res.* **32,** 2643–2650.

Lim, M., Liu, L. F., Jacobson-Kram, D., and Williams, J. R. (1986). Induction of sister chromatid exchanges by inhibitors of topoisomerases. *Cell Biol. Toxicol.* **2,** 485–494.

Liu, L. F. (1983a). HeLa topoisomerase I. *In* "Methods in Enzymology" (R. Wu, L. Grossman, and K. Moldave, eds.), Vol. 100, pp. 133–137.

Liu, L. F. (1983b). DNA topoisomerases—enzymes that catalyze the breaking and rejoining of DNA. *CRC Crit. Rev. Biochem.* **15,** 1–24.

Liu, L. F. (1989). DNA topoisomerase poisons as antitumor drugs. *Annu. Rev. Biochem.* **58,** 351–375.

Liu, L. F. (1990). Anticancer drugs that convert DNA topoisomerases into cellular DNA poisons. *In* "DNA topology and its biological effects," (N. Cozzarelli and J. Wang, eds.), Cold Spring Harbor, New York, in press.

Liu, L. F., and Miller, K. G. (1981). Eukaryotic DNA topoisomerases. Two forms of type I DNA topoisomerases from HeLa cell nuclei. *Proc. Natl. Acad. Sci. U.S.A.* **78,** 3487–3491.

Liu, L. F., and Wang, J. C. (1987). Supercoiling of the DNA template during transcription. *Proc. Natl. Acad. Sci. U.S.A.* **75,** 2098–2102.

Liu, L. F., Liu, C. C., and Alberts, B. M. (1980). Type II DNA topoisomerases. Enzymes that can unknot a topologically knotted DNA molecule via a reversible double-strand break. *Cell (Cambridge, Mass.)* **19,** 697–707.

Liu, L. F., Rowe, T. C., Yang, L., Tewey, K. M., and Chen, G. L. (1983). Cleavage of DNA by mammalian DNA topoisomerase II. *J. Biol. Chem.* **258,** 15365–15370.

Lock, R. B., and Ross, W. E. (1987). DNA topoisomerases in cancer therapy. *Anti-cancer Drug Des.* **2,** 151–165.

Loike, J. D., and Horwitz, S. B. (1976). Effects of VP-16-213 on the intracellular degradation of DNA in HeLa cells. *Biochemistry* **15,** 5443–5448.

Long, B. H., Musial, S. T., and Brattain, M. G. (1984). Comparison of cytotoxicity and DNA breakage activity of congeners of podophyllotoxin including VP16-213 and VM26: A quantitative structure-activity relationship. *Biochemistry* **23,** 1183–1188.

Long, B. H., Musial, S. T., and Brattain, M. G. (1985). Single- and double-strand DNA breakage and repair in human lung adenocarcinoma cells exposed to etoposide and teniposide. *Cancer Res.* **45,** 3106–3112.

Long, B. H., Musial, S. T., and Brattain, M. G. (1986). DNA breakage in human lung carcinoma cells and nuclei that are naturally sensitive or resistant to etoposide and teniposide. *Cancer Res.* **46,** 3809–3816.

Markovits, J., Pommier, Y., Kerrigan, D., Covey, J. M., Tilchen, E. J., and Kohn, K. W. (1987). Topoisomerase II-mediated DNA breaks and cytotoxicity in relation to cell proliferation and the cell cycle in NIH 3T3 fibroblasts and L1210 leukemia cells. *Cancer Res.* **47,** 2050–2055.

Markovits, J., Linassier, C., Fosse, P., Couprie, J., Pierre, J., Jacquemin-Sablon, A., Saucier, J.-M., LePecq, J.-B. and Larsen, A. K. (1989). Inhibitory effects of the tyrosine kinase inhibitor genistein on mammalian DNA topoisomerase II *Cancer Res.* **49,** 5111–5117.

Marshall, B., and Ralph, R. K. (1982a). The nature of DNA breakage by 4′-(9-acridinylamino)methanesulfon-*m*-anisidide. *FEBS Lett.* **145,** 187–190.

Marshall, B., and Ralph, R. K. (1982b). A reassessment of the mechanism of action of 4′-(9-acridinylamino)methanesulfon-*m*-anisidide. *Eur. J. Cancer Clin. Oncol.* **18,** 553–557.

Marshall, B., and Ralph, R. K. (1982c). A simple method for detecting drug effects on the DNA of mammalian cells. *Anal. Biochem.* **125,** 91–95.

Marshall, B., and Ralph, R. K. (1985). The mechanism of action of *m*AMSA. *Adv. Cancer Res.* **44,** 267–293.

Marshall, B., Ralph, R. K., and Hancock, R. (1983). Blocked 5′-termini in the fragments of chromosomal DNA produced in cells exposed to the antitumour drug 4′-(9-acridinylamino)methanesulfon-*m*-anisidide. *Nucleic Acids Res.* **11,** 4251–4256.

Miller, K. G., Liu, L. F., and Englund, P. T. (1981). A homogeneous type II DNA topoisomerase from HeLa cell nuclei. *J. Biol. Chem.* **256,** 9334–9339.

Minford, J., Pommier, Y., Filipski, J., Kohn, K. W., Kerrigan, D., Mattern, M., Michaels, S., Schwartz, R., and Zwelling, L. A. (1986). Isolation of intercalator-dependent protein-linked DNA strand cleavage activity from cell nuclei and identification as topoisomerase II. *Biochemistry* **25,** 9–15.

Miskimins, R., Miskimins, W. K., Bernstein, H., and Shimizu, N. (1983). Epidermal growth factor-induced topoisomerase(s). Intracellular translocation and relation to DNA synthesis. *Exp. Cell Res.* **146,** 53–62.

Moertel, C. G., Schutt, A. J., Reitemeier, R. J., and Hahn, R. G. (1972). Phase II study of camptothecin (NSC-100880) in the treatment of advanced gastrointestinal cancer. *Cancer Chemother. Rep.* **56,** 95–101.

Muggia, F. M., Creaven, P. J., Hansen, H. H., Cohen, M. H., and Selawry, O. S. (1972). Phase I clinical trial of weekly and daily treatment with camptothecin (NSC-100880): Correlation with preclinical studies. *Cancer Chemother. Rep.* **56,** 515–521.

Muller, M. T., Pfund, W. P., Mehta, V. B., and Trask, D. K. (1985). Eukaryotic type I topoisomerase is enriched in the nucleolus and catalytically active on ribosomal DNA. *EMBO J.* **4,** 1237–1243.

Muller, M. T., Spitzner, J. R., DiDonato, J. A., Mehta, V. B., Tsutsui, K., and Tsutsui, K. (1988). Single-strand DNA cleavages by eukaryotic topoisomerase II. *Biochemistry* **27,** 8369–8379.

Neidle, S., and Waring, M. J. (1983). "Molecular Aspects of Anti-Cancer Drug Action." Macmillan, London.

Neil, G. L., and Homan, E. R. (1973). The effects of dose interval on the survival of L1210 leukemic mice treated with DNA synthesis inhibitors. *Cancer Res.* **33,** 895–901.

Nelson, E. M., Tewey, K. M., and Liu, L. F. (1984). Mechanism of antitumor drugs. Poisoning of mammalian DNA topoisomerase II on DNA by an antitumor drug *m*-AMSA. *Proc. Natl. Acad. Sci. U.S.A.* **81,** 1361–1365.

Newport, J. (1987). Nuclear reconstitution in vitro: Stages of assembly around protein-free DNA. *Cell (Cambridge, Mass.)* **48,** 205–217.

Newport, J., and Spann, T. (1987). Disassembly of the nucleus in mitotic extracts: Membrane vesicularization, lamin disassembly and chromosome condensation are independent processes. *Cell (Cambridge, Mass.)* **48,** 219–230.

Nitiss, J., and Wang, J. C. (1988). DNA topoisomerase-targeting antitumor drugs can be studied in yeast. *Proc. Natl. Acad. Sci. U.S.A.* **85,** 7501–7505.

Okura, A., Arakawa, H., Oka, H., Yoshinary, T. and Monden, Y. (1988). Effect of genistein on topoisomerase activity and on the growth of [VAL12]Ha-ras-transformed NIH3T3 cells. *Biochem. Biophys. Res. Commun.* **157,** 183–189.

Per, S. R., Mattern, C. K., Drake, F. H., Johnson, R. K., and Crooke, S. T. (1987). Characterization of a subline of P388 leukemia resistant to amsacrine: Evidence of altered topoisomerase II function. *Mol. Pharmacol.* **32,** 17–25.

Pommier, Y., Zwelling, L. A., Kao-Shan, C.-S., Whang-Peng, J., and Bradley, M. O. (1985). Correlations between intercalator-induced DNA strand breaks and sister chromatid exchanges, mutations, and cytotoxicity in Chinese hamster cells. *Cancer Res.* **45,** 3143–3149.

Pommier, Y., Kerrigan, D., Schwartz, R. E., Swack, J. A., and McCurdy, A. (1986). Altered DNA topoisomerase II activity in Chinese hamster cells resistant to topoisomerase II inhibitors. *Cancer Res.* **46,** 3075–3081.

Pommier, Y., Kerrigan, D., Covey, J. M., Kao-Shan, C.-S., and Whang-Peng, J. (1988). Sister chromatid exchanges, chromosomal aberrations, and cytotoxicity produced by antitumor topoisomerase II inhibitors in sensitive (DC3F) and resistant (DC3F/9-OHE) Chinese hamster cells. *Cancer Res.* **48,** 512–516.

Potmesil, M., Hsiang, Y.-H., Liu, L. F., Bank, B., Grossberg, H., Kirschenbaum, S., Penziner, A., Kanganis, D., Knowles, D., Traganos, F., and Silber, R. (1988). Resistance of human leukemic and normal lymphocytes to drug-induced DNA cleavage and low levels of DNA topoisomerase II. *Cancer Res.* **48,** 3537–3543.

Pulleyblank, D. E., and Ellison, M. J. (1982). Purification and properties of type I topoisomerase from chicken erythrocytes: Mechanism of eukaryotic topoisomerase action. *Biochemistry* **21,** 1155–1161.

Ralph, R. K. (1980). On the mechanism of action of 4′-(9-acridinylamino)methanesulfone-*m*-anisidide. *Eur. J. Cancer Clin. Oncol.* **16,** 595–600.

Ralph, R. K., and Hancock, R. (1985). Chromosomal DNA fragments from mouse cells exposed to an intercalating agent containing a 175 kd terminal polypeptide. *Can. J. Biochem. Cell Biol.* **63,** 780–783.

Ralph, R. K., and Schneider, E. (1987). DNA topoisomerase and anti-cancer drugs. *In* "Integration and Control of Metabolic Processes: Pure and Applied Aspects" (O. L. Kon, ed.), pp. 373–388. ICSU Press, Cambridge, U.K.

Ralph, R. K., Marshall, B., and Darkin, S. (1983). Anti-cancer drugs which intercalate into DNA: How do they act? *Trends Biochem. Sci.* **8,** 212–214.

Richter, A., and Strausfeld, U. (1988). Effects of VM26, a specific inhibitor of type II DNA topoisomerase, on SV40 chromatin replication *in vitro*. *Nucleic Acids Res.* **16,** 10119–10129.

Richter, A., Strausfeld, U., and Knippers, R. (1987). Effects of VM-26 (teniposide), a specific inhibitor of type II DNA topoisomerase, on SV40 replication *in vivo*. *Nucleic Acids Res.* **15,** 3455–3478.

Riordan, J. R., and Ling, V. (1986). Genetic and biochemical characterization of multidrug resistance. *Pharmacol. Ther.* **28,** 51–75.

Riou, J. F., Multon, E., Vilarem, M. J., Larsen, C. J., and Riou, G. (1986a). *In vivo* stimulation by antitumour drugs of the topoisomerase II-induced cleavage sites in c-myc protooncogene. *Biochem. Biophys. Res. Commun.* **137,** 154–160.

Riou, J. F., Vilarem, M. J., Larsen, C. J., and Riou, G. (1986b). Characterization of the topoisomerase II-induced cleavage site in the c-myc protooncogene. *In vitro* stimulation by the antitumour intercalating drug *m*AMSA. *Biochem. Pharmacol.* **35,** 4409–4413.

Robbie, M. A., Baguley, B. C., Denny, W. A., Gavin, J. B., and Wilson, W. R. (1988). Mechanism of resistance of non-cycling mammalian cells to 4′-(9-acridinylamino)methanesulfon-*m*-anisidide: Comparison of uptake, metabolism and DNA breakage in log-phase and plateau-phase Chinese hamster fibroblast cell cultures. *Cancer Res.* **48,** 310–319.

Ross, W. E. (1985). DNA topoisomerases as targets for cancer therapy. *Biochem. Pharmacol.* **34,** 4191–4195.

Ross, W. E., and Bradley, M. O. (1981). DNA double-strand breaks in mammalian cells after exposure to intercalating agents. *Biochim. Biophys. Acta* **654,** 129–134.

Ross, W. E., and Smith, M. C. (1982). Repair of deoxyribonucleic acid lesions caused by adriamycin and ellipticine. *Biochem. Pharmacol.* **31,** 1931–1935.

Ross, W. E., Glaubiger, D. L., and Kohn, K. W. (1978). Protein-associated DNA breaks in cells treated with adriamycin or ellipticine. *Biochim. Biophys. Acta* **519,** 23–30.

Ross, W. E., Glaubiger, D., and Kohn, K. W. (1979). Qualitative and quantitative aspects of intercalator-induced DNA strand breaks. *Biochim. Biophys. Acta* **562,** 41–50.

Ross, W. E., Rowe, T. C., Glisson, B., Yalowich, J., and Liu, L. F. (1984). Role of topoisomerase II in mediating epipodophyllotoxin-induced DNA cleavage. *Cancer Res.* **44,** 5857–5860.

Rowe, T. C., Chen, G. L., Hsiang, Y.-H., and Liu, L. F. (1986a). DNA damage by antitumor acridines mediated by mammalian DNA topoisomerase II. *Cancer Res.* **46,** 2021–2026.

Rowe, T. C., Wang, J. C., and Liu, L. F. (1986b). In vivo localization of DNA topoisomerase II cleavage sites on *Drosophila* heat-shock chromatin. *Mol. Cell. Biol.* **6,** 985–992.

Rowe, T. C., Couto, E., and Kroll, D. J. (1987). Camptothecin inhibits Hsp 70 heat-shock transcription and induces DNA strand breaks in hsp 70 genes in *Drosophila. NCI Monogr.* **4,** 49–53.

Sahyoun, N., Wolf, M., Bestermann, J., Hsieh, T. S., Sanders, M., LeVine, H., III, Chang, K. J., and Cuatrecasas, P. (1986). Protein kinase C phosphorylates topoisomerase II: Topoisomerase activation and its possible role in phorbol ester-induced differentiation of HL-60 cells. *Proc. Natl. Acad. Sci. U.S.A.* **83,** 1603–1607.

Schmitt, B., Buhre, U., and Vosberg, H. P. (1984). Characterization of size variants of type I DNA topoisomerase isolated from calf thymus. *Eur. J. Biochem.* **144,** 127–134.

Schneider, E., Darkin, S. J., Robbie, M. A., Wilson, W. R., and Ralph, R. K. (1988a). Mechanism of resistance of non-cycling mammalian cells to 4′-[9-acridinylamino]methanesulphon-*m*-anisidide: Role of DNA topoisomerase II in log- and plateau-phase CHO cells. *Biochim. Biophys. Acta* **949,** 264–272.

Schneider, E., Hutchins, A. M., Darkin, S. J., Lawson, P. A., and Ralph, R. K. (1988b). Relationship between sensitivity to 4′-(9-acridinylamino)methanesulfon-*m*-anisidide and DNA topoisomerase II in a cold-sensitive cell-cycle mutant mastocytoma cell line. *Biochim. Biophys. Acta* **951,** 85–97.

Schneider, E., Lawson, P. A., and Ralph, R. K. (1989). Inhibition of protein synthesis reduces the cytotoxicity of 4′-(9-acridinylamino)methanesulfon-*m*-anisidide without affecting DNA breakage and DNA topoisomerase II in a murine mastocytoma cell line. *Biochem. Pharmacol.* **38,** 263–269.

Siedlecki, J., Zimmermann, W., and Weissbach, A. (1983). Characterization of a prokaryotic topoisomerase I activity in chloroplast extracts from spinach. *Nucleic Acids Res.* **11,** 1523–1536.

Singh, B., and Gupta, S. (1983). Mutagenic responses of thirteen anticancer drugs on mutation induction at multiple genetic loci and on sister chromatid exchanges in Chinese hamster ovary cells. *Cancer Res.* **43,** 577–584.

Snapka, R. M. (1986). Topoisomerase inhibitors can selectively interfere with different stages of simian virus 40 DNA replication. *Mol. Cell. Biol.* **6,** 4221–4227.

Spadari, S., Pedraly-Noy, G., Focher, F., Montecucco, A., Bordoni, T., Geroni, C., Guilani, F. C., Ventrella, G., Arcamone, F., and Ciarrocchi, G. (1986). DNA polymerases and DNA topoisomerases as targets for the development of anticancer drugs. *Anticancer Res.* **6,** 935–940.

Spataro, A., and Kessel, D. (1972). Studies on camptothecin-induced degradation and apparent reaggregation of DNA from L1210 cells. *Biochem. Biophys. Res. Commun.* **48,** 643–648.

Stewart, A. F., and Schutz, G. (1987). Camptothecin-induced *in vivo* topoisomerase I cleavages in the transcriptionally active tyrosine aminotransferase gene. *Cell (Cambridge, Mass.)* **50,** 1109–1117.

Sullivan, D. M., Glisson, B. S., Hodges, P. K., Smallwood-Kentro, S., and Ross, W. E. (1986). Proliferation dependence of topoisomerase II mediated drug action. *Biochemistry* **25,** 2248–2256.

Sullivan, D. M., Latham, M. D., and Ross, W. E. (1987). Proliferation-dependent topoisomerase II content as a determinant of antineoplastic drug action in human mouse and Chinese hamster ovary cells. *Cancer Res.* **47,** 3973–3980.

Taudou, G., Mirambeau, G., Lavenot, C., Garabedian, A., Vermeersch, J., and Duguet, M. (1984). DNA topoisomerase activities in concanavalin A stimulated lymphocytes. *FEBS Lett.* **176,** 431–435.

Tewey, K. M., Chen, G. L., Nelson, E. M., and Liu, L. F. (1984a). Intercalative antitumor drugs interfere with the breakage-reunion reaction of mammalian DNA topoisomerase II. *J. Biol. Chem.* **259,** 9182–9187.

Tewey, K. M., Rowe, T. C., Yang, L., Halligan, B. C., and Liu, L. F. (1984b). Adriamycin-induced DNA damage mediated by mammalian DNA topoisomerase II. *Science* **226,** 466–468.

Trask, D. K., and Muller, M. T. (1983). Biochemical characterization of topoisomerase I purified from avian erythrocytes. *Nucleic Acids Res.* **11,** 2779–2800.

Tsai-Pflugfelder, M., Liu, L. F., Liu, A. A., Tewey, K. M., Whang-Peng, J., Knutsen, T., Huebner, K., Croce, C. M., and Wang, J. C. (1988). Cloning and sequencing of cDNA encoding human DNA topoisomerase II and localization of the gene to chromosome 17q21-22. *Proc. Natl. Acad. Sci. U.S.A.* **85,** 7177–7181.

Tsao, Y. P., Wu, H.-Y., and Liu, L. F. (1989). Transcription-driven supercoiling of DNA: Direct biochemical evidence from *in vitro* studies. *Cell (Cambridge, Mass.)* **56,** 111–118.

Tse-Dinh, Y. C., Wong, T. W., and Goldberg, A. R. (1984). Virus- and cell-encoded tyrosine protein kinases inactivate DNA topoisomerases *in vitro*. *Nature (London)* **312,** 785–786.

Udvardy, A., Schedl, P., Sander, M., and Hsieh, T. S. (1985). Novel partitioning of DNA cleavage sites for *Drosophila* topoisomerase II. *Cell (Cambridge, Mass.)* **40,** 933–941.

Udvardy, A., Schedl, P., Sander, M., and Hsieh, T. S. (1986). Topoisomerase II cleavage in chromatin. *J. Mol. Biol.* **191,** 231–246.

Ueda, K., Cornwell, M. M., Gottesman, M. M., Pastan, I., Roninson, I. B., Ling, V., and Riordan, J. R. (1986). The mdr1 gene, responsible for multidrug resistance, codes for P-glycoprotein. *Biochem. Biophys. Res. Commun.* **141,** 956–962.

Uemura, T., and Yanagida, M. (1984). Isolation of type I and II DNA topoisomerase mutants from fission yeast: Single and double mutants show different phenotypes in cell growth and chromatin organization. *EMBO J.* **3,** 1737–1744.

Uemura, T., and Yanagida, M. (1986). Mitotic spindle pulls but fails to separate chromosomes in type II DNA topoisomerase mutants: uncoordinated mitosis. *EMBO J.* **5,** 1003–1010.

Uemura, T., Morino, K., Uzawa, S., Shiozaki, K., and Yanagida, M. (1987a). Cloning and sequencing of *Schizosaccharomyces pombe* DNA topoisomerase I gene, and effect of gene disruption. *Nucleic Acids Res.* **15,** 9727–9739.

Uemura, T., Ohkura, H., Adachi, Y., Morino, K., Shiozaki, K., and Yanagida, M. (1987b). DNA topoisomerase II is required for condensation and separation of mitotic chromosomes in *S. pombe*. *Cell (Cambridge, Mass.)* **50,** 917–925.

Utsugi, T., Demuth, S., and Hanna, N. (1989). Synergistic antitumor effects of topoisomerase inhibitors and natural cell-mediated cytotoxicity. *Cancer Res.* **49,** 1429–1433.

Vosberg, H. P. (1985). DNA topoisomerases: Enzymes that control DNA conformation. *Curr. Top. Microbiol. Immunol.* **114,** 19–102.

Wang, J. C. (1985). DNA topoisomerases. *Annu. Rev. Biochem.* **54,** 665–697.

Wang, J. C., and Liu, L. F. (1979). DNA topoisomerases. Enzymes that catalyze the concerted breaking and rejoining of DNA bonds. *In* "Molecular Genetics" (J. H. Taylor, ed.), Part 3, pp. 65–88. Academic Press, New York.

Waring, M. J. (1981). DNA modification and cancer. *Annu. Rev. Biochem.* **50,** 159–192.

Wilson, W. R., and Whitmore, G. F. (1981). Cell-cycle-stage specificity of 4′-(9-acridinylamino)methanesulfon-*m*-anisidide (*m*-AMSA) and interaction with ionizing radiation in mammalian cell cultures. *Radia. Res.* **87,** 121–136.

Wilson, W. R., Baguley, B. C., Wabelin, L. P. G., and Waring, M. J. (1981). Interaction of the antitumour drug 4′-(9-acridinylamino)methanesulfon-*m*-anisidide. *Mol. Pharmacol.* **20,** 404–414.

Wozniak, A. J., and Ross, W. E. (1983). DNA damage as a basis for 4′-demethyl epipodohyllotoxin-9-(4,6-O-ethylidene-β-D-glucopyranoside) (etoposide) cytotoxicity. *Cancer Res.* **43,** 120–124.

Wu, H.-Y., Shyy, S. H., Wang, J. C., and Liu, L. F. (1988). RNA transcription generates negatively and positively supercoiled domains in the template. *Cell (Cambridge, Mass.)* **53,** 433–440.

Wyllie, A. H. (1987). Apoptosis: Cell death in tissue regulation. *J. Pathol.* **153,** 313–316.

Yamagishi, M., and Nomura, M. (1988). Deficiency in both type I and II DNA topoisomerase activities differentially affects rRNA and ribosomal protein synthesis in *Schizosaccharomyces pombe*. *Curr. Genet.* **13,** 305–314.

Yang, L., Rowe, T. C., and Liu, L. F. (1985). Identification of DNA topoisomerase II as an intracellular target of antitumor epipodophyllotoxins in SV40 infected monkey cells. *Cancer Res.* **45,** 5872–5876.

Yang, L., Wold, M. S., Li, J. J., Kelly, T. J., and Liu, L. F. (1987). Roles of DNA topoisomerases in simian virus 40 DNA replication *in vitro*. *Proc. Natl. Acad. Sci. U.S.A.* **84,** 950–954.

Zhang, H., Wang, J. C., and Liu, L. F. (1988). Involvement of DNA topoisomerase I in the transcription of human ribosomal RNA genes. *Proc. Natl. Acad. Sci. U.S.A.* **85,** 1060–1064.

Zwelling, L. A. (1985). DNA Topoisomerase II as a target of antineoplastic drug therapy. *Cancer Metastasis Rev.* **4,** 263–276.

Zwelling, L. A., Michaels, S., Erickson, L. C., Ungerleider, R. S., Nichols, M., and Kohn, D. W. (1981). Protein-associated deoxyribonucleic acid strand breaks in L1210 cells treated with the deoxyribonucleic acid intercalating agents 4′(9-acridinylamino)methanesulfon-*m*-anisidide and adriamycin. *Biochemistry* **20,** 6553–6563.

Zwelling, L. A., Kerrigan, D., and Michaels, S. (1982a). Cytotoxicity and DNA strand breaks by 5-iminodaunorubicin in mouse leukemia L1210 cells: Comparison with adriamycin and 4′-(9-acridinylamino)methanesulfon-*m*-anisidide. *Cancer Res.* **42,** 2687–2691.

Zwelling, L. A., Michaels, S., Kerrigan, D., Pommier, Y., and Kohn, K. W. (1982b). Protein-associated deoxyribonucleic acid strand breaks produced in mouse leukemia L1210 cells by ellipticine and 2-methyl-9-hydroxyellipticinium. *Biochem. Pharmacol.* **31,** 3261–3267.

Zwelling, L. A., Estey, E., Silbermann, L., Doyle, S., and Hittelman, W. (1987). Effect of cell proliferation and chromatin conformation on intercalator-induced protein-associated DNA cleavage in human brain tumour cells and human fibroblasts. *Cancer Res.* **47,** 251–257.

Multidrug Resistance and Chemosensitization: Therapeutic Implications for Cancer Chemotherapy

Elias Georges,* Frances J. Sharom,† and Victor Ling*

**The Ontario Cancer Institute and the Department of Medical Biophysics University of Toronto Toronto, Canada*

†Guelph-Waterloo Centre for Graduate Work in Chemistry Department of Chemistry and Biochemistry University of Guelph Guelph, Canada

I. Introductory Remarks

Studies using multidrug resistant (MDR) tumor cell lines have provided compelling evidence that a membrane protein of 170 kDa (P-glycoprotein) is causative of the MDR phenotype. Cells over-expressing P-glycoprotein have been characterized by their ability to exclude a variety of apparently unrelated drugs in an energy-dependent manner. The role of P-glycoprotein as a drug-efflux pump has been proposed from its structural homology to a number of bacterial transport proteins. Other mechanisms of MDR, e.g. alteration in DNA topoisomerase activity or in glutathione metabolism, have been proposed (Pommier *et al.*, 1986; Sinha *et al.*, 1987; Tew and Clapper, 1987), but to date, P-glycoprotein remains the best understood mechanism of MDR with potential clinical relevance.

A major impetus for research into the mechanism of P-glycoprotein-mediated MDR is the possibility that MDR tumor cells can arise during tumor progression in human malignancies, and that the outgrowth of MDR tumor cells could eventually limit a patient's response to anticancer drugs. This hypothesis has been strengthened by recent reports demonstrating that relatively high levels of P-glycoprotein are observed in different cancers. Although further studies will be required to determine if the presence of P-glycoprotein-containing tumor cells is prognostic of response to chemotherapy, there is nonetheless optimism that this line of investigation will ultimately lead to a more rational approach to the development and use of anticancer drugs. A particularly exciting finding is that a group of structurally diverse compounds is able to reverse the P-glycoprotein-mediated MDR phenotype. Such compounds, labeled collectively as "chemosensitizers," include calcium channel blockers, calmodulin inhibitors, steroids, and other lipophilic agents. The mechanism by which these chemosensitizers modulate the MDR phenotype is poorly understood, but their use with conventional chemotherapy has yielded promising results in some previously nonresponsive tumors. The future application of chemosensitizers will likely provide new insight into cancer chemotherapy.

This review focuses on our current understanding of chemosensitization of the P-glycoprotein-mediated MDR phenotype, and discusses some of the hypotheses proposed to account for their mode of action. The interested reader may wish to consult a number of recent reviews for detailed discussion of the biochemistry and genetics of MDR and P-glycoprotein (Bradley *et al.*, 1988; Endicott and Ling, 1989).

II. The MDR Phenotype and P-Glycoprotein

A. Clinical Observations

The development of resistance to multiple chemotherapeutic drugs is a major obstacle in the clinical treatment of many human cancers. It has been suggested that chemotherapeutic treatment of cancer may result in the selection of drug-resistant cells from a heterogeneous population of tumor cells and thus the outgrowth of a drug-resistant tumor. In this respect, malignancies including multiple myeloma, breast cancers, ovarian cancers, and childhood neuroblastoma and leukemia may initially respond well to chemotherapy, resulting in a period of remission, only to be followed by the development of drug resistance, and subsequent regrowth of the tumor. Other tumors, primarily adenocarcinomas of the kidney and colon, are largely resistant to neoplastic agents, resulting in a lack of response to chemotherapeutic treatment at the outset. These drug-resistant tumors are often found to be resistant not only to the drugs used for treatment, but also to a broad range of structurally unrelated drugs that were not included in the original treatment regimen. Such tumors are said to be multidrug-resistant.

B. MDR Cell Lines

Investigation of the molecular basis of multidrug resistance has been greatly advanced by the development of cell lines selected for resistance to cytotoxic drugs. Cells resistant to a particular drug, such as colchicine, *Vinca* alkaloids, doxorubicin, or actinomycin D, have been derived by stepwise selection in increasing concentrations of the selecting agent. Clonal isolates selected for resistance to one drug frequently show cross-resistance to other apparently unrelated drugs. However, the cross-resistance profiles of multidrug-resistant cell clones derived from the same parental line may vary considerably. The molecular basis for these differences in drug cross-resistance patterns is currently unclear. Multidrug-resistant cell lines that have been studied intensively over the last 10 years include colchicine-selected Chinese hamster ovary lines (CHO) (Ling and Thompson, 1974), vinblastine-selected human carcinoma KB lines (Akiyama *et al.*, 1985), vincristine-selected Chinese hamster lung DC-3F lines (Meyers *et al.*, 1985), vinblastine-selected human ovarian carcinoma SKOV3 lines (Bradley *et al.*, 1989), and a variety of vinblastine-selected leukemic CEM lines (Beck, 1983). Such studies have revealed that these multidrug-resistant cell lines display a complex pleiotropic phenotype. A wide array of biochemical changes have been identified that distinguish drug-resistant cells from their drug-sensitive parents. Some of the common characteristics of these cell lines are listed in Table I.

Chemotherapeutic drugs that fall into the multidrug-resistance spectrum include the *Vinca* alkaloids (vinblastine and vincristine), the anthracyclines (doxorubicin and daunorubicin), epipodophyllotoxins (etoposide and teniposide), and

Table I

Characteristics of the Multidrug Resistance Phenotype

Increase in resistance to unrelated cytotoxic drugs
Decreased cellular accumulation of drugs
Overexpression of a 170- to 180-kDa membrane glycoprotein (P-glycoprotein)
Enhanced drug efflux
Collateral sensitivity to membrane-active agents
Reversal by chemosensitizers

actinomycin D. Figure 1 depicts the structures of some of the most widely used chemotherapeutic drugs involved in the MDR phenotype. These compounds are lipophilic, heterocyclic natural products of fungal, bacterial, or plant origin. However, these drugs have different modes of action and cellular targets, and until now no obvious common functional moieties have been identified.

Most multidrug-resistant cell lines characterized to date have been shown to accumulate lower total cellular amounts of drug than the drug-sensitive parent line, and this has been presumed to account for their resistance. Drugs involved in the multidrug-resistance spectrum are believed to enter the cell by simple diffusion, since influx is generally nonsaturable. Several groups have shown that multidrug-resistant cells have an enhanced ability to expel or pump out drugs, and that this efflux is energy-dependent, since it can be blocked by metabolic inhibitors, such as 2-deoxyglucose and azide, or by glucose deprivation (for a review, see Riordan and Ling, 1985). Extensive characterization of many multi-

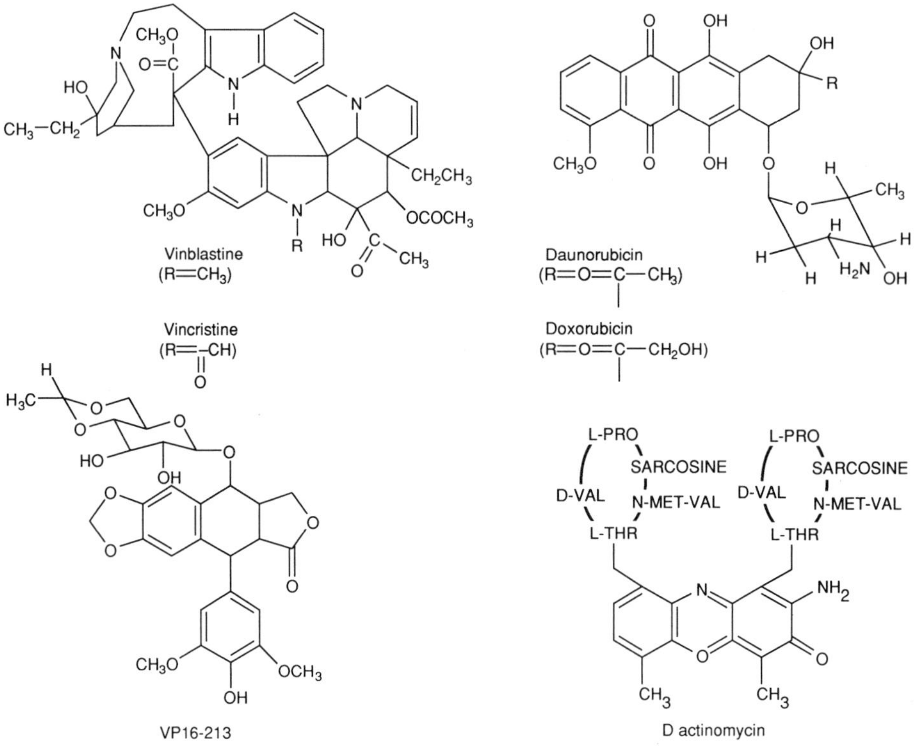

Vinblastine (R=CH_3)

Vincristine (R=CHO)

Daunorubicin (R=$-C(=O)-CH_3$)

Doxorubicin (R=$-C(=O)-CH_2OH$)

VP16-213

D actinomycin

Fig. 1 The molecular structures of some anticancer drugs such as vinblastine, vincristine, daunorubicin, doxorubicin, VP16-213 (4-dimethylepipodophyllotoxin), and actinomycin D.

drug-resistant cell lines isolated *in vitro* has revealed a consistent striking alteration in the expression of proteins in the cell membrane.

Ling and co-workers first reported that multidrug resistance in CHO cells correlated with an increase in a 170-kDa membrane glycoprotein, which they named P-glycoprotein (Juliano and Ling, 1976). Subsequently, P-glycoprotein, normally produced in barely detectable amounts in drug-sensitive cells, has been shown to be overexpressed in numerous independently derived multidrug-resistant cell lines. Recently, as described below, DNA-mediated transfection of drug-sensitive cells with cloned P-glycoprotein cDNAs from different sources indicates that an increased expression of P-glycoprotein is sufficient to produce a multidrug-resistance phenotype (Gros *et al.*, 1986c; Ueda *et al.*, 1987). In addition, structural features of the P-glycoprotein molecule are consistent with an energy-dependent drug-efflux pump protein. It is therefore envisioned that an increased level of P-glycoprotein in MDR cells leads to a reduced drug accumulation and thus to drug resistance.

Although the overexpression of P-glycoprotein appears to be the major change causing multidrug resistance, other secondary alterations are also seen in drug-resistant cells as compared to their drug-sensitive parent. A survey of these secondary changes is included in a recent review (Bradley *et al.*, 1988). One or more of these secondary alterations may result from gene amplification. For example, genes physically linked to those encoding P-glycoprotein have been found to be simultaneously coamplified in multidrug-resistant cell lines (Van der Bliek *et al.*, 1986). At least eight genes, including the P-glycoprotein genes, are linked in one large (>1000 kb) amplicon (Jongsma *et al.*, 1987). Thus amplification of the gene(s) for P-glycoprotein can lead to fortuitous coamplification of a variable number of flanking genes depending on the size of the amplicon. A flanking gene coding for a small (19–22 kDa) cytosolic Ca^{2+}-binding protein named sorcin (or V19) has been identified. It is coamplified with one or more P-glycoprotein genes in several multidrug-resistant cell lines (de Bruijn *et al.*, 1986; Jongsma *et al.*, 1987). In some multidrug-resistant cell lines the sorcin gene is not coamplified with the P-glycoprotein genes, and this suggests that sorcin is not required for multidrug resistance. Nevertheless, increased levels of sorcin may well contribute to the complex phenotype of some multidrug-resistant cell lines.

It is conceivable that a host of changes may occur in multidrug-resistant cells in response to the presence of increased levels of P-glycoprotein in the plasma membrane. The structure and function of the plasma membrane may be perturbed by abnormally high levels of P-glycoprotein, which can make up as much as 10% of the total membrane protein in some cell lines. These physical and biochemical perturbations may lead to the pleiotropic changes observed in the plasma membrane of drug-resistant cells. Two different multidrug-resistant cell lines show a large increase in the intramembranous particle density on freeze-fracture, demonstrating a major change in membrane ultrastructure and morphology (Arsenault *et al.*, 1988). Changes in the activity of a number of membrane-bound enzymes have also been associated with drug resistance. Membrane lipid composition and the pattern of glycolipids are also altered, and an increased rate of plasma membrane trafficking has been noted. Mountford and Wright (1988) have reported recently that the plasma membrane of some multidrug-resistant cells contains a novel lipoprotein particle with triglyceride as a major component. This nonbilayer structure has also been associated with metastatic tumor cells. Probes of the physical state of the bilayer have shown changes in the fluidity of the plasma membrane in several multidrug-resistant cell lines. Resistance to multiple drugs is also associated with increased sensitivity (collateral sensitivity) to membrane-active agents such as nonionic detergents, local anesthetics, and steroid hormones. Multidrug-resistant cells also show altered susceptibility to natural killer-cell-mediated cytotoxicity (Woods *et al.*, 1988).

It is clear that while these secondary changes do not by themselves cause multidrug resistance, they may be important in determining the overall phenotype and responses of multidrug-resistant cells. It remains a challenge to delineate the molecular basis of such changes.

III. P-Glycoprotein: Molecular Biology and Biochemistry

A. Cloning of the P-Glycoprotein Genes

The P-glycoprotein gene family has three gene classes (I, II, and III) in rodents (hamster and mouse), and two classes (I and III) in human (see Table II; Ng *et al.*, 1989). Several methods have been used to clone the P-glycoprotein genes. In hamster, P-glycoprotein-specific monoclonal antibodies were used to screen a λgt11 cDNA expression library prepared from a colchicine-resistant Chinese

Table II

P-Glycoprotein Gene Family in Human and Rodent[a]

Species	P-Glycoprotein gene classes		
	I	II	III
Hamster	*pgp1*	*pgp2*	*pgp3*
Mouse	*mdr3*	*mdr1*	*mdr2*
Human	*mdr1* (*MDR1*)	—	*mdr3* (*MDR2*)

[a] Relationships of the three hamster *pgp* genes to the mouse and human *mdr* genes are based on direct comparisons of the nucleotide sequence of their 3′ untranslated regions (Modified from Ng *et al.*, 1989).

hamster cell line (CH^R B30). A cDNA clone (pCHP1) was isolated and used as a probe to screen a second cDNA library prepared from the parental (drug-sensitive) cells (Endicott *et al.*, 1987; Riordan *et al.*, 1985). This work led to the isolation of other cDNA clones, which fell into three distinct classes based on homology in their nucleotide and protein sequences (Endicott *et al.*, 1987). The cDNA clones encoded three different classes of P-glycoprotein genes. In hamster, these are the class I (*pgp1*), class II (*pgp2*), and class III (*pgp3*) genes (Ng *et al.*, 1989). The class I and II P-glycoprotein genes are more homologous to each other than either one is to the class III genes.

Roninson *et al.* (1984) isolated a large amplified genomic DNA fragment from CH^{R}C5 and LZ/ADR hamster MDR cells using the technique of in-gel renaturation. Using this genomic probe, Gros *et al.* (1986b) isolated full-length cDNA clones from a drug-sensitive mouse pre-B cell line (BALB/c mouse cells). The human full-length cDNA sequence was isolated from KB/VLB human carcinoma cells by piecing together overlapping cDNA clones (Chen *et al.*, 1986). The sequences of the human *mdr1* and mouse *mdr1* (λDR11) genes were shown to be homologous to the hamster class I (*pgp1*) and class II (*pgp2*) genes, respectively (Endicott *et al.*, 1987). A full-length human *mdr3* gene, the homolog of the hamster class III (*pgp3*) gene was cloned from a cDNA library prepared from normal liver (Van der Bliek *et al.*, 1988).

B. MDR Expression

Initial transfection studies using genomic DNA from hamster CH^{R}C5 drug-resistant cells into drug-sensitive mouse LTA cells resulted in the transfer of the hamster P-glycoprotein gene(s) and the acquisition of the MDR phenotype (Deuchars *et al.*, 1987). Although these experiments demonstrated that the transfer and expression of an amplified P-glycoprotein gene(s) to drug-sensitive cells can result in the acquisition of the MDR phenotype, the possibility of cotransfection of other non-P-glycoprotein genes could not be entirely excluded from these studies. Gros *et al.* (1986c) provided conclusive evidence that the overexpression of a single gene product (P-glycoprotein) can confer the MDR phenotype on otherwise drug-sensitive cells. The transfection of a single full-length cDNA clone encoding the mouse *mdr1* (class II) gene isolated from mouse sensitive pre-B cells into hamster LR73 cells, and subsequent selection under nonpermissive drug concentrations, resulted in transfected cells which express the MDR phenotype. Similar results have also been obtained with the human *mdr1* cDNA (class I) gene (Ueda *et al.*, 1987). Recent studies using retrovirus expression vectors containing mouse *mdr1* or human *mdr1* (class II, and class I genes, respectively) cDNA clones demonstrate that it is possible to express the MDR phenotype in infected cells without selection in drugs (Guild *et al.*, 1988; Pastan *et al.*, 1988).

In contrast, transfection of class III full-length mouse (*mdr2*) and human (*mdr3*) cDNAs does not confer a detectable drug resistance phenotype (Gros *et al.*, 1988; P. Borst, personal communication). Analysis of the human class III transfectant clones using a monoclonal antibody that recognizes the class III gene product demonstrated the presence of P-glycoprotein by Western blotting and immunohistochemical staining (P. Borst, personal communication). In summary, experimental evidence thus far suggests that while overexpression of the class I and II *pgp* genes can confer the multidrug-resistance phenotype, overexpression of the class III gene cannot.

Southern blot analysis of genomic DNA can be used to identify the presence of P-glycoprotein gene(s) in distantly related species. For example, monkey, chicken, rabbit, and *Drosophila* all appear to have two P-glycoprotein genes. It is tempting to speculate that these members are two distinct functional classes, such as the class I and III of the human P-glycoprotein gene family (L. Veinot-Drebot and V. Ling, unpublished results). Other species contain three or more P-glycoprotein genes. For example, the P-glycoprotein gene family in pig is apparently made up of as many as five gene members. However, it is not yet known if all five genes encode functional P-glycoproteins, or whether some are pseudogenes (L. Veinot-Drebot and V. Ling, unpublished results).

The identification of P-glycoprotein-like genes in malaria parasites and yeast suggests that this protein is involved in functions that are fundamental to living systems and, thus, its structure is conserved throughout evolution. The amplification of P-glycoprotein genes in chloroquine-resistant strains of *Plasmodium falciparum* has been independently described by two groups (Foote *et al.*, 1989; Wilson *et al.*, 1989). A comparison of the amino acid sequences for these genes (*pfmdr*) and the murine *mdr1* gene (class II gene) suggests that they are homologous to the mammalian P-glycoprotein gene family. Another P-glycoprotein-like gene (*STE-6*) has been isolated from the yeast *Saccharomyces cerevisiae*, and shown to be homologous to the human *MDR1* gene (McGrath and Varshavsky, 1989). In addition it has been shown that the yeast P-glycoprotein is a transport protein involved in the export of the *a*-factor mating pheromone.

Other proteins, such as the bacterial transport proteins, have been found to share extensive homology with P-glycoprotein. These proteins include the bacterial transport proteins MalK (maltose), PstB (phosphate), HisP (histidine), HlyB (hemolysin), and ChvA (polysaccharide) (for reviews, see Ames, 1986; Endicott and Ling, 1989). The HlyB protein, which is half the length of a P-glycoprotein molecule, shares the highest degree of sequence and structural similarity to P-glycoprotein (Gros *et al.*, 1986a; Gerlach *et al.*, 1986; see Section III,C). Given the highly conserved nature of the P-glycoprotein gene family, it is possible to compare the coding and noncoding sequences for the three hamster *pgp* genes and generate a genealogy for the P-glycoprotein gene family (Ng *et al.*, 1989). It is speculated that an ancestral hemolysin B-like gene gave rise to a primitive P-glycoprotein gene by a gene duplication event. The primitive P-glycoprotein gene in turn was duplicated to give rise to two homologous P-glycoprotein genes: classes I and III. In rodents, however, the class I gene underwent a second gene duplication event to give rise to the class I and II isoforms.

In summary, it appears that P-glycoprotein arose early in evolution and has been conserved in diverse organisms. Although its normal function is currently not known, the different isoforms are likely to have different roles. The structural conservation of these membrane transport proteins suggests a function of fundamental importance.

C. P-Glycoprotein Structure–Function

An analysis of the amino acid sequences encoded by P-glycoprotein cDNA clones reveals that P-glycoprotein is made up of two tandemly duplicated halves, separated by a stretch of 60 amino acids (see Fig. 2). Each half of P-glycoprotein is divided into two domains, consisting of a hydrophobic and a hydrophilic region. The sequence of the hydrophobic domain encodes six putative transmembrane regions, while the hydrophilic domain contains a consensus sequence for an ATP-binding motif (Fig. 2) (Gros *et al.*, 1986a; Chen *et al.*, 1986; Gerlach *et al.*, 1986). Indirect immunofluorescence staining of MDR cells with monoclonal antibodies against different epitopes has localized the hydrophilic ATP-binding domain to the cytoplasmic side of the plasma membrane (Kartner *et al.*, 1985).

Biochemical evidence in support of the existence of the predicted ATP binding domains has come from photoaffinity cross-linking experiments using an analog of ATP, 8-azido-[α^{32}P]ATP. P-Glycoprotein cross-linked to 8-azido-[α-^{32}P]ATP *in vitro* can be immunoprecipitated with the P-glycoprotein-specific monoclonal antibodies MRK-16 and C219 (Cornwell *et al.*, 1987; Schurr *et al.* 1989; E. Georges and V. Ling, unpublished results). In addition, a low level of ATPase activity can be detected in immunopurified P-glycoprotein from K562/ADM human MDR cells (Hamada and Tsuruo, 1988). Recent transfection studies have shown that full-length mouse *mdr1* (class II) and human *mdr1* (class I) genes containing a single point mutation in either one of the ATP binding domains do not confer the MDR phenotype, suggesting that both domains may be required for P-glycoprotein function (Rothenberg and Ling, 1989).

The role of P-glycoprotein as an energy-dependent efflux pump has been proposed from its structural homology to the bacterial transport proteins, particularly HlyB (Gerlach *et al.*, 1986; Gros *et al.*, 1986a). However, unlike most other bacterial and eukaryotic transport proteins, P-glycoprotein exhibits very broad substrate specificity. Attempts to reconcile the cross-resistance phenotype, characteristic of MDR cells, with the role of P-glycoprotein as an efflux pump have led to a proposal that P-glycoprotein transports a carrier molecule with

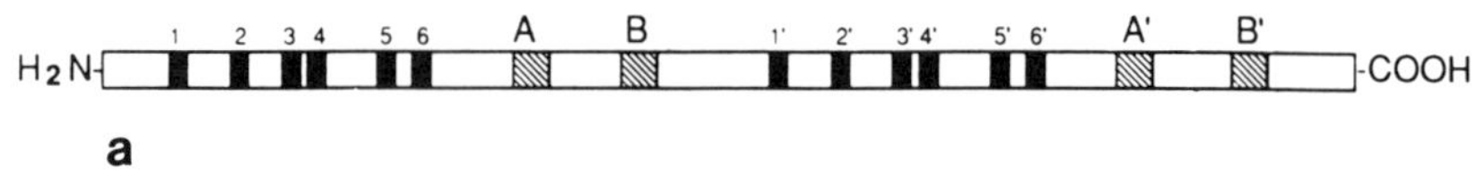

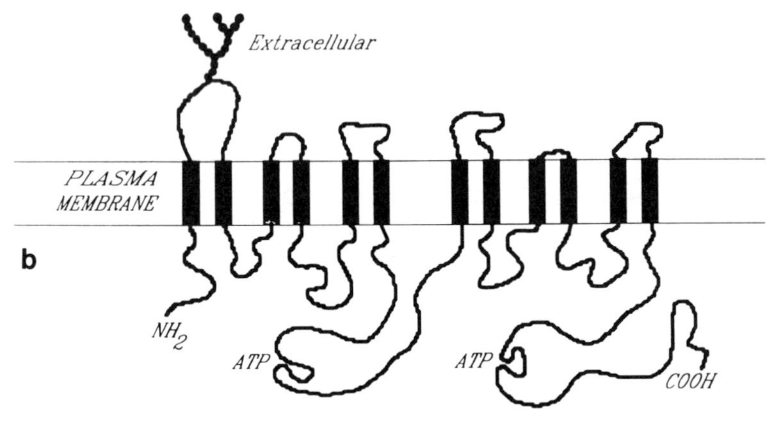

Fig. 2 A schematic model of the P-glycoprotein molecule. The solid boxes represent the 12 putative transmembrane domains in P-glycoprotein (a). The two ATP binding domains are located in the large cytoplasmic domains indicated here by shaded boxes, lettered A and B (a). The site(s) of N-linked oligosaccharides chains, represented by the solid circles, are found on the first extracellular domain from the N terminus (b). The schematic drawing shows proposed orientation of P-glycoprotein in the plasma membrane of cells (b). This model is based on the compiled sequence information for the human, hamster, and mouse P-glycoprotein genes, see text.

multiple drug binding sites (Gerlach *et al.*, 1986). Although this hypothesis appears plausible, no experimental evidence in favor of a carrier protein(s) has been reported to date. In contrast, evidence for the direct binding of anthracyclines to P-glycoprotein *in vitro* has been presented (Cornwell *et al.*, 1986), as will be detailed below. Thus, it appears that anticancer drugs effluxed by MDR cells are transported by direct interaction with P-glycoprotein. At present, it is not understood how a limited number of P-glycoprotein isoforms can mediate the efflux of many structurally unrelated drugs. However, a number of mechanisms have been suggested.

One mechanism involves mutations in the P-glycoprotein sequence which may lead to a subtle or gross change in the drug binding pattern. A spontaneous point mutation in the human *mdr1* (class I) gene has been proposed as a possible mechanism to account for a difference in the cross-resistance pattern of human KB MDR cells (Choi *et al.*, 1988). In this study, two MDR cell lines were separately derived from wild-type human KB cells by selection with either colchicine or vinblastine. These mutant lines both displayed a high level of resistance toward the selecting agent and a lower level of cross-resistance toward the other drug. Analysis of the *mdr1* (class I) cDNA from each cell line revealed that a spontaneous point mutation had occurred at position 185 of the amino acid sequence of P-glycoprotein in the colchicine-selected line. The *mdr1* gene from the colchicine-selected mutant contained valine at position 185, while the vinblastine-selected cells contained a glycine at this position. Transfection studies using the cDNA clones encoding either valine or glycine resulted in transfectant cells with higher levels of resistance to colchicine or vinblastine, respectively (Choi *et al.*, 1988). It is not yet possible to determine whether such a mechanism can account for all of the observed variability in cross-resistance patterns seen in MDR cells. However, the identification of other point mutations in P-glycoprotein may allow for a better understanding of what role such mutations may play in determining the cross-resistance pattern.

An alternative mechanism for generating structurally and functionally altered forms of P-glycoprotein may result from differential splicing of P-glycoprotein mRNAs. Van der Bliek *et al.* (1987) described the isolation of two altered class III cDNA clones from normal human liver and from HepG2 cells in addition to a "wild-type" sequence. The altered clones contained either an insertion of 7 amino acid residues in the cytoplasmic ATP binding domain, or a deletion of 21 amino acid residues corresponding to the fifth putative transmembrane domain in the C-terminal half of P-glycoprotein. However, no experimental data are presently available as to how such amino acid deletions or insertions might affect the cross-resistance pattern of MDR cells. To date, no evidence has been reported of similar deletions or insertions in P-glycoprotein genes isolated from MDR cells selected *in vitro*. Thus, further studies are needed to determine the role of such genetic alterations in the MDR phenotype.

In summary, P-glycoprotein has structural features compatible with a pore-forming protein that may function as a drug-efflux pump in MDR cells (Fig. 2). It appears that drugs effluxed by MDR cells do so by interacting directly with P-glycoprotein. The basis for the broad substrate specificity of P-glycoprotein is not presently understood; however, there has been a suggestion that certain alterations in the amino acid sequence of P-glycoprotein may modulate the cross-resistance phenotype. These regions may represent drug binding domains.

D. Posttranslational Modification of P-Glycoprotein

Biochemical analysis has demonstrated that P-glycoprotein is highly glycosylated, with carbohydrates accounting for approximately 20–40 kDa of its apparent molecular mass (Kartner *et al.*, 1985; Greenberger *et al.*, 1987, 1988). The drug resistance patterns of MDR cells have been examined under conditions that

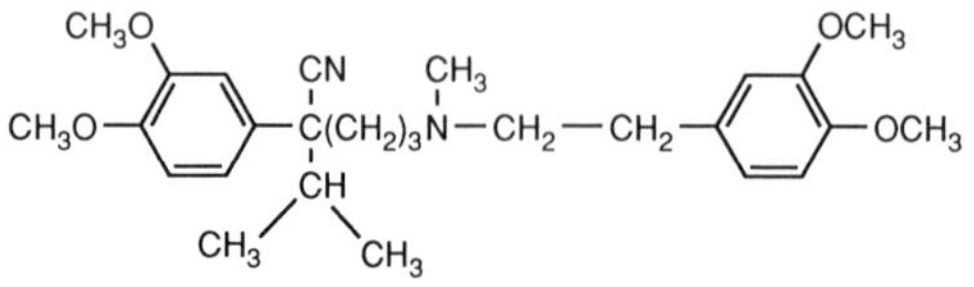

Verapamil

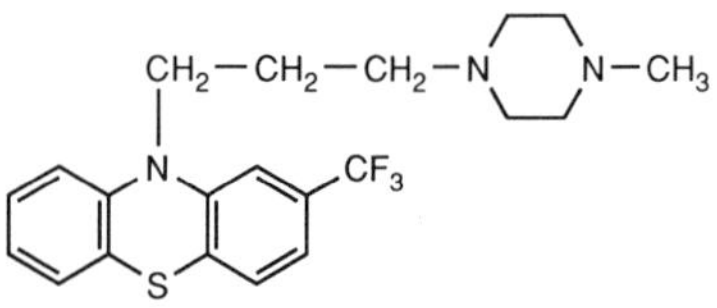

Trifluoperazine

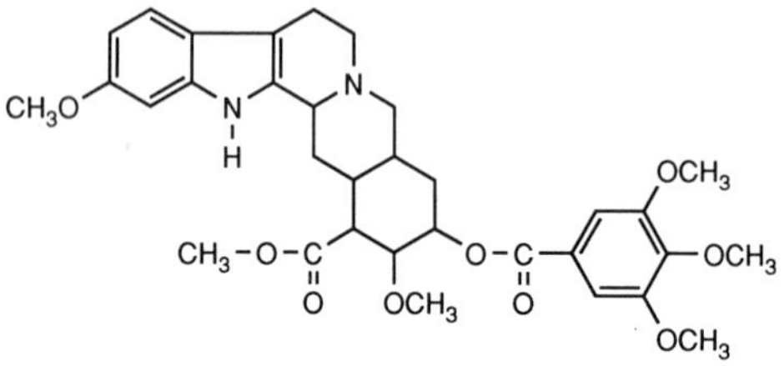

Reserpine

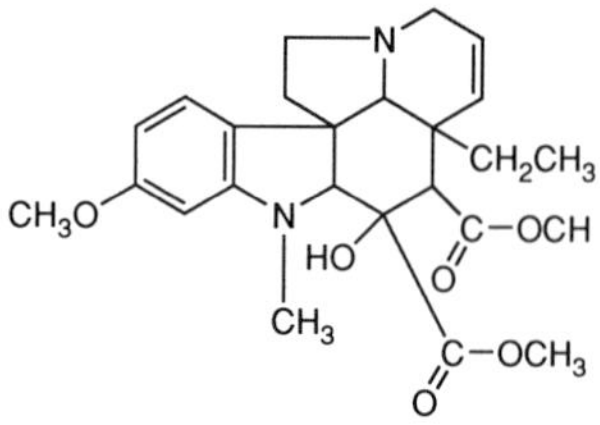

Vindoline

Fig. 3 The molecular structures of the chemosensitizing agents verapamil, trifluoperazine, reserpine, and vindoline.

modulate the glycosylation of cellular glycoproteins. The loss of the oligosaccharide moieties from P-glycoprotein occurs when drug-resistant cells are grown in the presence of tunicamycin (Beck and Cirtain, 1982), and a glycosylation-deficient mutant cell line has been selected by growing drug-resistant CH^RC5 cells in the presence of *Phaseolus vulgaris* phytohemagglutinin (Ling *et al.*, 1983). In both cases, the drug resistance pattern was not affected, suggesting that the oligosaccharide chains of P-glycoprotein are not directly involved in the expression of drug resistance.

P-Glycoprotein is phosphorylated *in vivo* at serine residues in mouse, human, and hamster MDR cells (Hamada *et al.*, 1987; Schurr *et al.*, 1989; E. Georges and V. Ling, unpublished observations). Drug-resistant cells incubated in the presence of agents known to modulate the MDR phenotype show changes in the sites and extent of P-glycoprotein phosphorylation. The phosphorylation level of P-glycoprotein has been shown to increase in the presence of agents that stimulate the activities of protein kinases A and C, or Ca^{2+}/calmodulin-dependent protein kinase (Hamada *et al.*, 1987; Nishizuka, 1984). For example, P-glycoprotein is hyperphosphorylated in the presence of either forskolin, phorbol esters, verapamil, or trifluoperazine. It is not clear whether the phosphorylation level of P-glycoprotein is increased through a direct interaction with these agents, or by the activation/inhibition of specific kinase/phosphatase proteins. Further work is required to clarify the effect of this posttranslational modification on the function of P-glycoprotein. It is not known whether phosphorylation is important in determining the cross-resistance patterns of MDR cells.

IV. *In Vitro* Chemosensitization of MDR Cells

A. Observation of Chemosensitization

A diverse group of structurally dissimilar compounds is capable of sensitizing resistant cells to multiple drugs *in vitro*. These compounds include Ca^{2+}-channel blockers, calmodulin inhibitors, cyclosporin A, quinidine, and noncytotoxic drug analogs (see Fig. 3). The process by which these agents circumvent multidrug resistance is referred to as pharmacological chemosensitization.

In the presence of increasing concentrations of a chemosensitizer such as verapamil, drug cytotoxicity is greatly potentiated in drug-resistant lines. The IC_{50} under these conditions will often approach that of drug-sensitive cells. The *in vitro* sensitization of resistant cells by verapamil was shown to result in an increased drug accumulation in P388/VCR cells (Tsuruo, 1983). Similar observations were made with daunorubicin-resistant Ehrlich ascites carcinomas (Slater *et al.*, 1982), and in adriamycin-resistant ovarian human cancer cell lines (Ozols, 1985). It is generally observed that Ca^{2+}-channel antagonists at nontoxic levels can completely sensitize tumor cell lines that are moderately resistant (3- to 10-fold resistance) to cytotoxic drugs, while only a partial reversal is observed in highly resistant cells (150-fold resistance) (Tsuruo *et al.*, 1985).

The ability of chemosensitizers to potentiate drug toxicity varies for different drugs. Verapamil at a given concentration was observed to reverse resistance to *Vinca* alkaloids selectively, but not resistance to anthracyclines, colchicine, or epipodophyllotoxins in multidrug-resistant human leukemic lymphoblasts (Beck *et al.*, 1986; Tsuruo *et al.*, 1983a). A similar observation was reported in human sarcoma cells (Harker *et al.*, 1986). In a colchicine-resistant CHO cell line, the accumulation of daunomycin and vinblastine was enhanced by verapamil, while that of colchicine was effectively unchanged even at high concentrations of chemosensitizer (Cano-Gauci and Riordan, 1987). The basis for this differential sensitization of cells is not understood.

Chemosensitizing agents that modulate drug resistance can be used to identify P-glycoprotein-associated MDR in nonmammalian cells. For instance, the drug-resistant strain of the malaria parasite *Plasmodium falciparum* was shown to respond to chloroquine in the presence of verapamil or desipramine (Bitonti *et al.*, 1988; Martin *et al.*, 1987). These results suggested the presence of a similar mechanism responsible for the multidrug resistance of these malaria strains, and predicted the presence of a P-glycoprotein-like gene prior to the cloning of the *pfmdr* genes (Foote *et al.*, 1989; Wilson *et al.*, 1989).

1. Drug Transport

Multidrug-resistant cells display altered drug transport properties relative to the parent line. The resistant cells show very rapid drug efflux with a half-time on the order of a minute or less, while sensitive cells display very low rates of efflux, often retaining drugs for periods of several hours. The level of drug accumulation is often inversely correlated with the degree of drug resistance. Unfortunately, because of the complexity of the system, it is very difficult to measure the kinetics of drug transport directly in intact cells. Processes such as "instantaneous" adsorption of drug to the cell surface, intracellular drug metabolism, binding to intracellular targets, and intracellular sequestration of drug make it virtually impossible to estimate the intracellular free drug concentration, or the initial rates of drug influx/efflux across the plasma membrane (Riordan and Ling, 1985). Thus, most investigators have measured the time course of the total cellular drug accumulation, using either radiolabeled or autofluorescent compounds. Drug accumulation can follow linear or nonlinear kinetics, and is usually concentration-dependent, so that studies of this type carried out in different laboratories under different conditions may be difficult to compare directly.

Both radiolabeled and fluorescent drugs can be used to quantitate drug efflux. The anthracycline class of compounds is fluorescent, and both single-cell photometry and flow cytometry have been used to quantitate their accumulation (Krishan *et al.*, 1986; Willingham *et al.*, 1986). These methods have the advantage of being rapid, and they can be used for analyzing the kinetics and extent of drug uptake in individual intact cells. Fluorescence microscopy can also be used to examine the intracellular compartmentalization of drug. However, fluorescence measurements of this type suffer from the disadvantage that they do not measure nonfluorescent drug metabolites and that quenching of drug fluorescence may occur following binding to intracellular targets. The nuclear accumulation of fluorescence resulting from anthracycline uptake was found to be low in drug-resistant lines when compared to sensitive cells, but was greatly increased by the presence of 10 μM verapamil (Willingham *et al.*, 1986).

Certain intracellular stains and vital dyes also appear to use a P-glycoprotein-mediated efflux mechanism. Colchicine-resistant CHO sublines showed reduced nuclear fluorescence relative to wild-type cells after staining with the DNA-binding fluorescent dye Hoechst 33342 (Lalande *et al.*, 1981). Dye retention could be increased to wild-type levels by treatment with chemosensitizers such as trifluoperazine or verapamil. Rhodamine-123 also appears to be effluxed by P-glycoprotein (Lampidis *et al.*, 1985). For example, multidrug-resistant cells incubated with rhodamine-123 effluxed the dye within a few minutes after transfer to drug-free media. In contrast, loss of rhodamine-123 from drug-sensitive cells took place over several hours. Interestingly, P-glycoprotein may efflux both rhodamine-123 and phosphine-3R (an acridine dye that stains nuclei) in drug-sensitive cells. Treatment of various nominally drug-sensitive cell lines, including hamster and mouse fibroblasts, with verapamil, trifluoperazine or reserpine blocked the slow efflux of both dyes by 60–80% (Neyfakh *et al.*, 1988). These cell lines are likely to contain low levels of P-glycoprotein (Kartner *et al.*, 1985). Thus, structurally dissimilar dye molecules appear to be transported by the P-glycoprotein efflux pump in both drug-sensitive and -resistant cells. The use of dyes that are effluxed by P-glycoprotein may provide a useful means for rapid screening of new chemosensitizing agents.

It has been suggested that chemosensitizing agents may also be substrates for the P-glycoprotein-mediated efflux system. Cano-Gauci and Riordan (1987) measured the uptake of [^{3}H]verapamil by resistant and sensitive CHO cell lines, and found that it showed the same pattern as the uptake of anticancer drugs. At 1 μM verapamil, resistant cells accumulated almost none of the compound intracellularly, while sensitive cells showed much greater uptake. Likewise, the accumulation of the chemosensitizer cyclosporin A by colchicine-resistant CHO cells was reduced relative to that of sensitive cells. Cyclosporin levels in resistant cells could be increased by treatment with verapamil (Goldberg *et al.*, 1988). Thus the cellular accumulation of chemosensitizers may be controlled, at least in part, by their interaction with P-glycoprotein.

Although metabolic inhibitors can arrest the efflux of cytotoxic drugs from MDR cells, the role of ATP binding and/or hydrolysis in this process is not understood in detail. Using radiolabeled vinblastine, increased drug binding to membrane vesicles isolated from KB/VBL MDR cells was observed when compared to vesicles prepared from the parent drug-sensitive cells (Cornwell *et al.*, 1986). A later study (Naito *et al.*, 1988) confirmed this result, and demonstrated that drug binding was dependent on the presence of ATP (Naito *et al.*, 1988). Some binding was also observed in the presence of GTP, while no increase in drug binding was seen when exogenous ADP or adenosine 5′-O-(3-thio) triphosphate was added. These results suggest that ATP hydrolysis is required for drug binding. Drug-resistant cells have a marked increase in cellular ATP consumption (Broxterman *et al.*, 1988b). This increase is verapamil inducible, and saturates at 1 μM of verapamil. Verapamil has also recently been shown to stimulate the ATPase activity associated with P-glycoprotein immunopurified from K652/ADM cells (Naito and Tsuruo, 1989). These results suggest that the concentration of verapamil, and possibly other cytotoxic drugs in the cell, is maintained at low levels at the expense of ATP hydrolysis.

In summary, the accumulated results from drug transport studies using whole cells have suggested that drug-resistant cells accumulate less cytotoxic drugs than parental lines, presumably because of an enhanced energy-dependent drug-efflux mechanism. However, further analysis of this mechanism in whole cells is difficult. A simpler transport system consisting of membrane vesicles or a reconstituted system is needed. To date, only two transport studies have been reported using membrane vesicles. Horio *et al.* (1988) have demonstrated an ATP-dependent drug transport using membrane vesicles from KB/VCR cells. A more recent study using inside-out membrane vesicles isolated from normal liver, which expresses relatively high levels of P-glycoprotein (see Section V,A), has also demonstrated ATP-dependent drug transport that can be inhibited by verapamil (Kamimoto *et al.*, 1989).

2. Verapamil Hypersensitivity

Some multidrug-resistant cell lines display greater susceptibility to verapamil cytotoxicity, i.e., they are collaterally sensitive to verapamil. For example, a drug-sensitive CHO cell line grew successfully in 80 μM verapamil, while concentrations as low as 2 μM were cytotoxic to multidrug-resistant clones (Cano-Gauci and Riordan, 1987). This result is remarkable, since the drug-resistant clones accumulated greatly reduced amounts of verapamil. It was suggested that this cytotoxic effect of verapamil, which is also a property of other Ca^{2+}-channel blockers, may be due to a direct interaction with the cell surface. Warr *et al.* (1988) reported that two MDR CHO lines selected with vincristine were 100-fold more sensitive to the cytotoxic effects of verapamil than the parent line. Reversion of vincristine resistance was correlated with reversion of verapamil hypersensitivity, suggesting a common underlying mechanism. The drug-resistant cells were also highly hypersensitive to other Ca^{2+}-channel blockers such as diltiazem and nicardipine, and were moderately hypersensitive to quinidine. Verapamil hypersensitivity has also been reported for a multidrug-resistant small cell lung cancer line (Twentyman *et al.*, 1986). However, not all MDR cell lines show this type of response to verapamil. For example, resistant CCRF/CEM cells show only a slight inhibition of cell growth at 10 μM verapamil (Beck, 1984). Schmidt and co-workers (1988) demonstrated that verapamil, in a dose-dependent fashion, rapidly and reversibly inhibits the proliferation of a variety of brain tumor cell lines. The concentration of verapamil (100 μM) required to inhibit cell growth completely was about 100-fold higher than that needed to enhance the toxicity of anti-cancer drugs. The cytotoxic and antiproliferative effects of verapamil on multidrug-resistant lines and tumor cells appear to be unrelated to its ability to block Ca^{2+} channels.

It should be noted that, although there is a link between the ability of chemosensitizers to reverse drug resistance and their ability to increase cellular drug accumulation, in many cases enhanced drug retention alone may not fully explain their effects. For example, in mouse L1210 leukemia cells with less than 50-fold levels of resistance, the large increase in doxorubicin cytotoxicity in combination with trifluoperazine could not be accounted for by either the modest increase in intracellular drug levels or the small changes in drug efflux (Ganapathi and Grabowski, 1988). The chemosensitizing potency of verapamil also did not correlate well with intracellular accumulation of doxorubicin in a resistant human sarcoma cell line (Harker *et al.*, 1986). Cyclosporin A completely reverses both primary resistance to vincristine and cross-resistance to daunorubicin in human T-ALL cells, without apparently changing either the measured uptake or efflux of the drug (Slater *et al.*, 1986).

The subcellular distribution of anthracyclines appears to be different in resistant and sensitive HL-60 cells. Drug accumulates in an intralysosomal compartment in the former, and is homogeneously distributed in the latter (Hindenburg *et al.*, 1987). Verapamil appears to alter the subcellular distribution of these compounds, changing it from the punctate pattern normally observed in resistant cells to the diffuse pattern seen for sensitive cells. These observations have led to the suggestion that part of verapamil's chemosensitizing action on resistant cells may lie in its ability to modify the subcellular drug distribution. It is not known, however, whether P-glycoprotein has a direct role in determining the subcellular drug distribution.

B. Molecular Basis for Chemosensitization

Ideally, chemosensitizers are noncytotoxic compounds that completely reverse the resistance of MDR cells to the cytotoxic action of anticancer drugs. Several classes of compounds have been identified which meet the above criteria. These include noncytotoxic drug analogs, Ca^{2+}-channel blockers, calmodulin inhibitors, lysosomotropic agents, and cyclosporin A. The molecular basis of chemosensitization is generally not well understood. However, competition experiments using cytotoxic drugs and reversing agents suggest a possible mechanism in which they directly compete for one or more drug binding sites on P-glycoprotein. Evidence for direct interaction between P-glycoprotein and cytotoxic drugs has come from the use of photoaffinity analogs of anthracycline and vinblastine (Safa *et al.*, 1986). Two photoactive radioactive analogs of vinblastine, *N*-(*p*-azido-3,5-[^{3}H]benzoyl)-*N*′-β-aminoethyl vindesine and *N*-(*p*-azido-3-[^{125}I]salicyl)-*N*′-β-aminoethyl vindesine (^{125}I-NASV), labeled P-glycoprotein in plasma membrane vesicles from MDR cell lines (Cornwell *et al.*, 1986; Safa *et al.*, 1986). A dose-dependent inhibition of P-glycoprotein photolabeling was demonstrated with vinblastine, vincristine, and verapamil but not with colchicine or dexamethasone. The capacity of various compounds to reverse the MDR phenotype was compared to their ability to inhibit the photoaffinity labeling of P-glycoprotein by ^{125}I-NASV (Akiyama *et al.*, 1988). This study suggested that many, but not all, reversing agents can inhibit the photolabeling of P-glycoprotein by ^{125}I-NASV. Thus, it may be possible to use a photoaffinity labeling inhibition assay similar to that used by Akiyama *et al.* (1988) to mass screen for reversing agents of the MDR phenotype.

The physicochemical properties of compounds that modulate the MDR phenotype were examined by Zamora *et al.* (1988) to determine if there are any common features shared by these chemosensitizing agents. It was concluded that general properties such as lipid solubility at physiological pH, cationic charge, and similar values of molar refractivity (which reflects the fundamental property of molecular volume) are common to these reversing agents. The recent study by Pearce *et al.* (1989) extended the above conclusion. They suggested that substructural domains (a basic nitrogen atom and two planar aromatic rings) may be common features of many chemosensitizing agents. Experiments using analogs of reserpine and yohimbine containing these well-defined substructural domains suggested that the relative disposition of these domains correlates with their capacity to reverse MDR and compete with ^{125}I-NASV for binding to P-glycoprotein.

In summary, although the prediction of physicochemical commonalities, such as lipid solubility and cationic charge, is in agreement with other independent studies (Burke *et al.*, 1988), they are insufficient to explain the mechanism by which some very effective chemosensitizing agents (e.g., cyclosporin A) reverse the MDR phenotype. It is possible that different classes of chemosensitizers may differ in their mechanisms of action.

1. Drug Analogs

The initial use of these compounds as chemosensitizers was based on the hypothesis that noncytotoxic drug analogs may be substrates for the drug-efflux system found in resistant cells. Thus, by competing for a similar binding site(s) on P-glycoprotein, they could lead to an increase in the accumulation of cytotoxic drugs. *N*-Acetyldaunorubicin (*N*-acetyl-DNR), a noncytotoxic analog of daunorubicin (DNR), was used to potentiate the cytotoxicity of daunorubicin in resistant tumor cell lines (Skovsgaard, 1980). When both DNR and *N*-acetyl-DNR were added to Ehrlich ascites tumor cells the active efflux of DNR was greatly reduced. Later studies with a larger number of noncytotoxic analogs of anthracyclines and *Vinca* alkaloids (Inaba *et al.*, 1984) have demonstrated a similar effect on drug accumulation and efflux in P388/ADR and P388/VCR resistant leukemic cells. Three synthetic anthracycline analogs were shown to potentiate the activity of vincristine and doxorubicin on resistant cells *in vitro*. Similarly, six natural analogs of the *Vinca* alkaloids were found to potentiate the effect of vincristine and doxorubicin on resistant P388 leukemic cells (Inaba and Nagashima, 1986). These studies also determined that the effective concentration of the *Vinca* alkaloid analogs (10 μg/ml) is greater than that of the *N*-acetyl-DNR (1 μg/ml) analogs, suggesting that the latter group of compounds may be more effective competitors. These results show that more systematic work is required to identify the most effective drug analogs.

2. Calcium Channel Blockers

The inhibitory effect of this group of compounds on the calcium channel in muscle fibers *in vitro* and *in vivo* is well documented (Ferry *et al.*, 1985; Garcia *et al.*, 1986; Snyder and Reynolds, 1985). However, the exact molecular mechanism by which these agents exert their effects on calcium channels has not yet been defined. Tsuruo *et al.* (1981) reported the sensitization of MDR P388 leukemic cells to vinblastine when the cells were simultaneously incubated with both vinblastine and verapamil (a class II calcium channel blocker). Verapamil caused a reversal in the MDR phenotype *in vitro* in P388/VCR leukemic cells, and *in vivo* in daunorubicin-resistant Ehrlich ascites tumor cells. Kessel and Wilberding (1985), using tiapamil and its analogs (tiapamil is related to verapamil), have identified compounds that are 10-fold more effective than verapamil at potentiating anthracycline (e.g., daunorubicin) accumulation in P388/ADR cells. One of the tiapamil analogs at a concentration of 0.8 μM was able to reverse daunorubicin resistance completely in P388/ADR cells, while a concentration of 2–6 μM verapamil was necessary to produce the same effect. This study indicates that the ability of these analogs to sensitize MDR cells does not necessarily correlate with their ability to block the calcium channel.

Both direct and indirect evidence suggests that the effect of verapamil on MDR cells is distinct from its previously established role as a calcium channel blocker. The demonstration that both D and L enantiomers of verapamil are equally effective in reversing drug resistance and increasing cellular accumulation of vincristine in leukemic cells (Gruber *et al.*, 1988) is in contrast to the stereospecific interaction of only L-verapamil with the calcium channel receptor (Triggle and Swamy, 1983; Echizen *et al.*, 1985). Furthermore, the mode of action of verapamil on MDR cells has been shown to be independent of calcium ion transport (Gruber *et al.*, 1988; Kessel and Wilberding, 1985). An independent study using whole cells and the single channel patch–clamp technique supported this conclusion (Lee *et al.*, 1988). No significant differences in the type and number of ion channels in MDR and parental T cell leukemia clones were found. Furthermore, sensitive CEM and resistant CEM/VLB_{100} cells have no measurable calcium channels. Thus, it is not immediately obvious how verapamil exerts its chemosensitizing effect on these cells. One possibility is that verapamil directly interacts with a membrane component at the cell surface, presumably P-glycoprotein. Evidence in support of this possibility has been obtained by direct labeling of P-glycoprotein with photoactive analogs of verapamil, *N*-(*p*-azido[3,5-^{3}H]benzoyl)aminomethyl verapamil and *N*-(*p*-azido[3-^{125}I]salicyl)aminomethyl verapamil) (Safa, 1988). The two verapamil analogs were shown to cross-link covalently to P-glycoprotein in plasma membrane vesicles isolated from vincristine-resistant KB cells (Safa, 1988). The labeling of P-glycoprotein with a photoactive verapamil derivative could be inhibited competitively by *Vinca* alkaloids (e.g., vinblastine) and anthracyclines (e.g., daunorubicin), as well as a large number of calcium antagonists (see Table III).

The class I calcium channel antagonist azidopine (1,4-dihydropyridine arylazide) has also been shown to interact with P-glycoprotein in plasma membrane isolated from drug-resistant cells (Safa *et al.*, 1987). Azidopine photolabeled the 150 to 180-kDa P-glycoprotein band in plasma membranes isolated from DC-3F/VCRd-5L and DC-3F/ADX cells. This labeling was completely inhibited by excess verapamil, other calcium channel antagonists, and vinblastine. No inhibition of azidopine labeling was observed when excess molar concentrations of doxorubicin, colchicine, and methotrexate were present. Other

Table III

Chemosensitizing Agents and Interaction with P-Glycoprotein

Sensitization of MDR cells	Binding to P-Glycoprotein	References
Calcium antagonists		
Verapamil	[a]	Safa (1988)
Azidopine	[a]	Safa *et al.* (1987)
Tiapamils	nd[b]	Kessel and Wilberding (1985)
Calmodulin antagonists		
Trifluoperazine	[c]	Akiyama *et al.* (1988)
Chlorpromazine	[c]	Akiyama *et al.* (1988)
Lysosomotropic agents		
Chloroquine	[c]	Beck *et al.* (1988)
Triton WR-1339	nd	Klohs and Steinkampe (1988a)
Drug analogs		
Vindoline	nd	Inaba and Nagashima (1986)
Anthracycline analogs (ID-8279)	nd	Inaba *et al.* (1984)
Other compounds		
Cyclosporins	[a]	Foxwell *et al.* (1989)
Progesterone	[d]	Yang *et al.* (1989)
Reserpine	[c]	Akiyama *et al.* (1988)
AHC-52	nd	Shinoda *et al.* (1989)
SDB-ethylenediamine	[c]	Akiyama *et al.* (1988)
Quinidine	[c]	Cornwell *et al.* (1987)

[a] Direct binding of photoactive analogs with P-glycoprotein.

[b] nd, Not determined.

[c] Indirect binding, compete with ^{125}I-NASV for binding to P-glycoprotein.

[d] Indirect binding, compete with [$^{3+}$H]azidopine for binding to P-glycoprotein.

studies have demonstrated the azidopine labeling of a 130 to 150-kDa membrane glycoprotein (P-glycoprotein) in murine J774.2/Col, J774.2/VLB, and taxol-resistant cell lines (Yang *et al.*, 1988). Labeling was inhibited in the presence of excess amounts (1000 μM) of some classes of calcium antagonists, while other calcium antagonists showed a stimulatory effect (25–50%). A number of steroids have been identified as possible chemosensitizers by their ability to compete with azidopine photolabeling of P-glycoprotein (Yang *et al.*, 1989). These include dexamethasone, hydrocortisone, testosterone, and progesterone. In this group, progesterone was most effective in reversing the MDR phenotype and it showed the greatest ability to inhibit photolabeling of P-glycoprotein by azidopine. It was also suggested that among these selected steroids the degree of their inhibition of azidopine photolabeling correlated with their hydrophobicity index (Yang *et al.*, 1989). A recent study by Nogae (1989) aimed to determine the structural features of 1,4-dihydropyridine which are important in the reversal of MDR. Dihydropyridine analogs were examined for (1) their ability to inhibit vincristine efflux in drug-resistant cells, and (2) inhibition of P-glycoprotein photolabeling by ^{125}I-NASV. Although it was not possible to determine the precise structural moiety(ies) essential for their interaction with P-glycoprotein, there was a correlation between the reversal of drug resistance and the inhibition of photolabeling.

Efforts to determine the azidopine binding domain on P-glycoprotein have resulted in the identification of one, or possibly two, major tryptic fragments that contain the majority of the azidopine label (Yang *et al.*, 1988). Thus, only a limited number of sites on P-glycoprotein interact with azidopine. One may speculate that other drugs that can compete with azidopine for labeling of P-glycoprotein are likely to interact with such a site(s) (directly or indirectly). It is noteworthy that while this approach may be useful in identifying the peptide sequence that is cross-linked to the azido group of the photoaffinity ligand, the actual drug binding domain may be distant from this labeled peptide. The labeling of a particular peptide region with azidopine in itself does not identify the actual drug binding site (Glossmann *et al.*, 1987).

3. Lysosomotropic Agents

Certain membrane-active agents, especially lysosomotropic species, are able to chemosensitize multidrug-resistant cells. The detergent Triton WR-1339 accumulates preferentially in the lysosomes and may also interfere with exocytosis. Klohs and Steinkampf (1988a) have shown that this detergent can increase the cytotoxicity and accumulation of doxorubicin, and block drug efflux in murine leukemic P388 cells. At nontoxic concentrations, Triton WR-1339 was as effective as verapamil. Other membrane-active agents at equivalent concentrations, such as the detergent deoxycholate and the pore-forming polyene antibiotics filipin and amphotericin B, had no effect on cytotoxicity, drug uptake, or efflux. Thus, the ability of agents to interact with the plasma membrane is not by itself sufficient for chemosensitization.

Increased rates of plasma membrane traffic (exo- and endocytosis) and a large increase in the size of the endosomal compartment have been shown to be features of multidrug-resistant Ehrlich ascites and P388 leukemia cells (Sehested *et al.*, 1987a,b). The proton ionophores monensin and nigericin block drug efflux from these cells, and also prove to be highly effective chemosensitizers of multidrug resistance (Sehested *et al.*, 1988). These ionophores are known to increase the pH of acidic intracellular compartments, disrupt vesicular traffic, and inhibit the secretion of proteins from the cell. On the other hand, permeant amines such as ammonium chloride and methylamine, which only produce changes in intravesicular pH, have no effect on drug accumulation or efflux. Thus the same agents that potentiate drug cytotoxicity and inhibit efflux also block secretion, suggesting that the primary effect of the ionophore chemosensitizers may be at the level of exocytosis and secretion. It has been proposed that weakly basic drugs such as doxorubicin and vinblastine become trapped by protonation in acidic compartments, perhaps the lysosomes or the vesicles of the trans-Golgi network. Migration of these drug-loaded vesicles to the plasma membrane, followed by fusion, could lead to drug efflux (Beck, 1987). Verapamil has also been shown to inhibit plasma membrane traffic significantly in resistant Ehrlich ascites tumor cells (Sehested *et al.*, 1987a), raising the possibility that this chemosensitizer may act, at least in part, at the level of increasing endosomal drug trapping and decreasing vesicle exocytosis. This suggests a new mechanism for drug efflux which utilizes membrane vesicles as vehicles for extruding cytotoxic drugs. It is not clear what role P-glycoprotein would play in this process. However, it may be speculated that P-glycoprotein acts as an influx pump, concentrating cytotoxic drugs into vesicles of the endoplasmic reticulum (ER) which are destined to the plasma membrane for exocytosis. Alternatively, P-glycoprotein may be a recognition site for vesicle fusion on the plasma membrane.

4. Calmodulin Antagonists

Calmodulin antagonists represent a group of antipsychotic drugs and related compounds which bind to calmodulin in a calcium-dependent manner (Hait and DeRosa, 1988). Some of these drugs (e.g., trifuoperazine, prenylamine, and clomipramine), though not the most potent calmodulin antagonists, can increase the cytotoxic effects of vincristine and doxorubicin on MDR cells (Tsuruo *et al.*, 1982, 1983b). Chemosensitization of P388/VCR and K562/DOX leukemic cells *in vitro* by calmodulin inhibitors caused an increase in drug accumulation which was presumed to be due to the inhibition of drug efflux (Tsuruo *et al.*, 1983b; Ganapathi and Grabowski, 1983; Ganapathi *et al.*, 1984).

It is of interest that phenothiazine calmodulin inhibitors accumulate in the brain, whereas most cytotoxic drugs cannot pass through the blood–brain barrier. Given this property of calmodulin inhibitors, a recent review on the use of calmodulin as a target for chemotherapy has suggested the use of trifluoperazine in combination with bleomycin in the treatment of malignant astrocytomas (Hait, 1985).

Calmodulin inhibitors are generally highly toxic at the levels required to show a complete reversal of the MDR phenotype. This may be due to the number of cellular events mediated by calmodulin (see review by Hait, 1985). Rhodamine-123, a calmodulin antagonist (Hait and DeRosa, 1988) which accumulates in the mitochondria of sensitive cells, is rapidly effluxed from resistant cells (see Section IV,A,1, above), probably through the P-glycoprotein pump. However, it is not known whether all calmodulin inhibitors sensitize MDR cells by interacting directly with P-glycoprotein. Further work with calmodulin antagonists and their analogs may identify mechanisms of chemosensitization other than that mediated by the direct interaction of drugs with P-glycoprotein. For example, it has been suggested that the calmodulin inhibitor trifluoperazine enhances the cytotoxicity of anthracyclines through posttranslational hyperphosphorylation of P-glycoprotein (Hamada *et al.*, 1987).

In summary, it has been demonstrated that calmodulin inhibitors may be used as chemosensitizers to circumvent MDR *in vitro* and to some extent *in vivo*. However, more work needs to be done with these agents to determine whether their chemosensitization effect is mediated through direct interaction with P-glycoprotein or through another biochemical pathway involving the action of calmodulin.

5. Cyclosporins

Cyclosporin A is a cyclic polypeptide of fungal origin. It is believed that its immunosuppressive activity on T cell growth and differentiation is at the transcriptional level, through its ability to inhibit interleukin 2 production. Cyclosporin A binds with high affinity to the cytosolic protein cyclophilin. A lower binding affinity of cyclosporin toward calmodulin has been recently observed (Colombani *et al.*, 1989). The initial study by Slater *et al.* (1986) demonstrated that cyclosporin A reverses vincristine resistance in L100/VCR human T cell acute lymphatic leukemia (ALL). This finding was of considerable interest, since relatively high levels of cyclosporin A can be achieved in patients. *In vitro*, cyclosporin A potentiated the cytotoxicity of etoposide and doxorubicin by inhibiting drug efflux in L1210 resistant leukemic cells (Osieka *et al.*, 1986). The sensitization of drug-resistant SKOV3 cells to vinblastine and adriamycin has been demonstrated in the presence of low concentrations of cyclosporin A. Figure 4 shows a D_{10} cytotoxicity assay that illustrates the complete reversal of vinblastine and adriamycin resistance in SKOV3 cells in the presence of 0.5–1.0 μg/ml of cyclosporin A (M. Duthie and V. Ling, unpublished results). Measurements of intracellular cyclosporin A have revealed a lower accumulation of cyclosporin in resistant P388 leukemic cells compared to the sensitive cells (Twentyman *et al.*, 1987). Moreover, coincubation of cells with increasing concentrations of daunorubicin did not restore cyclosporin accumulation in resistant cells. These results suggest that cyclosporin A is a substrate for the drug-effluxing pump and that its affinity for the pump is substantially higher than that of daunorubicin.

Recently, Foxwell *et al.* (1989) have demonstrated that P-glycoprotein binds cyclosporin A. A photoaffinity analog of cyclosporin A was covalently cross-linked to a 170-kDa protein that could be specifically immunoprecipitated with the anti-P-glycoprotein monoclonal antibody C219. The photoaffinity labeling of P-glycoprotein by cyclosporin A was inhibited in a dose-dependent manner in the

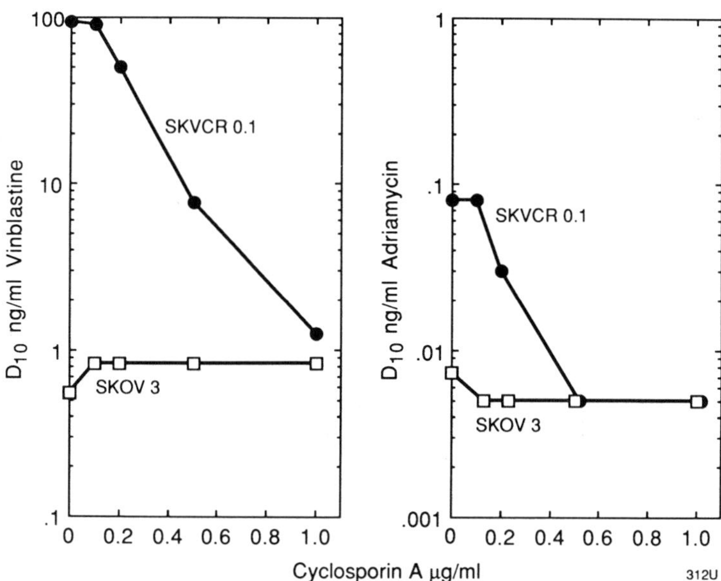

Fig. 4 Chemosensitization of multidrug-resistant (SKVCR 0.1) and drug-sensitive (SKCVR 0.3) human ovarian cells with cyclosporin A. D_{10} is the concentration of drug required to reduce the colony-forming ability of the cell line by 90%. Cyclosporin alone has no affect on colony-forming ability.

presence of excess vinblastine, verapamil, azidopine, or diltiazem, while high concentrations of colchicine had no effect. Twentyman *et al.* (1987) used three analogs of cyclosporin A (cyclosporin G, C, and H) to investigate the correlation between their immunosuppressive capacity and their ability to potentiate the cytotoxicity of vincristine and adriamycin in MDR cells. This study suggested a close correlation between the immunosuppressive efficiency and the chemosensitizing capacity of cyclosporin A analogs *in vitro*. Such a tight correlation was not observed in the study reported by Foxwell *et al.* (1989). The testing of more cyclosporin A analogs may yield a chemosensitizing agent with minimal immunosuppressive activity and high MDR sensitizing capacity.

6. Monoclonal Antibodies

Monoclonal antibodies directed against the extracellular domain(s) of P-glycoprotein have been shown to increase the accumulation of cytotoxic drugs in MDR cells (Hamada and Tsuruo, 1986). The monoclonal antibody MRK-16 was found to enhance the accumulation of vincristine, but not adriamycin, in a multidrug-resistant human ovarian carcinoma line (Broxterman *et al.*, 1988a). Similarly, the addition of the monoclonal antibody HYB-241 to resistant neuroblastoma cells (MC-1XC/VCR) caused a 3- to 8-fold increase in the accumulation of vincristine and actinomycin D (O'Brien *et al.* 1989). Incubation of resistant cells with verapamil in addition to either MRK-16 or HYB-241 monoclonal antibodies resulted in a greater increase in drug accumulation than that seen in the presence of either the monoclonal antibodies or verapamil alone. Antibodies against extracellular domains of P-glycoprotein may be conjugated to toxins. One such study using MRK-16 (FigzGerald *et al.*, 1987) coupled to *Pseudomonas* toxin showed selective killing of resistant cells expressing high levels of P-glycoprotein. Thus, it may be possible to use P-glycoprotein-specific monoclonal antibodies to inactivate P-glycoprotein specifically in MDR cells. Moreover, because of their binding specificity, P-glycoprotein-specific monoclonal antibodies may be highly specific sensitizers of MDR cells.

V. *In Vivo* Chemosensitization of MDR Cells

A. P-Glycoprotein Expression in Normal and Tumor Tissues

The role of P-glycoprotein as an efflux pump has been elucidated from studies of MDR cells selected *in vitro*. However, the normal physiological function of this protein is still undefined. In normal tissues of human and rodent, P-glycoprotein shows a restricted distribution (Fojo *et al.*, 1987a; Mukhopadhyay *et al.*, 1988; Sugawara *et al.*, 1988a; Georges *et al.*, 1990). High levels of P-glycoprotein mRNA have been detected in tissues with secretory functions, such as the adrenal gland, kidney, liver, and intestinal tract. In some of these tissues, immunohistochemical straining using P-glycoprotein-specific monoclonal antibodies showed that the expression of P-glycoprotein is polarized at the cellular level, being localized to the apical surface facing a lumen. For example, the staining of P-glycoprotein in liver tissue sections was localized to the biliary canalicular surface of hepatocytes, the apical surface of epithelial cells in the villi of the intestinal tract, and in the proximal renal tubule of the kidney (Fojo *et al.*, 1987b; Mukhopadhyay *et al.*, 1988; Thiebaut *et al.*, 1987). More recently, high levels of P-glycoprotein have been found in the endothelial cells of capillaries in the brain, and at other blood–tissue barriers, such as in the testes (Cordon-Cardo *et al.*, 1989). This result suggests that P-glycoprotein may be involved in regulating the entry of certain substances at these sites. It is interesting that both the brain and testes are known pharmacological sanctuaries for metastatic cancer.

A study of the differential expression of P-glycoprotein in mouse normal tissues, using gene-specific DNA probes and Northern blot analysis, demonstrated the predominant expression of the *mdr1* (class II) gene in the adrenal gland, the *mdr3* (class I) gene in the intestine, and the *mdr2* (class III) gene in muscle, spleen, and heart (Croop *et al.*, 1989). In most tissues at least two isoforms were detected. An independent study (Georges *et al.*, 1990), using a panel of epitope-specific monoclonal antibodies that discriminates between the different classes of P-glycoprotein isoforms, revealed a similar pattern of differential expression in normal hamster tissues. The immunohistochemical staining of tissue sections in the hamster study localized the expression of P-glycoprotein isoforms to a subset of specialized cells. For example, only a small subset of muscle fibers expressed the class III isoform, while the class II P-glycoprotein isoform was found only in the zona fasciculata and zona reticularis of the adrenal cortex. In addition, the expression of P-glycoprotein may be developmentally regulated in these cells since no P-glycoprotein was detected in fetal or neonatal adrenal gland using the MRK-16 monoclonal antibody (Sugawara *et al.*, 1988b).

P-Glycoprotein expression *in vivo* may be hormonally regulated. The induction of P-glycoprotein mRNA expression (class II isoform) (Croop *et al.*, 1989) in secretory epithelial cells in the gravid uterus of rodent was recently demonstrated (Arceci *et al.*, 1988; G. Bradley and V. Ling, unpublished results). High levels of P-glycoprotein expression were detected in carcinogen-induced hyperplastic nodules in rat liver, and in hepatocytes from regenerating liver (Fairchild *et al.*, 1987; Thorgeirsson *et al.*, 1987). The induction of P-glycoprotein in hyperplastic liver nodules may be a response to the presence of carcinogens, and may serve to protect these cells against the cytotoxic action of these agents, similar to that observed in MDR selected cells. It is interesting that the cells in these hyperplastic nodules are resistant not only to the transforming agent but also to a number of cytotoxic carcinogens (Parker and Gruenstein, 1976).

In summary, the tissue distribution of P-glycoprotein is consistent with its postulated role as a transport protein. Its polarized distribution in some normal tissues and organs has led to speculation that it may be involved in normal detoxification mechanisms that protect organisms from plant alkaloids and other xenobiotics (Klohs and Steinkampf, 1988). In other tissues it may be involved in the transport of normal lipophilic metabolites, such as hormones (Georges *et al.*, 1990). Moreover, the differential expression of the P-glycoprotein isoforms in normal tissues suggests that these isoforms may have specialized secretory functions. In this respect, it is interesting to note that only the class I and II P-glycoprotein isoforms confer the MDR phenotype *in vitro,* while the class III isoform apparently does not (see Section III,A).

The overexpression of P-glycoprotein has been observed in many tumor biopsies using monoclonal antibodies and DNA probes. Initial studies using Western blot analysis demonstrated an increased level of P-glycoprotein in biopsies obtained from patients with advanced nonresponsive ovarian cancer (Bell *et al.*, 1985), and in some sarcomas (Gerlach *et al.*, 1987). In one study, the sequential testing of ANLL leukemic cell samples from two patients with progressively nonresponsive disease showed an increase in the staining intensity and the proportion of tumor blast cells staining positively for P-glycoprotein with C219 monoclonal antibody (Ma *et al.*, 1987). Other studies (Fojo *et al.*, 1987a), including an extensive survey by Goldstein *et al.* (1988), also showed the presence of high P-glycoprotein mRNA levels using Southern blotting and RNA slot-blot analysis. It is interesting that, in many instances, significant levels of P-glycoprotein expression are seen in tumor biopsies taken prior to chemotherapy. It is possible that in these cases the tumor cells are expressing a differentiation phenotype typical of some tissue types as noted above.

Taken together, these results suggest that P-glycoprotein is likely to be expressed in most tumor types. It is not known at present if the presence of cells containing relatively high levels of P-glycoprotein in either treated or untreated tumors is a significant factor in a patient's response to chemotherapy. Further correlative studies are required to determine whether or not the expression of P-glycoprotein is prognostic of response to chemotherapy. It would not be surprising if the answer is different for different malignancies.

B. Animal Studies and Clinical Trials

The discovery of compounds that can reverse the MDR phenotype has generated significant interest in their potential clinical applications. In one study (Tsuruo *et al.*, 1981), the sensitizing effect of verapamil was tested by treating mice bearing P388/VCR resistant leukemic cells with vincristine or with a combination of vincristine and verapamil (75 mg/kg). The latter treatment resulted in a cure (survival beyond 6 months) of 10–60% of treated mice. Slater *et al.* (1982) have also demonstrated the potentiation of daunorubicin cytotoxicity in the presence of verapamil in mice inoculated with daunorubicin-resistant Ehrlich ascites cells. In both studies, it was concluded that verapamil was specific in potentiating the efficacy of the drug against resistant tumor cells. It is noteworthy that verapamil was less effective in the treatment of mice bearing transplantable drug-resistant solid tumors (Formelli *et al.* 1988). The reason for the lack of chemosensitization by verapamil in this mouse tumor system is not clear. However, it was suggested that a critical drug concentration in tumors must be reached before chemosensitization may be observed. In this respect, it is interesting that a greater number of mice bearing P388/VCR resistant cells were cured with verapamil when 2.0 mg/kg (versus 1.5 mg/kg) of vincristine was administered (Tsuruo *et al.*, 1985).

In summary, studies with animal model systems indicate that sensitization of resistant tumor cells using verapamil may be possible with some but not all tumor model systems. Although a number of studies have been designed to determine the efficacy of chemosensitizing agents using transplantable tumors, the pharmacokinetics of most chemosensitizers have not yet been examined. Further work to determine the pharmacokinetics may provide more insight as to how chemosensitization may be more effectively applied *in vivo.*

Initial studies using verapamil in the treatment of nonresponsive cancers have recently been described (Ozols *et al.*, 1987; Dalton *et al.*, 1989). In one study (Dalton *et al.*, 1989), patients with multiple myeloma failing treatment with VAD (vincristine, doxorubicin, and dexamethasone) were subsequently treated with VAD plus verapamil. Partial remission was seen with four of the five patients whose myeloma cells were P-glycoprotein-positive as determined by immunohistochemical staining with C219 monoclonal antibody. In the same study, patients with P-glycoprotein-negative myeloma cells showed no response to VAD plus verapamil. The chemosensitization results brought about by verapamil in this study are encouraging, and support the contention that P-glycoprotein mediates drug resistance in these nonresponsive myeloma cells, and that the presence of a chemosensitizer renders these cells drug-sensitive again. Significant side effects due to the cardiovascular activity of verapamil were observed in this trial in the majority of the patients; however, these side effects were reversible on the withdrawal of verapamil. More severe side effects of verapamil at higher doses have been observed in other clinical trials (Ozols *et al.*, 1987). Other sensitizing agents with minimal cardiovascular activities, such as AHC-52 or bepridil, are currently being investigated (Shinoda *et al.*, 1989; Schuurrhuis *et al.*, 1987).

In summary, the use of chemosensitizing agents in the treatment of some cancers refractory to chemotherapy has yielded encouraging results. The modest response seen with verapamil in the myeloma study suggests a correlation between the overexpression of P-glycoprotein and effective chemosensitization. Further studies with verapamil and other chemosensitizers in the treatment of nonresponsive tumors overexpressing P-glycoprotein are required to determine if the initial observation with myeloma is applicable to other cancers.

Acknowledgments

The authors would like to thank their colleagues at the Ontario Cancer Institute for helpful discussions, and especially Jane Endicott and Lela Veinot-Drebot for their critical reading of this review. The studies in the authors' laboratories were supported by the National Cancer Institute of Canada, Public Health Service Grant CA37130 from the National Institute of Health (V. Ling), and the Medical Research Council of Canada.

References

Akiyama, S.-I., Fojo, A., Hanover, J. A., Pastan, I., and Gottesman, M. M. (1985). Isolation and characterization of human KB cell lines resistant to multiple drugs. *Somatic Cell Mol. Genet.* **11,** 117–126.

Akiyama, S.-I., Cornwell, M. M., Kuwano, M., Pastan, I., and Gottesman, M. M. (1988). Most drugs that reverse multidrug resistance also inhibit photoaffinity labeling of P-glycoprotein by a vinblastine analog. *Mol. Pharmacol.* **33,** 144–147.

Ames, G. F.-L. (1986). Bacterial periplasmic transport systems: Structure, mechanism, and evolution. *Annu. Rev. Biochem.* **55,** 397–425.

Arceci, R. J., Croop, J. M., Horwitz, S. B., and Housman, D. (1988). The gene encoding multidrug resistance is induced and expressed at high levels during pregnancy in the secretory epithelium of the uterus. *Proc. Natl. Acad. Sci. U.S.A.* **85,** 4350–4354.

Arsenault, L., Ling, V., and Kartner, N. (1988). Altered plasma membrane ultrastructure in multidrug-resistant cells. *Biochim. Biophys. Acta* **938,** 315–321.

Beck, W. T. (1983). Vinca alkaloid-resistant phenotype in cultured human leukemic lymphoblasts. *Cancer Treat. Rep.* **67,** 875–882.

Beck, W. T. (1984). Cellular pharmacology of Vinca alkaloid resistance and its circumvention. *Adv. Enzyme Regul.* **22,** 207–227.

Beck, W. T. (1987). The cell biology of multiple drug resistance. *Biochem. Pharmacol.* **36,** 2879–2887.

Beck, W. T., and Cirtain, M. C. (1982). Continued expression of Vinca alkaloid resistance by CCRF-CEM cells after treatment with tunicamycin or pronase *Cancer Res.* **42,** 184–189.

Beck, W. T., Cirtain, M. C., Look, A. T., and Ashmun, R. A. (1986). Reversal of Vinca alkaloid resistance but not multiple drug resistance in human leukemic cells by verapamil. *Cancer Res.* **46,** 778–784.

Beck, W. T., Cirtain, M. C., Glover, J., Felsted, R. L., and Safa, A. R. (1988). Effect of indole alkaloids on multidrug resistance and labeling of P-glycoprotein by photoaffinity analog of vinblastine. *Biochem. Biophys. Res. Commun.* **152,** 552–558.

Bell, D. R., Gerlach, J. H., Kartner, N., Buick, R. N., and Ling, V. (1985). Detection of P-glycoprotein in ovarian cancer: A molecular marker associated with multidrug resistance. *J. Clin. Oncol.* **3,** 311–315.

Bitonti, A. J., Sjoerdsma, A., McCann, P. P., Kyle, D. E., Oduola, A. M. J., Rossan, R. N., Milhous, W. K., and Davidson, D. E. (1988). Reversal of chloroquine resistance in malaria parasite Plasmodium falciparum by desipramine. *Science* **242,** 1301–1303.

Bradley, G., Juranka, P. F., and Ling, V. (1988). Mechanism of multidrug resistance. *Biochim Biophys. Acta* **948,** 87–128.

Bradley, G., Naik, M., and Ling, V. (1989). P-Glycoprotein expression in multidrug-resistant human ovarian carcinoma cell lines. *Cancer Res.* **49,** 2790–2796.

Broxterman, H. J., Kuiper, C. M., Schuurhuis, G. J., Tsuruo, T., Pinedo, H. M., and Lankelma, J. (1988a). Increase of daunorubicin and vincristine accumulation in multidrug resistant human ovarian carcinoma cells by a monoclonal antibody reacting with P-glycoprotein. *Biochem. Pharmacol.* **37,** 2389–2393.

Broxterman, H. J., Pinedo, H. M., Kuiper, C. M., Kaptein, L. C. M., Schuurhuis, G. J., and Lankelma, J. (1988b). Induction by verapamil of a rapid increase in ATP consumption in multidrug-resistant tumor cells. *FASEB J.* **2,** 2278–2282.

Burke, T. G., Sartorelli, A. C., and Tritton, T. R. (1988). Selectivity of the anthracyclines for negatively charged model membranes: Role of the amino group *Cancer Chemother. Pharmacol.* **21,** 274–280.

Cano-Gauci, D. F., and Riordan, J. R. (1987). Action of calcium antagonists on multidrug resistant cells. *Biochem. Pharmacol.* **36,** 2115–2123.

Chen, C., Chin, J. E., Ueda, K., Clark, D. P., Pastan, I., Gottesman, M. M., and Roninson, I. B. (1986). Internal duplication and homology with bacterial transport proteins in the *mdr*1 (P-glycoprotein) gene from multidrug-resistant human cells. *Cell (Cambridge, Mass.)* **47,** 381–389.

Choi, K., Chen, C., Kriegler, M., and Roninson, I. B. (1988). An altered pattern of cross-resistance in multidrug-resistant cells results from spontaneous mutations in the mdr1 (P-glycoprotein) gene. *Cell (Cambridge, Mass.)* **53,** 519–529.

Colombani, P. M., Robb, A., and Hess, A. D. (1989). Cyclosporin A binding to calmodulin. A possible site of action on T lymphocytes. *Science* **228,** 337.

Cordon-Cardo, C., O'Brien, J. P., Casals, D., Rittman-Grauer, L., Biedler, J. L., Melamed, M., and Bertino, J. (1989). Multidrug-resistance gene (P-glycoprotein) is expressed by endothelial cells at blood-brain barrier sites. *Proc. Natl. Acad. Sci. U.S.A.* **86,** 695–698.

Cornwell, M. M., Safa, A. R., Felsted, R. L., Gottesman, M. M., and Pastan, I. (1986). Membrane vesicles from multidrug-resistant human cancer cells contain a specific 150- to 170-kDa protein detected by photoaffinity labeling. *Proc. Natl. Acad. Sci. U.S.A.* **83,** 3847–3850.

Cornwell, M. M., Tsuruo, T., Gottesman, M. M., and Pastan, I. (1987). ATP-binding properties of P-glycoprotein from multidrug-resistant KB cells. *FASEB J.* **1,** 51–54.

Croop, J. M., Raymond, M., Haber, D., Devault, A., Arceci, R. J., Gros, P., and Housman, D. E. (1989). The three mouse multidrug resistance (mdr) genes are expressed in a tissue specific manner in normal mouse tissues. *Mol. Cell. Biol.* **9,** 1346–1350.

Dalton, W. S., Grogan, T. M., Durie, B. G. M., Meltzer, P. S., Scheper, R. J., Taylor, C. W., Miller, T. W., and Salmon, S. E. (1989). Drug resistance in B-cell neoplasmas: Detection of P-glycoprotein and potential circumvention by addition of verapamil to chemotherapy. *J. Clin. Oncol.* **7,** 415–424.

de Bruijn, M. H. L., Van der Bliek, A. M., Biedler, J. L., and Borst, P. (1986). Differential amplification and disproportionate expression of five genes in three multidrug-resistant Chinese hamster lung cell lines. *Mol. Cell. Biol.* **6,** 4717–4722.

Deuchars, K. L., Du, R.-P., Naik, M., Evernden-Porelle, D., Kartner, N., Van der Bliek, A. M., and Ling, V. (1987). Expression of hamster P-glycoprotein and multidrug resistance in DNA-mediated transformants of mouse LTA cells. *Mol. Cell. Biol.* **7,** 718–724.

Echizen, H., Vogelegesang, B., and Eichelbaum, M. (1985). Effect of D-, L-verapamil on atrioventricular conduction in relation to its stereoselective first-pass metabolism. *Clin. Pharmacol. Ther.* **38,** 71–76.

Endicott, J. A., and Ling, V. (1989). The biochemistry of P-glycoprotein-mediated multidrug resistance. *Annu. Rev. Biochem.* **58,** 137–171.

Endicott, J. A., Juranka, P. F., Sarangi, F., Gerlach, J. H., Deuchars, K. L., and Ling, V. (1987). Simultaneous expression of two P-glycoprotein genes in drug-sensitive Chinese hamster ovary cells. *Mol. Cell. Biol.* **7,** 4075–4081.

Fairchild, C. R., Ivy, S. P., Rushmore, T., Lee, G., Koo, P., Goldsmith, M. E., Myers, C. E., Farber, E., and Cowan, K. H. (1987). Carcinogen-induced mdr over-expression is associated with xenobiotic resistance in rat preneoplastic liver nodules and hepatocellular carcinomas. *Proc. Natl. Acad. Sci. U.S.A.* **84,** 7701–7705.

Ferry, D. R., Kampf, K., Goll, A., and Glossmann, H. (1985). Subunit composition of skeletal muscle transverse tubule calcium channels evaluated with the 1,4-dihydropyridine photoaffinity probe. [^{3}H]azidopine. *EMBO J.* **4,** 1933–1940.

FitzGerald, D. J., Willingham, M. C., Cardarelli, C. O., Hamada, H., Tsuruo, T., Gottesman, M. M., and Pastan, I. (1987). A monoclonal antibody-Pseudomonas toxin conjugate that specifically kills multidrug-resistant cells. *Proc. Natl. Acad. Sci. U.S.A.* **84,** 4288–4292.

Fojo, A. T., Shen, D.-W., Mickley, L. A., Pastan, I., and Gottesman, M. M. (1987a). Intrinsic drug resistance in human kidney cancer is associated with expression of a human multidrug-resistance gene. *J. Clin. Oncol.* **5,** 1922–1927.

Fojo, A. T., Ueda, K., Slamon, D. J., Poplack, D. G., Gottesman, M. M., and Pastan, I. (1987b). Expression of a multidrug-resistance gene in human tumors and tissues. *Proc. Natl. Acad. Sci. U.S.A.* **84,** 265–269.

Foote, S. J., Thompson, J. K., Cowman, A. F., and Kemp, D. J. (1989). Amplification of the multidrug resistance gene in some chloroquine-resistant isolates of P. falciparum. *Cell (Cambridge, Mass.)* **57,** 921–930.

Formelli, F., Cleris, L, and Carsana, R. (1988). Effect of verapamil on doxorubicin activity and pharmacokinetics in mice bearing resistant and sensitive solid tumors. *Cancer Chemother. Pharmacol.* **21,** 329–336.

Foxwell, B. M. J., Mackie, A., Ling, V., and Ryffel, B. (1989). Identification of the multi-drug resistance related, P-glycoprotein as a cyclosporine binding protein. *Mol. Pharmacol.* **36,** 543–546.

Ganapathi, R., and Grabowski, D. (1983). Enhancement of sensitivity to adriamycin in resistant P388 leukemia by the calmodulin inhibitor trifluoperazine. *Cancer Res.* **43,** 3696–3699.

Ganapathi, R., and Grabowski, D. (1988). Differential effect of the calmodulin inhibitor trifluoperazine in modulating cellular accumulation, retention and cytotoxicity of doxorubicin in progressively doxorubicin resistant L1210 mouse leukemia cells. *Biochem. Pharmacol.* **37,** 185–193.

Ganapathi, R., Grabowski, D., Turinic, R., and Valenzuela, R. (1984). Correlation between potency of calmodulin inhibitors and effects on cellular levels and cytotoxic activity of doxorubicin (adriamycin) in resistant P388 mouse leukemia cells. *Eur. J. Cancer Clin. Oncol.* **20,** 799–806.

Garcia, M. L., King, V. F., Siegl, P. K. S., Reuben, J. P., and Kaczorowski, G. J. (1986). Binding of Ca^{2+} entry blockers to cardiac sarcolemmal membrane vesicles. *J. Biol. Chem.* **261,** 8146–8157.

Georges, E., Bradley, G., Gariepy, J., and Ling, V. (1990). Detection of P-glycoprotein isoforms by gene specific monoclonal antibodies. *Proc. Natl. Acad. Sci. U.S.A.* **87,** 152–156.

Gerlach, J. H., Endicott, J. A., Juranka, P. F., Henderson, G., Sarangi, F., Deuchars, K. L., and Ling, V. (1986). Homology between P-glycoprotein and a bacterial haemolysin transport protein suggests a model for multidrug resistance. *Nature (London)* **324,** 485–489.

Gerlach, J. H., Bell, D. R., Karakousis, C., Slocum, H. K., Kartner, N., Rustum, Y. M., Ling, V., and Baker, R. M. (1987). P-Glycoprotein in human sarcoma: Evidence for multidrug resistance. *J. Clin. Oncol.* **5,** 1452–1460.

Glossmann, H., Ferry, D. R., Striessnig, J., Goll, A., and Moosburger, K. (1987). Resolving the structure of the Ca^{2+} channel by photoaffinity labelling. *Trends Pharmacol. Sci.* **8,** 95–100.

Goldberg, H., Ling, V., Wong, P. I., and Skorecki, K. (1988). Reduced cyclosporin accumulation in multidrug-resistant cells. *Biochem. Biophys. Res. Commun.* **152,** 552–558.

Goldstein, L., Galski, H., Fojo, A., Willingham, M., Green, A., Crist, W., Gottesman, M., and Pastan, I. (1988). Expression of a multidrug-resistance gene in human tumors. *Proc. Am. Assoc. Cancer Res.* **29,** 298.

Greenberger, L. M., Williams, S. S., and Horwitz, S. B. (1987). Biosynthesis of heterogeneous forms of multidrug resistance-associated glycoproteins. *J. Biol. Chem.* **262,** 13685–13689.

Greenberger, L. M., Williams, S. S., Georges, E., Ling, V., and Horwitz, S. B. (1988). Electrophoretic analysis of P-glycoproteins produced by mouse J774.2 and Chinese hamster ovary multidrug-resistant cells. *J. Natl. Cancer Inst.* **80,** 506–510.

Gros, P., Croop, J., and Housman, D. (1986a). Mammalian multidrug resistance gene: Complete cDNA sequence indicates strong homology to bacterial transport proteins. *Cell (Cambridge, Mass.)* **47,** 371–380.

Gros, P., Croop, J., Roninson, I., Varshavsky, A., and Housman, D. E. (1986b). Isolation and characterization of DNA sequences amplified in multidrug resistant hamster cells. *Proc. Natl. Acad. Sci. U.S.A.* **83,** 337–341.

Gros, P., Neriah, Y. B., Croop, J. M., and Housman, D. E. (1986c). Isolation and expression of a complementary DNA that confers multidrug resistance. *Nature (London)* **323,** 728–731.

Gros, P., Raymond, M., Bell, J., and Housman, D. (1988). Cloning and characterization of a second member of the mouse mdr gene family. *Mol. Cell. Biol.* **8,** 2770–2778.

Gruber, A., Peterson, C., and Reizenstein, P. (1988). D-Verapamil and L-verapamil are equally effective in increasing vincristine accumulation in leukemic cells in vitro. *Int. J. Cancer* **41,** 224–226.

Guild, B., Mulligan, R. C., Gros, P., and Houseman, D. (1988). Retroviral transfer of a murine cDNA for multidrug resistance confers pleiotropic drug resistance to cells without prior drug selection. *Proc. Natl. Acad. Sci. U.S.A.* **85,** 1595–1599.

Hait, W. N. (1985). Pre-clinical and phase I-II studies of bleomycin (BLEO) with calmodulin-antagonists (CaM- A). *Proc. Am. Assoc. Cancer Res.* **26,** 326.

Hait, W. N., and DeRosa, W. T. (1988). Calmodulin as a target for new chemotherapeutic strategies. *Cancer Invest.* **6**(5), 499–511.

Hamada, H., and Tsuruo, T. (1986). Functional role for the 170- to 180-kDA glycoprotein specific to drug-resistant tumor cells as revealed by monoclonal antibodies. *Proc. Natl. Acad. Sci. U.S.A.* **83,** 7785–7789.

Hamada, H., and Tsuruo, T. (1988). Purification of the 170- to 180-kilodalton membrane glycoprotein associated with multidrug resistance. *J. Biol. Chem.* **263,** 1454–1458.

Hamada, H., Hagiwara, K.-I., Nakajima, T., and Tsuruo, T. (1987). Phosphorylation of the Mr 170,000 to 180,000 glycoprotein specific to multidrug-resistant tumor cells: Effects of verapamil, trifluoperazine, and phorbol esters. *Cancer Res.* **47,** 2860–2865.

Harker, W. G., Bauer, D., Etiz, B. B., Newman, R. A., and Sikic, B. I. (1986). Verapamil-mediated sensitization of doxorubicin-selected pleiotropic resistance in human sarcoma cells: Selectivity for drugs which produce DNA scission. *Cancer Res.* **46,** 2369–2373.

Hindenburg, A. A., Baker, M. A., Gleyzer, E., Stewart, V. J., Case, N., and Taub, R. N. (1987). Effect of verapamil and other agents on the distribution of anthracyclines and on the reversal of drug resistance. *Cancer Res.* **47,** 1421–1425.

Horio, M., Gottesman, M. M., and Pastan, I. (1988). ATP-dependent transport of vinblastine in vesicles from human multidrug-resistant cells. *Proc. Natl. Acad. Sci. U.S.A.* **85,** 3580–3584.

Inaba, M., and Nagashima, K. (1986). Non-antitumor Vinca alkaloids reverse multidrug resistance in P388 leukemia cells in vitro. *Jpn. J. Cancer Res.* **77,** 197–204.

Inaba, M., Nagashima, K., Sakurai, Y., Fukui, M., and Yanagi, Y. (1984). Reversal of multidrug resistance by non-antitumor anthracycline analogs. *Gann* **75,** 1049–1052.

Jongsma, A. P. M., Spengler, B. A., Van der Bliek, A. M., Borst, P., and Biedler, J. L. (1987). Chromosomal localization of three genes coamplified in the multidrug-resistant CHRC5 Chinese hamster ovary cell line. *Cancer Res.* **47,** 2875–2878.

Juliano, R. L., and Ling, V. (1976). A surface glycoprotein modulating drug permeability in Chinese hamster ovary cell mutants. *Biochim. Biophys. Acta* **455,** 152–162.

Kamimoto, Y., Gatmaitan, Z., Hsu, J., and Arias, I. (1989). The function of Gp170, the multidrug resistance gene product, in rat liver canalicular membrane vesicles. *J. Biol. Chem.* **264,** 11693–11698.

Kartner, N., Evernden-Porelle, D., Bradley, G., and Ling, V. (1985). Detection of P-glycoprotein in multidrug-resistant cell lines by monoclonal antibodies. *Nature (London)* **316,** 820–823.

Kessel, D., and Wilberding, C. (1985). Promotion of daunorubicin uptake and toxicity by the calcium antagonist tiapamil and its analogs. *Cancer Treat. Rep.* **69,** 673–676.

Klohs, W. D., and Steinkampe, R. W. (1988a). The effect of lysosomotropic agents and secretory inhibitors on anthracycline retention and activity in multiple drug-resistant cells. *Mol. Pharmacol.* **34,** 180–185.

Klohs, W. D., and Steinkampf, R. W. (1988b). Possible link between the intrinsic drug resistance of colon tumors and a detoxification mechanism of intestinal cells. *Cancer Res.* **48,** 3025–3030.

Krishan, A., Sauerteig, A., Gordon, K., and Swinkin, C. (1986). Flow cytometric monitoring of cellular anthracycline accumulation in murine leukemic cells. *Cancer Res.* **46,** 1768–1773.

Lalande, M. E., Ling, V., and Miller, R. G. (1981). Hoechst 33342 dye uptake as a probe of membrane permeability changes in mammalian cells. *Proc. Natl. Acad. Sci. U.S.A.* **78,** 363–367.

Lampidis, T. J., Munck, J.-N., Kreshan, A., and Tapiero, H. (1985). Reversal of resistance to rhodamine 123 in adriamycin-resistant Friend leukemia cells. *Cancer Res.* **45,** 2626–2631.

Lee, S. C., Deutsch, C., and Beck, W. T. (1988). Comparison of ion channels in multidrug-resistant and -sensitive human leukemic cells. *Proc. Natl. Acad. Sci. U.S.A.* **85,** 2019–2023.

Ling, V., and Thompson, L. H. (1974). Reduced permeability of CHO cells as a mechanism of resistance to colchicine. *J. Cell. Physiol.* **83,** 103–116.

Ling, V., Kartner, N., Sudo, T., Siminovitch, L., and Riordan, J. R. (1983). The multidrug resistance phenotype in Chinese hamster ovary cells. *Cancer Treat. Rep.* **67,** 869–874.

Ma, D. D., Davey, R. A., Harman, D. H., Isbister, J. P., Scurr, R. D., Mackertich, S. M., Dowden, G., and Bell, D. R. (1987). Detection of a multidrug resistant phenotype in acute non-lymphoblastic leukemia. *Lancet* **1,** 135–137.

Martin, S. K., Oduola, A. M. J., and Milhous, W. K. (1987). Reversal of chloroquine resistance in Plasmodium falciparum by verapamil. *Science* **235,** 899–901.

McGrath, J. P., and Varshavsky, A. (1989). The yeast STE6 gene encodes a homologue of the mammalian multidrug resistance P-glycoprotein. *Nature (London)* **340,** 400–404.

Meyers, M. B., Spengler, B. A., Chang, T. D., Melera, P. W., and Biedler, J. L. (1985). Gene amplification-associated cytogenetic aberrations and protein changes in vincristine-resistant Chinese hamster, mouse, and human cells. *J. Cell Biol.* **100,** 588–597.

Mountford, C. E., and Wright, L. C. (1988). Organization of lipids in the plasma membranes of malignant and stimulated cells: A new model. *Trends Biochem. Sci.* **13,** 172–177.

Mukhopadhyay, T., Batsakis, J. G., and Kuo, M. T. (1988). Expression of the mdr (P-glycoprotein) gene in Chinese hamster digestive tracts. *J. Natl. Cancer Inst.* **80,** 269–275.

Naito, M., and Tsuruo, T. (1989). Competitive inhibition by verapamil of ATP-dependent high affinity vincristine binding to the plasma membrane of multidrug-resistant K562 cells without calcium ion involvement. *Cancer Res.* **49,** 1452–1455.

Naito, M., Hamada, H., and Tsuruo, T. (1988). ATP/Mg^{2+}-dependent binding of vincristine to the plasma membrane of multidrug-resistant K562 cells. *J. Biol. Chem.* **263,** 11887–11891.

Neyfakh, A. A., Dmitrevskaya, T. V., and Serpinskaya, A. S. (1988). The membrane transport system responsible for multidrug resistance is operating in non-resistant cell. *Exp. Cell. Res.* **178,** 513–517.

Ng, W. F., Sarangi, F., Zastawny, R. L., Veinot-Drebot, L., and Ling, V. (1989). Identification of members of the P-glycoprotein multigene family. *Mol. Cell. Biol.* **9,** 1224–1232.

Nishizuka, Y. (1984). The role of protein kinase C in cell surface signal transduction and tumour promotion. *Nature (London)* **308,** 693–698.

Nogae, I. (1989). Analysis of structural features of dihydropyridine analogs needed to reverse multidrug resistance and to inhibit photoaffinity labeling of P-glycoprotein. *Biochem. Pharmacol.* **38,** 519–527.

O'Brien, J. P., Spengler, B. A., Rittman-Grauer, L., Bertino, J. R., and Biedler, J. L. (1989). Collateral sensitivity of human multidrug-resistant cells to verapamil is potentiated by the monoclonal antibody HYB-241 recognizing P-glycoprotein. *Proc. Am. Assoc. Cancer Res.* **30,** 505 (abstr.).

Osieka, R., Seeber, S., Pannenbiacker, R., Sall, D., Glatte, P., and Schmidt, C. G. (1986). Enhancement of etoposide-induced cytotoxicity by cyclosporin A. *Cancer Chemother. Pharmacol.* **18,** 298–202.

Ozols, R. F. (1985). Pharmacological reversal of drug resistance in ovarian cancer. *Semin. Oncol.* **12,** 7–11.

Ozols, R. F., Cunnion, R. E., Klecker, R. W., Jr., Hamilton, T. C., Ostchega, Y., Parrillo, J. E., and Young, R. C. (1987). Verapamil and adriamycin in the treatment of drug-resistant ovarian cancer patients. *J Clin. Oncol.* **5,** 641–647.

Parker, F. E., and Gruenstein, M. (1976). The resistance of putative premalignant liver cell populations, hyperplastic nodules, to acute cytotoxic effects of some hypatocarcinogens. *Cancer Res.* **36,** 3879–3887.

Pastan, I., Gottesman, M. M., Ueda, K., Lovelace, E., Rutherford, A. V., and Willingham, M. C. (1988). A retrovirus carrying an MDR1 cDNA confers multidrug resistance and polarized expression of P-glycoprotein in MDCK cells. *Proc. Natl. Acad. Sci. U.S.A.* **85,** 4486–4490.

Pearce, H. L., Safa, A. R., Bach, N. J., Winter, M. A., Cirtain, M. C., and Beck, W. T. (1989). Essential features of P-glycoprotein pharmacophore as defined by a series of reserpine analogs that modulate multidrug resistance. *Proc. Natl. Acad. Sci. U.S.A.* **86,** 5128–5132.

Pommier, Y., Schwartz, R. E., Zwelling, L. A., Kerrigan, D., Mattern, M. R., Charcossct, J. Y., Jacquemin-Sablon, A., and Kohn, K. W. (1986). Reduced formation of protein-associated DNA strand breaks in Chinese hamster cells resistant to topoisomerase II inhibitors. *Cancer Res.* **46,** 611–616.

Riordan, J. R., and Ling, V. (1985). Genetic and biochemical characterization of multidrug resistance. *Pharmacol. ther.* **28,** 51–75.

Riordan, J. R., Deuchars, K., Kartner, N., Alon, N., Trent, J., and Ling, V. (1985). Amplification of P-glycoprotein genes in multidrug-resistant mammalian cell lines. *Nature (London)* **316,** 817–819.

Roninson, I. B., Abelson, H. T., Housman, D. E., Howell, N., and Varshavsky, A. (1984). Amplification of specific DNA sequences correlates with multi-drug resistance in Chinese hamster cells. *Nature (London)* **309,** 626–628.

Rothenberg, M., and Ling, V. (1989). Multidrug resistance: Molecular biology and clinical relevance. *J. Natl. Cancer Inst.* **81,** 907–910.

Safa, A. R. (1988). Photoaffinity labeling of the multidrug-resistance-related P-glycoprotein with photoactive analogs of verapamil. *Proc. Natl. Acad. Sci. U.S.A.* **85,** 7187–7191.

Safa, A. R., Glover, C. J., Meyers, M. B., Biedler, J. L., and Felsted, R. L. (1986). Vinblastine photoaffinity labeling of a high molecular weight surface membrane glycoprotein specific for multidrug-resistant cells. *J. Biol. Chem.* **261,** 6137–6140.

Safa, A. R., Glover, C. J., Sewell, J. L., Meyers, M. B., Biedler, J. L., and Felsted, R. L. (1987). Identification of the multidrug resistance-related membrane glycoprotein as an acceptor for calcium channel blockers. *J. Biol. Chem.* **262,** 7884–7888.

Schmidt, W. F., Huber, K. R., Ettinger, R. S., and Neuberg, R. W. (1988). Antiproliferative effect of verapamil alone on brain tumor cells in vitro. *Cancer Res.* **48,** 3617–3621.

Schurr, E., Raymond, M., Bell, J. C., and Gros, P. (1989). Characterization of the multidrug resistance protein expressed in cell clones stably transfected with the mouse mdrl cDNA. *Cancer Res.* **49,** 2729–2733.

Schuurrhuis, G. J., Broxterman, H. J., van der Hoeven, J. J. M., Pinedo, H. M., and Lankelma, J. (1987). Potentiation of doxorubicin cytotoxicity by the calcium antagonist bepridil in anthracycline-resistant and -sensitive cell lines. *Cancer Chemother. Pharmacol.* **20,** 285–290.

Sehested, M., Skovsgaard, T., van Deurs, B., and Winther-Nielsen, H. (1987a). Increased plasma membrane traffic in daunorubicin resistant P388 leukemic cells. *Br. J. Cancer* **56,** 747–751.

Sehested, M., Skovsgaard, T., van Deurs, B., and Winther-Nielsen, H. (1987b). Increase in nonspecific adsorptive endocytosis in anthracycline and Vinca alkaloid resistant Ehrlich ascites tumor cell lines. *JNCI J. Natl. Cancer Inst.* **78,** 171–179.

Sehested, M., Skovsgaard, T., and Roed, H. (1988). The carboxylic ionophore monensin inhibits active drug efflux and modulates *in vitro* resistance in daunorubicin resistant Ehrlich ascites tumor cells. *Biochem. Pharmacol.* **37,** 3305–3310.

Shinoda, H., Inaba, M., and Tsuruo, T. (1989). In vivo circumvention of vincristine resistance in mice with P388 leukemia using a novel compound, AHC-52. *Cancer Res.* **49,** 1722–1726.

Sinha, B. K., Katki, A. G., Batist, G., Cowan, K. H., and Myers, C. E. (1987). Adriamycin-stimulated hydroxyl radical formation in the human breast tumor cells. *Biochem. Pharmacol.* **36,** 793–796.

Skovsgaard, T. (1980). Circumvention of resistance to daunomycin by N-acetyldaunorubicin in Ehrlich ascites tumor. *Cancer Res.* **40,** 1077–1083.

Slater, L. M., Murray, S. L., Wetzel, M. W., Wisdom, R. M., and Duval, E. M. (1982). Verapamil restoration of daunorubicin responsiveness in daunorubicin-resistant Ehrlich ascites carcinoma. *J. Clin. Invest.* **70,** 1131–1134.

Slater, L. M., Sweet, P., Stupecky, M., and Gupta, S. (1986). Cyclosporin A reverses vincristine and daunorubicin resistance in acute lymphatic leukemia in vitro. *J. Clin. Invest.* **77,** 1405–1408.

Snyder, S. H., and Reynolds, I. J. (1985). Calcium-antagonist drugs. *N. Engl. J. Med.* **313,** 995–1002.

Sugawara, I., Kataooka, I., Morishita, Y., Hamada, H., Tsuruo, T., Itoyama, S., and Mori, S. (1988a). Tissue distribution of P-glycoprotein encoded by a multidrug-resistant gene as revealed by a monoclonal antibody, MRK 16. *Cancer Res.* **48,** 1926–1929.

Sugawara, I., Nakahama, M., Hamada, H., Tsuruo, T., and Mori, S. (1988b). Apparent stronger expression in the human adrenal cortex than in the human adrenal medulla of Mr 170,000–180,000 P-glycoprotein. *Cancer Res.* **48,** 4611–4614.

Tew, K. D., and Clapper, M. L. (1987). Glutathione S-transferases and anticancer drug resistance. *In* "Mechanisms of Drug Resistance in Neoplastic Cells" (P. V. Wooley and K. D. Tew, eds.), pp. 141–157. Academic Press, Orlando.

Thiebaut, T., Tsuruo, T., Hamada, H., Gottesman, M. M., Pastan, I., and Willingham, M. C. (1987). Cellular localization of the multidrug-resistance gene product P-glycoprotein in normal human tissues. *Proc. Natl. Acad. Sci. U.S.A.* **84,** 7735–7738.

Thorgeirsson, S. S., Huber, B. E., Sorrell, S., Fojo, A., Pastan, I., and Gottesman, M. M. (1987). Expression of the multidrug-resistant gene in hepatocarcinogenesis and regenerating rat liver. *Science* **236,** 1120–1122.

Triggle, D. J., and Swamy, V. C. (1983). Calcium antagonists. Some chemical-pharmalogical aspects. *Circ. Res.* **52,** 17–28.

Tsuruo, T. (1983). Reversal of acquired resistance to Vinca alkaloids and anthracycline antibiotics. *Cancer Treat. Rep.* **67,** 889–894.

Tsuruo, T., Iida, H., Tsukagoshi, S., and Sakurai, Y. (1981). Overcoming of vincristine resistance in P388 leukemia in vivo and in vitro through enhanced cytotoxicity of vincristine and vinblastine by verapamil. *Cancer Res.* **41,** 1967–1972.

Tsuruo, T., Iida, H., Tsukagoshi, S., and Sakurai, Y. (1982). Increased accumulation of vincristine and adriamycin in drug-resistant P388 tumor cells following incubation with calcium antagonists and calmodulin inhibitors. *Cancer Res.* **42,** 4730–4733.

Tsuruo, T., Iida, H., Nojiri, M., Tsukagoshi, S., and Sakurai, Y. (1983a). Circumvention of vincristine and adriamycin resistance in vitro and in vivo by calcium influx blockers. *Cancer Res.* **43,** 2905–2910.

Tsuruo, T., Iida, H., Nojiri, M., Tsukagoshi, S., and Sakurai, Y. (1983b). Potentiation of chemotherapeutic effect of vincristine in vincristine resistant tumor bearing mice by calmodulin inhibitor clomipramine. *J. Pharm. Dyn.* **6,** 145–147.

Tsuruo, T., Iida, H., Tsukagoshi, S., and Sakurai, Y. (1985). Cure of mice bearing P388 leukemia by vincristine in combination with a calcium channel blocker. *Cancer Treat. Rep.* **69,** 523–525.

Twentyman, P. R., Fox, N. E., Wright, K. A., and Bleehen, N. M. (1986). Derivation and preliminary characteristics of adriamycin resistant lines of human lung cancer cells. *Br. J. Cancer* **53,** 529–537.

Twentyman, P. R., Fox, N. E., and White, D. J. G. (1987). Cyclosporin A and its analogues as modifiers of adriamycin and vincristine resistance in a multi-drug resistance human lung cancer cell line. *Br. J. Cancer* **56,** 55–59.

Ueda, K., Pastan, I., and Gottesman, M. M. (1987). Isolation and sequence of the promoter region of the human multidrug-resistance (P-glycoprotein) gene. *J. Biol. Chem.* **262,** 17432–17436.

Van der Bliek, A. M., Van der Velde-Koerts, T., Ling, V., and Borst, P. (1986). Over-expression and amplification of five genes in a multidrug-resistant Chinese hamster ovary cell line. *Mol. Cell. Biol.* **6,** 1671–1678.

Van der Bliek, A. M., Baas, F., Ten Houte de Lange, T., Kooiman, P. M., Van der Velde-Koerts, T., and Borst, P. (1987). The human mdr3 gene encodes a novel P-glycoprotein homologue and gives rise to alternatively spliced mRNAs in liver. *EMBO J.* **6,** 3325–3331.

Van der Bliek, A. M., Kooiman, P. M., Schneider, C., and Borst, P. (1988). Sequence of the mdr3 cDNA, encoding a human P-glycoprotein. *Gene* **30,** 401–411.

Warr, J. R., Anderson, M., and Fergusson, J. (1988). Properties of verapamil-hypersensitive multidrug-resistant Chinese hamster ovary cells. *Cancer Res.* **48,** 4477–4483.

Willingham, M. C., Cornwell, M. M., Cardarelli, C. O., Gottesman, M. M., and Pastan, I. (1986). Single cell analysis of daunomycin uptake and efflux in multidrug-resistant and -sensitive KB cells: Effects of verapamil and other drugs. *Cancer Res.* **46,** 5941–5946.

Wilson, G. M., Serrano, A. E., Wasley, A., Bogenschutz, M. P., Shankar, A. H., and Wirth, D. F. (1989). Amplification of a gene related to mammalian mdr genes in drug-resistant Plasmodium falciparum. *Science* **244,** 1184–1186.

Woods, G., Lund, L. A., Naik, M., Ling, V., and Ochi, A. (1988). Resistance of multidrug-resistant lines to natural killer-like cells-mediated cytotoxicity. *FASEB J.* **2,** 2791–2796.

Yang, C.-P. H., Mellado, W., and Horwitz, S. B. (1988). Azidopine photoaffinity labeling of multidrug resistance-associated glycoproteins. *Biochem. Pharmacol.* **37,** 1417–1421.

Yang, C.-P. H., DePinho, S. G., Greenberger, L. M., Arceci, R. J., and Horwitz, S. B. (1989). Progesterone interacts with P-glycoprotein in multidrug-resistant cells and in the endometrium of gravid uterus. *J. Biol. Chem.* **264,** 782–788.

Zamora, J. M., Pearce, H. J., and Beck, W. T. (1988). Physical-chemical properties shared by compounds that modulate multidrug resistance in human leukemic cells. *Mol. Pharmacol.* **33,** 454–462.

Peptides: Chemistry, Biology, and Pharmacology

Amrit K. Judd* and Gary K. Schoolnik†

**Bio-Organic Chemistry Laboratory*
Life Sciences Division
SRI International
Menlo Park, California 94025

†Howard Hughes Medical Institute
Stanford University
Stanford, California 94305

I. Introduction

Peptides are small proteins composed of fewer than 50 amino acids. Unlike most globular proteins, peptides frequently have modified amino (N) and carboxyl (C) termini, contain D-amino acids and multiple disulfide bridges, or exist in cyclic forms with linked N and C termini. These features not only contribute to the functional role of these compounds, but also confer stability in physiological environments, specifically by preventing proteolytic degradation. The number of naturally occurring peptides that have been identified and structurally characterized has grown substantially in the past decade as a result of improved protein purification and sequencing techniques and through the isolation of cDNAs encoding putative peptidelike structures. However, the functions of many of these compounds have not been defined, although the tissues in which they are

Advances in Pharmacology, Volume 21

concentrated have been identified and, in some instances, their pharmacological properties have been determined by *in vitro* and *in vivo* studies. These kinds of investigations have led to the recognition that peptides can be assigned to one of four functional categories: hormones, neurotransmitters, antibiotics, and toxins. The production of synthetic derivatives of these compounds, including competitive antagonists and potent agonists, the use of these agents in increasingly refined physiological studies, and the identification of their cellular receptors are gradually clarifying their functional role. These advances are described in this article by focusing on the structural features of a broad range of naturally occurring peptides and their recognized physiological and pharmacological properties, particularly where these properties, when altered by specific modifications of the natural product, have led to a deeper understanding of structure–function relationships.

A second and quite distinctive line of investigation during the past decade has been the use of synthetic peptides as immunological reagents, particularly as "predetermined" sequence-specific vaccines. This effort was stimulated by the availability of a large number of amino acid sequences—some deduced from the corresponding gene sequence, others derived directly from the amino acid sequence—and by the capacity to synthesize substantial amounts of the immunizing peptide chemically using Merrifield's solid-phase techniques. Optimistic reports soon appeared describing the properties of antibodies to synthetic peptides that were elicited when studied by *in vitro* immunoassays. These were followed in turn by reports describing the failure of many such vaccines to confer protection in relevant animal models. As this area of study matured, attention shifted to the characterization of the immunological properties of peptides per se and particularly to the structural features of B and T cell epitopes. The major findings of these studies and the current status of synthetic peptide vaccines are summarized in the last section of this article.

II. Peptide Synthesis

Synthetic peptides structurally related to their native counterparts are effective tools to probe the relationship between peptide structure and biological activity. Syntheses have not only provided these rare compounds in quantity but have facilitated the study of their mode of action and advanced our understanding of the role of structure in determining biological function. In certain instances, synthesis has been used to elucidate the sequence of a naturally occurring peptide or to confirm a proposed sequence. From a pharmacological point of view it is of particular interest that synthetic analogs of biologically active peptides (e.g., hormones) may exhibit unique properties such as superpotency, altered biological specificity, and long-lasting activity. Thus, synthetic peptides may be required for therapeutic purposes, particularly if they are not easily obtainable in sufficient quantities from the natural source.

Another novel application of synthetic peptide chemistry is in the production of peptides to be used as immunogens in the generation of antisera specific for proteins. Furthermore, synthetic peptide studies may be performed simply for the sake of methodological progress.

The formation of a peptide bond, in principle, can be reduced to four steps: (1) Protection of the α-amino and carboxyl and side-chain functional groups, (2) activation of the carboxyl component, (3) coupling of the carboxyl component and the amino component to form a peptide linkage, (4) removal of the protecting groups *in toto,* if the synthesis is completed, or selective cleavage of the α-amino or carboxyl protecting groups.

At present the most frequently used methods of peptide synthesis are (a) conventional solution method, and (b) solid-phase method. It is not intended to give here a thorough discussion of the techniques (e.g., coupling methods, protecting groups, deprotecting techniques) of peptide synthesis. Several reviews have been published in recent years that cover the growing literature of this field. The series *The Peptides* edited by Gross and Meienhofer (1978–1985), a volume by Bodanszky (1984), and a review by Erickson and Merrifield (1976) are excellent for their treatment. The laboratory techniques related to solid-phase peptide synthesis are the subject of a book by Stewart and Young (1984). This chapter considers several of the more common approaches to peptide synthesis and gives a few examples of each synthetic methodology.

A. Solution Synthesis

The solution synthesis method involves the condensation of an N^{α}-protected amino acid with activated carboxyl group (carboxyl component) with another amino acid that has free N^{α} and protected carboxyl function (amino component) to produce a protected peptide (Fig. 1). The most commonly used amino protecting groups are the benzyloxycarbonyl group or CBZ, the *tert*-butyloxycarbonyl group or t-Boc, and modification of these groups. For carboxyl protection, methyl, ethyl, benzyl, and *tert*-butyl esters are most frequently employed. In addition, side-chain protection often is required for trifunctional amino acids. For peptide bond formation, four efficient methods have found wide and general application: the azide method, the mixed anhydride method, the dicyclohexylcarbodiimide method, and the active ester method (*N*-hydroxysuccinimide, *p*-nitrophenyl, pentachlorophenyl, and pentafluorphenyl). The synthesis is carried out in homogeneous phase. Intermediate products are purified by crystallization or chromatographic techniques. On completion of the synthesis, the terminal- and side-chain protecting groups are removed and the peptide is purified by crystallization or by employing chromatographic techniques.

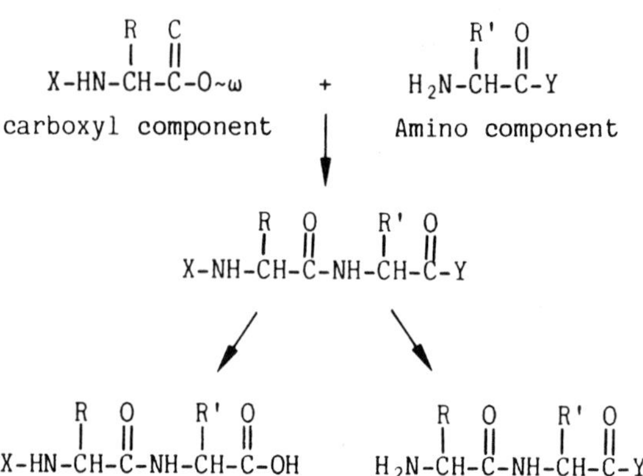

Fig. 1 General scheme for solution synthesis. X, α-amino protecting group; Y, carboxyl protecting group; R and R′, side chains of amino acid residues; ω, carboxyl activating moiety.

The choice of protecting groups, of coupling method, and of deprotection procedures is regarded as the *tactics* of peptide synthesis. The pattern of assembling all amino acid residues into the desired peptide sequence is referred to as the *strategy*. The peptide sequence can be built up by incremental stepwise elongation procedure, i.e., the successive incorporation of one amino acid residue at a time starting from the C terminus. Alternatively, peptide chains may be constructed by fragment condensation, i.e., the joining of small peptides with the appropriate partial sequences to form larger intermediate fragments for final assembly of the target structure (Fig. 2). The stepwise elongation method can be very conveniently used for the synthesis of peptides with up to 15 amino acid residues. For the construction of larger peptide chains, fragment condensation provides the most promising route. It allows for greater flexibility in the choice of protecting groups and coupling methods; however, the greatest advantage is the ease of purification. Stepwise procedure results in a complex mixture of closely related products that are difficult to separate even by the most sophisticated purification procedures. Separation of sizable fragments from a reaction mixture is a considerably easier task than separation of a family of closely similar complex peptides. Fragment condensation has been successfully applied to the synthesis of many peptide hormones with up to about 90 amino acid residues.

B. Solid-Phase Synthesis

The solid-phase peptide synthesis (SPPS) approach involves phase separation of the peptide from reagents, by-products, and side products. The growing peptide chain is kept covalently attached to an entirely insoluble support throughout all

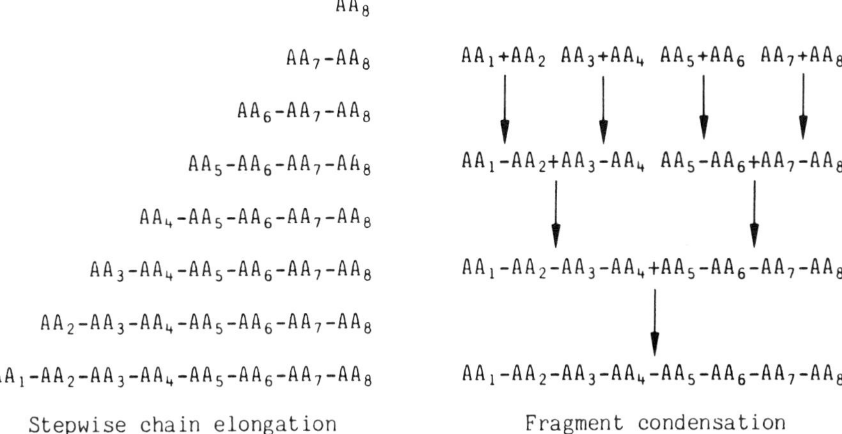

Fig. 2 Strategies for peptide chain assembly.

stages of the synthesis. The solid phase is in a form that allows rapid filtration for the removal of the liquid phase, containing the soluble reagents, by-products, and side products, from the solid phase. To be applicable for multistage syntheses of large polypeptides, 100% quantitative incorporation of each amino acid residue must be accomplished. Finally, the solid support is removed from the completed peptide without altering or degrading the desired product. Complete achievement of the above steps should provide a procedure for the rapid preparation of homogeneous peptides in high yields. The technique of solid-phase peptide synthesis is known as Merrifield's method of peptide synthesis.

The attractive characteristics of the solid-phase method—namely, simplicity, speed, avoidance of intermediate isolation, and, most noteworthy, automatization—opened new avenues in the field of synthetic oligopeptides and enabled scientists to cope with increasing challenges. Since Merrifield's method was first conceived (Merrifield, 1963), numerous modifications of the original polystyrene-derived insoluble support, of protecting groups, and coupling techniques have been suggested, aimed at solving various synthesizing difficulties and obtaining optimal conditions for synthesizing peptides with biological activity. As a consequence of these enormous efforts, the solid-phase methodology is generally the current method of choice in peptide chemistry and is particularly useful when a large number of peptides must be prepared for screening (e.g., bioactivity or immunogenicity) purposes.

The majority of solid-phase syntheses were carried out on polystyrene-derived supports and employed the t-Boc chemistry in which strong acids, e.g., trifluoroacetic acid (TFA) and anhydrous hydrofluoric acid (HF) or trifluoromethanesulfonic acid (TMSA), are primarily used, TFA for the N^{α} deprotection after each coupling step and HF or TMSA for the simultaneous cleavage of the completed peptide from the resin and side-chain protection (Fig. 3). Moreover, the growing peptide chain in the "conventional" Merrifield synthesis is vastly different in its polar nature from the hydrophobic polystyrene support. This may lead to incompletion of certain reactions. As an approach toward solving this drawback, Sheppard has suggested the use of supports whose solvation properties would be similar to those of the growing peptide chain (Arshady *et al.*, 1981; Atherton *et al.*, 1981). The syntheses are carried out on polar polydimethylacrylamide-derived supports, employing a polar solvent, dimethylformamide (DMF), a base-labile α-amino protecting group (fluoroenylmethoxycarbonyl; Fmoc) throughout the synthesis, and mild acidolysis [various concentrations of TFA in dichromethane (DCM)] for final cleavage of the peptide from the resin and for side-chain deprotection (Fig. 4). Efforts to optimize the coupling and cleavage conditions are still under way and the method has been found to be of only limited use.

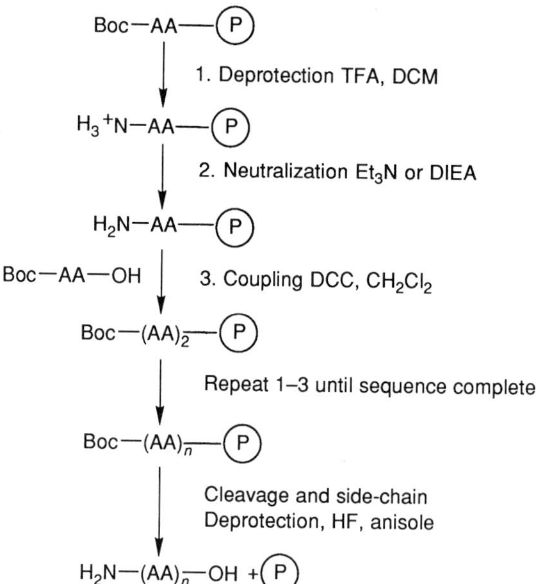

Fig. 3 Solid-phase synthesis using t-BOC chemistry. Boc, *tert*-butyloxycarbonyl; TFA, trifluoroacetic acid; DCM, dichromethane; HF, anhydrous hydrofluoric acid; Et_3N, triethylamine; DCC, dicyclohexylcarbodiimide.

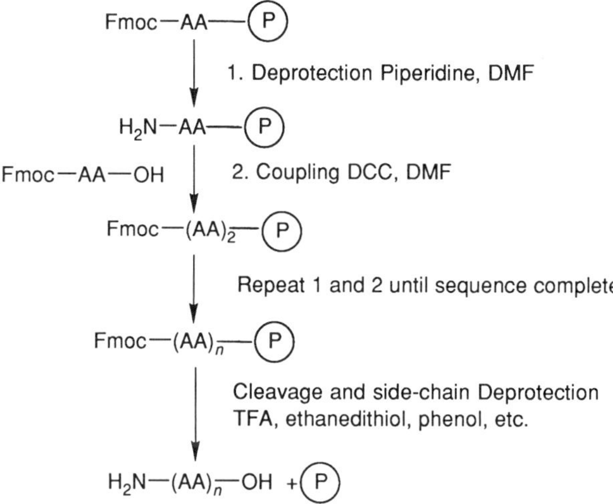

Fig. 4 Solid-phase synthesis using Fmoc chemistry.

III. Peptide Hormones

Peptide hormones have been isolated from a variety of sources and have a multitude of biological activities. They have been derived from brain, pituitary, hypothalamus, pancreas, intestine, gastrointestinal (GI) tract, gonad, and various other sources. We have divided peptide hormones arbitrarily into two groups, namely, gastrointestinal peptides and neuropeptides.

A. Gastrointestinal Peptides

Gastrointestinal peptides were originally demonstrated to occur in the pancreas or in the GI tract, but they have also been recognized in the brain. In the past 10 years, over 50 new peptides have been identified in the central nervous system (CNS) or GI tract. In almost every case, a peptide identified in the gut was subsequently found in the brain and vice versa. Some of these peptides are described below.

1. Substance P

Substance P (SP) was discovered by von Euler and Gaddum (1931) in ethanol extracts of rabbit and horse intestines and brain and was shown to be a smooth-muscle contracting and hypotensive factor. The sequence of SP was determined by Chang *et al.* (1971) and Tregear *et al.* (1971) confirmed its structure by synthesis.

Structurally, SP is related to a group of peptides of nonmammalian origin, called tachykinins, that induce a rapid contraction of the guinea pig ileum (GPI). Eledoisin, a tachykinin isolated from salivary glands of cephalopods, represents the earliest stage in the evolution, whereas SP, which occurs only in mammals, represents the latest stage. Amino acid sequences of various tachykinins are shown in Table I.

The structural correspondence of the tachykinins is mainly restricted to the respective C-terminal pentapeptide sequences, which are regarded as the minimal part necessary for full biological activity. This is in accordance with the principle that the sequence region is indispensable for the function to remain stable during evolution.

SP can be distinguished from the other tachykinins by a diminished potency toward selected smooth-muscle preparations or by an increased effect in lowering blood pressure *in vivo* (Otsuka *et al.*, 1975). The most notable feature of SP, however, is its role in the CNS, where it is located in the neurons of the brain stem and the spinal cord. The possible physiological and regulatory role of SP in the CNS (Skrabanek and Powell, 1977) can be attributed to the following: (1) the occurrence of SP in synapses and its release by K^+, (2) the accumulation of SP in the spinal cord and in ganglia of the dorsal roots, (3) synapses and interactions between SP-ergic and catecholaminergic neurons, (4) depolarization of spinal motoneurons by SP, (5) SP–endorphin interactions in pain transmission, and (6) inhibition of K^+-induced enkephalin release by SP (Jessel and Iversen, 1977). The release of SP from the GPI as a result of nerve stimulation (Franco *et al.*, 1979) suggests that SP is also an intrinsic neuroregulatory factor in the gut. The C-terminal pentapeptide of SP (Phe-Phe-Gly-Leu-Met-NH_2) is structurally similar to the N-terminal pentapeptide of endorphin and Met-enkephalin (Tyr-Gly-Gly-Phe-Met) except that in SP the C-terminal methionine is amidated. Both are

Table I

Amino Acid Sequences of Various Tachykinins

Tachykinin	Sequence
Substance P	Arg-Pro -Lys -Pro -Gln -Gln-Phe-Phe-Gly-Leu-Met-NH_2
Neurokinin A	His -Lys -Thr-Aps-Ser -Phe-Val -Gly-Leu-Met-NH_2
Neurokinin B	Asp-Met-His -Asp-Phe-Phe-Val -Gly-Leu-Met-NH_2
Eledoisin	pGlu-Pro -Ser -Lys-Asp-Ala-Phe-Ile -Gly-Leu-Met-NH_2
Uperolein	pGLu-Pro -Asp-Pro -Asn-Ala-Phe-Tyr-Gly-Leu-Met-NH_2
Physalaemin	pGlu-Ala -Asp-Pro -Asn-Lys-Phe-Tyr -Gly-Leu-Met-NH_2
Kassinin	Asp-Val-Pro -Lys -Ser -Asp-Gln-Phe-Val -Gly-Leu-Met-NH_2

of hydrophobic character and represent the minimal active part of the corresponding CNS peptide (Stewart and Channabasavaiah, 1979).

Over the past few years a large number of SP analogs have been synthesized to study their structure–activity relationships (SAR). Amino acid exchanges in SP undecapeptide were carried out mainly in positions 1, 8, and 11 in order to influence enzymatic degradation, to obtain precursors for ^{3}H- and ^{125}I-labeling, and to avoid side reactions of the Met^{11} residue during the synthesis. SP analogs with Tyr^{8} and an N-terminal Tyr were iodinated and used for radioimmunoassay (Yanaihara *et al.*, 1977). Dehydroproline^{2,4} and *p*-chlorophenylalanine^{7,8} analogs of [Nle^{11}]-SP are suitable precursors for tritiation (Yanaihara *et al.*, 1977; Bienert *et al.*, 1979a), as these alterations do not markedly influence the smooth-muscle activity of SP. In SAR studies, however, variations of the C-terminal part of the molecule give more information about peptide–receptor interactions. [D-Leu^{8}, D-Phe^{9}]-SP has been reported to be antagonist without any agonism (Leban *et al.*, 1979), and this opens up a new perspective for SP research. The successive addition of amino acid residues to the C-terminal pentapeptide increases the activity in different bioassays (Franzen et al., 1981; Theodoropoulos *et al.*, 1981; Baizman *et al.*, 1983). The hexapeptides are almost fully active. With further elongation of the chain, the increase of activity reaches a maximum for the octapeptides. Cyclopeptides, which contain the intact hexapeptide structure SP (6–11), showed very weak biological activities, indicating the importance of flexibility (Neubert *et al.*, 1979). The increase of activity of the pentapeptide on spinal motoneurons by the addition of an N-terminal pyroglutamyl residue was also found in the vasodepressor response (Traczyk, 1977). Acetylated (7–11) pentapeptides and (6–11) hexapeptides have been found to exhibit a higher activity with the GPI than SP or nonacetylated fragments (Bienert *et al.*, 1979b). SP (6–11), like SP, in low doses, produces an analgetic effect that can be inhibited by pretreatment with naloxone (Stewart *et al.*, 1976; Oehme *et al.*, 1980). This indicates the mutual modulating effects of SP and endogenous opioids and reveals a dual function of this hormone in the CNS. Conformationally restrained and metabolically stable SP analogs have also been synthesized and studied (Rubini *et al.*, 1981; Ewenson *et al.*, 1985; Morgan *et al.*, 1988), but a specific inactivating protease with high affinity, as known for enkephalins, has not yet been found for SP.

2. Cholecystokinin

Cholecystokinin (CCK) is a brain/gut peptide that has been detected in the small intestine (Harper and Raper, 1943) as well as in the brain (Dockray, 1976). In the gut, CCK induces gall bladder contraction and the release of pancreatic enzymes (Mutt, 1976, 1980). The amino acid sequences of porcine CCK 58 (Mutt and Jorpes, 1971; Eng *et al.*, 1983) and rat CCK (Deschenes *et al.*, 1984) have been reported. Recently, Takahashi *et al.* (1985) reported the sequence of the human CCK gene.

CCK occurs in numerous molecular forms. The significance of this heterogeneity is not known. A number of these peptides have been purified and sequenced: CCK 8 from brain (Reeve *et al.*, 1984; Dockray *et al.*, 1978; Eng *et al.*, 1983), CCK 58 from brain and intestine (Eysselein *et al.*, 1982, 1984), N-terminal fragments of CCK 33 (Eng *et al.*, 1983), CCK 22 from rat intestine (Eng *et al.*, 1984), and a novel form of CCK 8 from guinea pig intestine (Zhou *et al.*, 1985). These studies have indicated that the major form of CCK-like immunoreactivity is CCK 8 sulfate, though small amounts of CCK 58-, CCK 33-, and CCK 4-like peptides have also been detected. The pattern in the gut is quite different, with high-molecular-weight forms like CCK 58 and intermediate forms like CCK 22 being detected, and with CCK 12 being more abundant than in brain.

The C-terminal octapeptide portion of CCK is able to exhibit the whole range of biological activities, the sequence being

$$\begin{array}{l}\quad\;\; SO_3H \\ \quad\quad | \\ \text{Asp-Tyr-Met-Gly-Trp-Met-Asp-Phe-}NH_2\end{array}$$

The results of SAR studies indicate that the sulfate ester moiety of the tyrosyl residue is critical for maximal biological activity in peripheral tissues, namely, guinea pig gall bladder and ileum (Gaudreau *et al.*, 1987). Among the N- and C-terminal fragments, the general order of potency in both smooth-muscle preparations is CCK 26-33 $>$ CCK 1-33 $>$ CCK 27-33 $>>>$ nonsulfated CCK 26-33 $>$ CCK 30-33.

For the past few years, numerous peptide and nonpeptide CCK receptor antagonists have been synthesized by various groups. Asperlicin represented a key breakthrough as a nonpeptide competitive and selective antagonist ($K_i = 600$ nM) at the CCK receptor (Chang *et al.*, 1985). Rosamond *et al.* (1988) synthesized a number of various CCK analogs and studied their satiety effect. Crawley and Beinfeld (1983) reported the most potent CCK 8 analog (U-67827E) related to satiety. Freidinger *et al.* (1988) described different approaches for designing antagonists of CCK. Rodriguez *et al.* (1988) studied the importance of peptide bonds in the C-terminal heptapeptide of CCK, and their studies indicated that analogs differed in their potencies toward pancreatic and brain CCK receptors.

3. Gastrin

The GI peptide hormone gastrin, which is the most potent stimulant of gastric hydrochloric acid secretion known, has been reported in aqueous extracts of cerebral cortex from a variety of mammalian species, including man (Vanderhaegen *et al.*, 1975). Like CCK, gastrin exists in multiple molecular forms, not all of which have been identified chemically. Gastrin 17 is the major form in the stomach (Renfeld, 1981) and gastrin 34 makes up about 60 to 70% of fasting plasma gastrin (Dockray and Taylor, 1976; Lamers *et al.*, 1979). The amino acid sequence of porcine gastrin 17 I and II was reported by Gregory and Tracy (1964). Other forms of gastrin that were isolated and sequenced later are "big gastrin" (gastrin 34 I and II) (Gregory and Tracy, 1972), "minigastrin" G 13 or G 14 (Gregory and Tracy, 1975), and gastrin 6 (Gregory *et al.*, 1983). The sequence of gastrin 17 is

```
                                                              R
                                                              |
Glu-Gly-Pro-Trp-Leu-Glu-Glu-Glu-Glu-Glu-Ala-Tyr-Gly-Trp-Met-Asp-Phe-NH2
```

where human gastrin I has R = H and human gastrin II has R = SO_3H (Bentley *et al.*, 1966). There is a considerable analogy in the C-terminal sequences of gastrin and CCK, as shown below:

```
              SO3H
              |
Gastrin      -Tyr-Gly-Trp-Met-Asp-Phe-NH2

                  SO3H
                  |
CCK          Asp-Tyr-Met-Gly-Trp-Met-Asp-Phe-NH2
```

It was recognized early that, of the 17 amino acid residues of the molecule, only the C-terminal tetrapeptide Trp-Met-Asp-Phe-NH_2 is required for the remarkable range of physiological effects displayed by the natural hormone (Tracy and Gregory, 1964). In the case of CCK, the C-terminal octapeptide is required for exhibiting the activities of whole natural hormone. Gastrin and CCK overlap in their activities.

Extensive SAR studies could be carried out more readily on this hormone than on CCK because the short active C-terminal sequence is quite amenable to synthetic experimentation. With the help of hundreds of analogs prepared for this purpose, Morley (1968a,b) could point out the important features of the active portion of the molecule. Several of the synthetic peptides were found to be quite active and a partially protected pentapeptide, *tert*-butyloxycarbonyl-β-alanyl-L-tryptophyl-L-methionyl-Laspartyl-L-phenylalanine amide (Peptovlon, ICI 50.123), became commercially available for physiological studies.

4. Bombesin

Bombesin (BN), a 14-amino acid peptide, was isolated from the skin of the European frog *Bombina bombina* by Anastasi *et al.* (1973). It stimulates the cat small intestinal and the rat uterine and urinary tract smooth muscle after intravenous infusion. In 1979, the mammalian equivalent of BN, a 27-amino acid peptide, was isolated from porcine nonantral stomach tissue. Because it was identified on the basis of its ability to stimulate gastrin secretion from the dog stomach, it was named gastrin-releasing peptide (GRP). Sequences of canine, chicken, and human GRP are now available. More recently, two 10-amino acid peptides were isolated from the porcine spinal cord based on their ability to stimulate rat uterus smooth-muscle preparations; they were named neuromedin B and neuromedin C (Minemino *et al.*, 1983, 1984). The sequences of BN-like peptides and GRP are shown in Table II.

Among the BN-like peptides, there is strong homology in the C-terminal decapeptide region of BN, neuromedins, and human GRP.

Endogenous BN-like peptides are present in discrete regions of the rat and human brain. These peptides are released from brain neurons by depolarizing stimuli and they may diffuse and activate receptors present on adjacent neurons. These receptors have been detected in discrete brain regions. Thus, BN-like peptides may function in a paracrine manner in the CNS.

In the periphery, BN-like peptides and receptors are present in high density in intrinsic neurons of the GI tract. BN functions as a satiety agent in the rodent as well as man and delays gastric emptying. Also, BN stimulates some hormones (particularly gastrin and secretin), stimulates smooth-muscle preparations, causes pancreatic secretion, and alters respiration.

BN-like peptides are associated with the disease small cell lung cancer (SCLC). Excessive amounts of BN-like peptides are produced and secreted from this tumor. BN also stimulates the growth of this tumor.

Numerous investigators have synthesized BN-like peptides and tested their biological activity in the CNS and periphery. In general, these studies have indicated that the C-terminal sequence of BN or GRP is essential for biological activity. Rivier and Brown (1978) synthesized a number of BN analogs and studied their effect on thermoregulation. Their data indicated that (Tyr^4)BN is the most potent analog as a hypothermic agent in a receptor-binding assay; (Lys^3)BN, BN,

Table II

Amino Acid Sequences of Bombesin-Like Peptides

Peptide	Sequence
BN	pGlu-Gln-Arg-Leu-Gly-Asn-Gln-Trp-Ala-Val-Gly-His-Leu-Met-NH_2
Neuromedin B	Gly-Asn-Leu-Trp-Ala-Thr-Gly-His-Phe-Met-NH_2
Neuromedin C	Gly-Asn-His-Trp-Ala-Val-Gly-His-Leu-Met-NH_2
Human GRP (18–27)	Gly-Asn-His-Trp-Ala-Val-Gly-His-Leu-Met

and GRP are slightly less potent. Leucine at the penultimate position of BN is preferred to induce hypothermia. (N-Ac-Gly^5)BN, which lacks the N-terminal tetrapeptide, is a potent agonist. (D-Ala^5)BN and (D-Ala^{11})BN were approximately as potent as BN. The C-terminal octapeptide of GRP (GRP 20–27) is twofold more potent than BN, indicating that the C-terminal eight amino acids of GRP are essential for full biological activity.

Putative SP antagonists antagonize the action of BN in the CNS and periphery (Jensen *et al.*, 1984a,b). However, the role of BN-like peptides in the CNS is not known with certainty.

5. VIP Family of Peptides

The VIP family of peptides includes vasoactive intestinal peptide (VIP), secretin, glucagon, and the peptide histidine isoleucine amide (PHI). VIP was first characterized by Said (1967) as a vasoactive peptide in extracts if mammalian lung and was subsequently isolated by Said and Mutt (1970) from porcine intestine. Secretin was the first gut hormone to be discovered (in hog intestine) and it revolutionized physiology because its discovery led to the concept of blood-borne chemical messengers. Glucagon was first discovered by Kimball and Murlin (1923) as a hyperglycemic substance in extracts of bovine pancreas. PHI, the newest member of the VIP peptide family, was originally isolated from the porcine intestinal tract by Tatemoto and Mutt (1980). Later studies indicated the structural similarities of the four peptides (Table III); of the four, PHI has the greatest sequence homology to VIP.

Secretin and glucagon are contained in both nerves and endocrine cells in the GI tract, whereas VIP and PHI are contained only in nerves. All four peptides, however, influence GI function. Studies of the biological actions of the peptides indicate a great deal of overlap in their functions, some of which might be explained by their structural similarities.

a. VIP Vasoactive intestinal peptide was isolated by Said and Mutt (1970) from pig small intestine on the basis of its powerful hypotensive and vasodilatory effects, and its sequence (Table III) indicated that it was related to secretin and glucagon (Mutt *et al.*, 1970). It has been detected by immunocytochemistry throughout the gut (Polak *et al.*, 1974), and more recently, high concentrations have been found (Larsson *et al.*, 1976) in the CNS, particularly the hypothalamus, and effects on hypothalamus-mediated release of growth hormones prolactin and luteinizing hormone (LH) have been observed (Kato *et al.*, 1978; Vijayan *et al.*, 1979). Elevated levels of VIP are present (Said and Porter, 1979) in hypophyseal portal blood, suggesting possible direct physiological effects on pituitary function.

VIP has been shown to function as both a central and a peripheral neurotransmitter and it is a potent bronchodilator. VIP-containing neurons innervate airway

Table III

Amino Acid Sequences of VIP Family of Peptides

Peptide	Sequence
VIP-28	H S D A V F T D N Y T R L R K Q M A V K K Y L N S I L N NH_2
PHI-27	H A D G V F T S D F S R L L G Q L S A K K Y L E S L I NH_2
Secretin-27	H S D G T F T S E L S R L R D S A R L Q R L L Q G L V NH_2
Glucagon-29	H S Q G T F T S D Y S K Y L D S R R A Q D F V Q W L M N T

smooth muscle and exocrine glands in the lung, and VIP has been shown to be a major endogenous component of airway smooth-muscle relaxation (Said *et al.*, 1974). It is postulated that aberrant VIP functioning may be responsible for the bronchoconstriction, edema, and mucous secretion found in bronchial asthma (Morice *et al.*, 1983; Barnes and Dixon, 1984). VIP has also been shown to induce sleep.

Initial *in vitro* and preliminary clinical results from studies on VIP have indicated its potential as a therapeutic agent for bronchial asthma. Bolin *et al.* (1988) synthesized analogs of VIP to study SAR. These studies indicated that the replacement of Met^{17} by norleucine increases the smooth-muscle relaxant activity on guinea pig tracheal rings. Secondary structural calculations predict the central portion of the molecule (12–20) to be helical. Replacement of residues within this region by helix-favoring residues enhanced potency. For example, replacement of Arg^{12} or Arg^{14} with Lys or Orn results in a 1.7- to 2.6-fold increase in potency. By synthesizing combinations of the most favorable changes, Bolin *et al.* (1988) found a series of analogs with larger increases in potency. The analog [Ac-His^{1}, Lys^{12}, Lys^{14}, Nle^{17}, Val^{26}, Thr^{28}]-VIP is 10-fold more potent than native VIP.

b. Secretin Secretin is widely distributed in the brain. In the GI tract it is found distal to the duodenum with a peak in the ileum (in rat). It is contained in endocrine cells in the superficial layers of the mucosa of the small intestine in various species and is located in secretory granules (Dodd *et al.*, 1979; Phillis and Kirkpatrick, 1979).

The major function of secretin appears to be to induce secretions important to digestion. Secretin increases the flow of hepatic bile, an action independent of the actions of secretin on the pancreas and intestines. It influences smooth-muscle function in the digestive tract and cardiovascular function. Injection of secretin causes diuresis in anesthetized dogs. In man, doses of secretin submaximal for pancreatic secretion increase renal excretion of water, sodium, and bicarbonate.

The biological activity of secretin requires the complete sequence of 27 amino acids. The omission of the N-terminal amino acid histidine (Mutt and Jorpes,

1967) or the replacement of aspartic acid in position 3 with asparagine or of C-terminal carboxamide with a free carboxyl group results in a drastic reduction in or a complete loss of potency. On the other hand, an active analog was obtained when the four arginine residues were replaced by ornithine.

c. Glucagon Glucagon-like peptides have been detected in the CNS tissue of several species; by radioimmunoassay (RIA), glucagon-like immunoreactivity was detected in human brain (Ghatei *et al.*, 1984), but the major source of glucagon is the pancreas. It is also found in the other organs of the GI tract; four different glucagon-like peptides have been identified in human distal intestine.

In rat brain, the binding sites for pancreatic glucagon are the olfactory tubercle, hippocampus, amygdala, and anterior pituitary. Binding sites for glucagon have also been identified in the liver, where they are associated with adenylate cyclase.

Glucagon is important in glucose homeostasis, stimulating glycogenolysis in the liver and gluconeogenesis in the liver and other tissues. Unger (1978) suggested that glucagon may be involved in the pathogenesis of diabetes mellitus.

A considerable number of studies have been devoted to the SAR and the conformational properties of glucagon. An X-ray crystal structure of glucagon has been determined (Sasaki *et al.*, 1975). In the crystal, glucagon is primarily α-helical, with only the N-terminal residue not participating in the helical structure. Helical structure is stabilized by interactions involving lipophilic residues at positions 22–29 and 6–14. On the basis of this and other structure–function data, these investigators suggested that the binding to the glucagon plasma membrane receptor involves similar interactions between monomeric helical glucagon and the lipophilic regions on the receptor. In view of the length of the helical glucagon molecule (about 40 Å), it is possible that glucagon binds to two symmetrically related regulatory subunits. In the crystal structure, the 1–4 region has a disordered structure and can change its conformation readily; it seems to be intimately involved in the biological message. In particular, the His^1 is important since it was found that [des-His^1]-glucagon is a partial agonist and the corresponding N^{ϵ}-phenylthiocarbamoyl derivative is an antagonist (Hruby, 1981). Further evidence that the N-terminal region contains primarily the biological message and the rest of the molecule the address is provided by studies showing that glucagon (1–21) and glucagon (1–6) are fully active biologically, but at reduced potencies (Wright and Rodbell, 1979; Wright *et al.*, 1978). Thus, glucagon inhibitors can be developed by appropriate modification of the N-terminal region and these would be of aid in understanding the mechanism of glucagon action on the liver. A few glucagon antagonists have been synthesized (Cote and Epand, 1979; Bregman and Hruby, 1979) by chemically modifying the α- and ϵ-amino positions of the hormone. Bregman *et al.* (1980) investigated the importance of these amino groups to biological function. It is shown that antagonists result from similar group modifications of the α- and/or ϵ-amino positions, resulting in a change in the monomeric structure of glucagon. Agonists result from hydrophilic modifications at the α- or ϵ-amino position, but differing effects on potency and agonistic ability of the analogs occur, depending on the modification. [1-N^{α}-Trinitrophenylhistidine, 12-homoarginine]glucagon is the most potent inhibitor tested (Bregman *et al.*, 1980).

Recent studies by Corvera *et al.* (1984) and Murphy *et al.* (1987) suggest that glucagon may mediate some of its actions independent of cyclic AMP (cAMP). To obtain further insight into the basis of these observations, McKee *et al.* (1988) examined both glucagon and one of their most potent synthetic glucagon antagonists (des-amino-His^{1}, D-Phe^{4}, Tyr^{5}, Arg^{12}, $Lys^{17,18}$, Glu^{21}-glucagon, [des-amino-fYRKKE]glucagon) for bioactivities throughout the glycogenolytic cascade. Using a nonrecirculatory perfusion technique with thin liver slices, McKee *et al.* (1988) investigated hepatic hormonal mechanisms by monitoring intracellular events and overall cellular processes simultaneously. They observed that glucagon at low concentrations and the adenylate cyclase antagonist [des-amino-fYRKKE]glucagon at high concentrations stimulated hepatic glycogenolysis independent of any intracellular cAMP accumulation or activation of the cAMP-dependent protein kinase. These results support the notion that glucagon can mediate physiological events independent of cAMP.

d. PHI Peptide histidine isoleucine amide, a 27-residue peptide (PHI-27), is the newest member of the VIP peptide family, originally isolated from the porcine intestinal tract (Tatemoto and Mutt, 1980, 1981). It was named peptide HI (PHI) on the basis of an N-terminal histidine (H) and a C-terminal isoleucine (I) amide. Later, Carlquist *et al.* (1984) isolated PHI from bovine upper intestine in a 40-fold higher yield. The bovine PHI differs from porcine PHI at position 10 and from human PHI at positions 10, 12, and 27. PHI has also been found in high concentration in nasal mucosa and urogenital system (Yiangou *et al.*, 1986). In human endocrine tumors (Bloom *et al.*, 1983; Itoh *et al.*, 1983), VIP and PHM, the human counterpart of PHI, are derived from a common precursor. PHI and VIP are coreleased by vagal stimulation in the dog (Yasui *et al.*, 1987). PHI has been found to be structurally homologous to VIP, glucagon, secretion, and growth hormone-releasing factor (GRF). However, in terms of activity, PHI possesses few similarities to GRF, glucagon, or secretin, but it has a number of biological activities in common with VIP. Both PHI and VIP are potent stimulants of pancreatic secretion (Dimaline and Dockray, 1980; Jensen *et al.*, 1981; Szecowka *et al.*, 1980) and intestinal secretion in several species (Ghiglione *et al.*, 1982; Anagnostides *et al.*, 1983a,b). In addition, it has been shown that PHI can displace VIP label bound to membrane receptors from lung (Robberecht *et al.*, 1982). However, unlike VIP, PHI is only a weak vasodilator (Lundberg and Tatemoto, 1982).

Brennan *et al.* (1982) were the first to suggest a possible physiological action of PHI in the gall bladder. They reported that PHI is capable of decreasing basal gall bladder pressure and that it reduces bilirubin and bile acid output in man.

Table IV

Amino Acid Sequences of Neuropeptide Y Family

Peptide	Sequence
NPY	Y P S K P D N P G E D A P A E D L A R Y Y S A L R H Y I N L I T R Q R Y NH_2
PYY	Y P A K P E A P G E D A S P E E L S R Y Y A S L R H Y L N L V T R Q R Y NH_2
PPP	A P L E P V Y P G D D A T P E Q M A Q Y A A E L R R Y I N M L T R P R Y NH_2

Other biological activities of PHI include release of insulin, glucagon, and prolactin. Ahren and Lundquist (1988) recently reported that PHI potentiates glucose-induced insulin secretion and carbachol-induced glucagon secretion in the mouse.

Moroder *et al.* (1981) chemically synthesized PHI to prove the proposed sequence and to define its physiological role. Robberecht *et al.* (1987) synthesized [D-Phe^4]PHI and reported that this analog was a highly selective VIP agonist of stimulus–effector coupling in rat pancreatic plasma membranes.

e. NPY, PYY, and PPP Neuropeptide Y (NPY) is an important neurotransmitter that regulates the cardiovascular system. The complete amino acid sequence of this 36-residue peptide amide was elucidated by Tatemoto (1982b), who had isolated it from porcine brain tissues. The sequence of NPY shows extensive homology to pancreatic polypeptide (PPP) (Kimmel *et al.*, 1975) and peptide YY (PYY) (Tatemoto, 1982a) (Table IV), isolated from porcine intestinal extract (Tatemoto and Mutt, 1980).

NPY, PYY, and PPP are capable of inhibiting exocrine pancreatic secretion stimulated by secretin and CCK (Tatemoto *et al.*, 1982). PYY has a vasoconstrictory action and inhibits jejunal and colonic motility; it is localized in gut endocrine cells of several mammalian species, including man. NPY also has potent vasoconstrictory properties, being more potent than PPP but less potent than PYY. Balasubramaniam *et al.* (1987) and Kiyama *et al.* (1987) succeeded in synthesizing NPY. Synthetic NPY caused prolonged increase of systemic arterial blood pressure and decreased pancreatic blood flow in dogs (Kiyama *et al.*, 1987). Recently, Ishiguro *et al.* (1988) synthesized fragments of NPY for use in studying the structure–activity in relation to inhibition of calmodulin-stimulated phosphodiesterase; they reported that the carboxy-half fragments of NPY were more potent than NPY in this regard.

6. Motilin

Motilin is a 22-amino acid residue polypeptide isolated from porcine intestine (Brown *et al.*, 1970). Immunohistochemical mapping of motilin demonstrates that motilin is also present in several brain areas. The structure of motilin is

Phe-Val-Pro-Ile-Phe-Thr-Tyr-Gly-Glu-Leu-Gln-Arg-Met-Glu-Glu-Lys-Glu-Arg-Asn-Lys-Gly-Gln

When injected intravenously into dogs, motilin induces powerful motor activity increases in the fundic gland area and antral pouches of the stomach. These motor activity increases are accompanied by increases in pepsin output from the fundic gland area pouches, but with no increase in hydrogen ion output. Recent studies by Hashmonai *et al.* (1987) suggest that the receptors for motilin may be located outside the CNS.

Hirning and Burks (1986) examined the contractile effects of motilin in isolated canine small intestine segments. Their studies indicate that motilin produces increases in intraluminal pressure. Synthesis of motilin was achieved by Beyerman *et al.* (1979). Kuno *et al.* (1986) synthesized an analog of motilin (Gln^{15}-motilin); they found that this analog was as active as synthetic motilin in contracting rabbit duodenal muscles.

7. Galanin

Galanin is a novel 29-residue mammalian gut peptide that was discovered by the detection of its C-terminal amide structure in porcine intestinal extract. Tatemoto *et al.* (1983) reported the isolation, amino acid sequence, and some of the biological activities of this novel peptide amide, which they designated galanin from the N- and C-terminal residues glycine and alanine. Its structure is

Gly-Trp-Thr-Leu-Asn-Ser-Ala-Gly-Tyr-Leu-Leu-Gly-
Pro-His-Ala-Ile-Asp-Asn-His-Arg-Ser-Phe-His-Asp-
Lys-Tyr-Gly-Leu-Ala-NH_2

Galanin induces contractions of the fundus strip, ileum, colon, and urinary bladder (Tatemoto *et al.,* 1983). It also induces mild but sustained hyperglycemia. Recently, Yanaihara *et al.* (1988) performed structure–function studies of galanin and compared it with other synthetic peptides in terms of effect on glucose-induced insulin release in the isolated rat pancreas. They found that synthetic galanin suppressed the glucose-induced insulin release. *N*-Acetylgalanin showed significant suppressing effect, whereas galanin (2–29) had no more suppressing effect, thus suggesting the crucial role of the first amino acid, Gly, for the suppressing effect of galanin on glucose-induced insulin release. Further shortening the peptide chain gave peptides that, conversely, had potentiating effects, with maximum potency at the 15–29 length. This is the first demonstration that a peptide and its fragments possess opposite effects in action on a single biological system. From the secondary structure predictions of the analogs and fragments, high incidence of β-sheet structure in the N-terminal 1–11 sequence of galanin was suggested to be essential for the suppressing effect on glucose-induced insulin release in the isolated rat pancreas.

8. Insulin

The term "insulin" is usually associated with diabetes mellitus. The primary structure of this hormone is shown in Fig. 5. It consists of two polypeptide

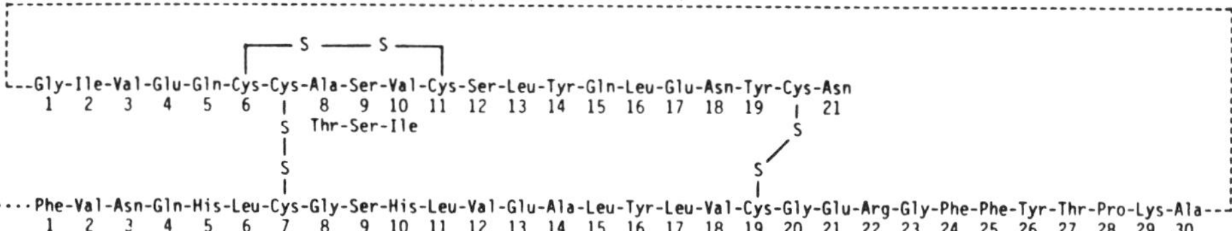

Fig. 5 The primary structure of bovine insulin.

chains, A and B, joined by two disulfide bridges. Insulin is secreted by the β cells of the islets of Langerhans of the pancreas. It can be readily crystallized as a zinc salt, although nickel, calcium, and cobalt also are effective. Insulin is essential for the proper metabolism of blood sugar (glucose) and for maintenance of the proper blood sugar level. Inadequate secretion of insulin results in improper metabolism of carbohydrates and fats and brings on diabetes, characterized by hyperglycemia and glycosuria. The secretion of insulin is primarily dependent on the concentration of blood glucose, with an increase of blood sugar bringing about an increase in the secretion of insulin.

The response of cells to insulin is initiated by the binding of insulin to its cell-surface receptor, an integral transmembrane glycoprotein composed of two α subunits and two β subunits. Because of the therapeutic value of insulin, remarkable progress has been made in the past few years in the development of synthetic and semisynthetic methods for the preparation of insulin and its analogs. To cover the entire work done in this regard is beyond the scope of this review. A few examples are mentioned below. Markussen *et al.* (1987) achieved the biosynthesis of human insulin in yeast. Riggs *et al.* (1979) prepared human insulin via recombinant DNA technology. Yang *et al.* (1988) chemically synthesized the A chain of insulin and succeeded in the partial synthesis of crystalline porcine insulin from the synthetic A chain and the natural B chain and studied the biological activity of their products. Markussen *et al.* (1988) synthesized substituted analogs of insulin by genetic engineering and tryptic transpeptidation and studied the influence of substitutions on the prolonged effect on blood glucose in rabbits. Brandenburg (1981) described various methods for the synthesis and semisynthesis of insulin.

Hefford *et al.* (1986) studied the SAR of insulin. Currently, the free monomeric unit of insulin is believed to be a biological species relevant to receptor binding, and the conformation of the monomeric unit of insulin is essentially the same in its free and associated states in solution. Davies *et al.* (1986) identified the cleavage sites of insulin by insulin proteinase.

B. Neuropeptides

Neuropeptides were originally isolated from brain tissue, but neither the origin nor the target of these neuropeptides is confined to the CNS. They are widely distributed throughout the body. As the gastrointestinal peptides were found to be located in the CNS, the neuropeptides originally isolated from brain tissue have now been shown to occur in certain enteric or pancreatic endocrine cells, e.g., somatostatin, neurotensin, thyrotropin-releasing hormone (TRH), enkephalin, endorphin, adrenocorticotropin (ACTH), and gonadotropin-releasing hormone (GRH). GRH has also been shown to be present in and produced by the human placenta. In addition, a number of these peptides have been found in peripheral nerves. We will only describe two classes of neuropeptides here, the hypothalamic peptides and the opioid peptides.

1. Hypothalamic Peptides

Neuropeptides in this group include luteinizing hormone-releasing hormone (LHRH), thyrotropin-releasing hormone (TRH), corticotropin-releasing factor (CRF), growth hormone-releasing factor (GRF), somatostatin, oxytocin, and vasopressin; they are all present in high concentrations in the hypothalamus. Evidence based on morphological, physiological, and pharmacological studies indicates that the role of these hypothalamic peptides is not restricted to that of releasing or release-inhibiting hormones; they may also act as neurotransmitters at extrahypothalamic sites.

a. LHRH Luteinizing hormone-releasing hormone (LHRH), also known as LRH or LRF, is a decapeptide and is the key mediator in the neuroregulation of the secretion of the gonadotropins luteinizing hormone (LH) and follicle-stimulating hormone (FSH). In addition to its role as a hypothalamic hypophysiotropic hormone, LHRH can modify sexual behavior (Pfaff, 1973; Moss and McCann, 1973) and is distributed in and exhibits electrophysiological effects in various neural regions. Its essential function in the regulation of gonadotropin secretion and in reproductive processes has been demonstrated by the marked reductions in plasma gonadotropin and sex steroid levels, gonadal atrophy, and inhibition of gametogenesis observed following active or passive immunoneutralization of LHRH.

pGlu-His-Trp-Ser-Tyr-Gly-Leu-Arg-Pro-Gly-NH_2

Research on LHRH in recent years has led to the discovery of highly potent agonists and antagonists. Both of these classes of compounds are being investigated as potential contraceptives—antagonists as ovulation inhibitors and superagonists as postcoital agents that interfere with implantation or maintenance of pregnancy. According to Nestor (1984), the substitution of hydrophobic D-amino acids in position 6 gave the most potent analog *in vivo*. This was attributed to a combination of factors, including increased receptor affinity, protection from proteolysis, and prolonged duration of action due to depositing of the analog in the body. Nestor *et al.* (1982, 1984, 1985) have reported a series of analogs that exhibit high biological activity. Hocart *et al.* (1987, 1988) studied the effect of introducing a variety of hydrophobic alkyl and aryl groups into the side chain of Lys in positions 6 (D) and 8 (L) in an attempt to reduce the histamine-releasing activity of the analogs.

b. TRH The characterization of thyrotropin-releasing hormone (TRH) as the tripeptide amide pGlu-His-Pro-NH_2 was a major advance in neuroendocrinology. TRH is distributed throughout the extrahypothalamic nervous system, the spinal cord, and the retina as well as other tissues and has been found to have a variety of effects in the CNS. The capacity of TRH to reverse the anesthetic effect of sedative–hypnotic compounds was among the first of its behavioral effects to be characterized. Prange *et al.* (1974) initially demonstrated that TRH antagonized pentobarbital-induced narcosis in mice. It was later shown to reverse the sedation induced by a number of other central depressant agents, including other barbiturates, alcohol, chlorpromazine, α-methyltyrosine, Δ^9-tetrahydrocannabinol, reserpine, diazepam, chloral hydrate, and ketamine. In contrast, it did not alter the anesthesia produced by morphine or halothane (Horita *et al.*, 1976a; Smith *et al.*, 1976). TRH has been shown to have a respiratory stimulant effect in both anesthetized and conscious mammals (Andry and Horita, 1977). Vijayan and McCann (1977) demonstrated that TRH suppresses food and water intake in the food-deprived rat. TRH increases gastrointestinal contraction, motility, and secretion. It has also been shown to have a vasopressor action and to induce cardiovascular changes (Beale *et al.*, 1977; Horita *et al.*, 1976b; Eriksson and Gordon, 1981; Koivusalo *et al.*, 1979). Many studies have shown that TRH improves survival after induction of circulatory shock by endotoxemia, hemorrhage, spinal cord trauma, or leukotriene D_4 (Faden *et al.*, 1981; Holaday *et al.*, 1981; Lux *et al.*, 1983).

The neuropharmacological effects of TRH and its antidepressant activity in man (Prange *et al.*, 1972) have attracted much interest. Morgan *et al.* (1979) synthesized a series of analogs of TRH having differing biological profiles. Their Dmp analog showed greatly increased neuropharmacological potency and a reduced ability to evoke release of prolactin. Nutt *et al.* (1979) synthesized TRH analogs and reported the reversal of the hypothermic action of chlorpromazine by one of them. Labroo *et al.* (1985) synthesized imidazole-substituted analogs of TRH and reported that three of them significantly raised the blood pressure and heart rate in conscious rats. Stezowski and Eckle (1983) carried out an extensive program of crystal structure analysis for TRH analogs in an effort to contribute to an understanding of the interrelationship between chemical structure, conformation, and CNS activity. They observed similarities in conformations of TRH analogs and the last three residues of a Leu^5-enkephalin molecule.

c. CRH Corticotropin-releasing hormone (CRH), also known as corticotropin-releasing factor (CRF), is a 41-amino acid straight-chain peptide first isolated by Vale and colleagues (1981) from sheep hypothalamic extracts.

Subsequent characterization of the active principles from rat, bovine, porcine, and human sources indicates that human and rat CRHs are identical and differ by seven amino acids from the ovine molecule first sequenced. The amino acid sequence of the human CRH is shown in Fig. 6.

CRH has as much as 50% homology with several other known peptides that share a number of similar physiological effects. Among these substances are sauvagine (40 amino acids), isolated from the skin of frogs, and urotensin I (38 amino acids), obtained from the urohypophysis of the sucker fish and other teleosts (Vale *et al.*, 1983; MacCannell and Lederis, 1983). CRH also shows homology with calmodulin and with angiotensinogen at the renin and converting enzyme cleavage sites (Vale *et al.*, 1983).

CRH has a stimulatory effect on the synthesis and release of adrenocorticotropin (ACTH) and other pro-opiomelanocortin-related peptides by anterior pituitary cells. The demonstration of the essential role played by endogenous CRF in modulating ACTH secretion was supported by the lowering of basal plasma ACTH levels of adrenalectomized rats or stress-induced ACTH release by intact animals following the administration of a CRF antiserum (Rivier *et al.*, 1982) or a specific CRF antagonist (Rivier *et al.*, 1984). This stimulatory effect initiated by binding of CRH to specific high-affinity receptors on the cell surface. Intracerebral administration of CRH markedly suppresses LH release in rats, with elevated levels of gonadotropin; however, there is no effect on FSH secretion (Rivier and Vale, 1984a, 1985; Ono *et al.*, 1984). Centrally administered CRH also suppresses growth hormone release in the rat (Ono *et al.*, 1984; Rivier and Vale, 1984b). CRH has been shown to have an antipyretic effect in the rabbit. Hyperglycemia is regularly seen in rats given CRH centrally. It also causes increased mean arterial blood pressure and heart rate in the dog and rat (Brown and Fischer, 1983, 1985; Fischer *et al.*, 1982). Diminished gastric acid secretion is seen after intracerebral microinjection of CRH in rats and dogs (Tache *et al.*, 1983; Lenz *et al.*, 1985).

Rivier *et al.* (1988) described the synthesis and biological characterization of several CRF analogs in an attempt to determine which conformational parameters were important for the biological response. Some of their CRF antagonists exhibited significantly higher biological potency than did α-helical CRF (9–41) in both *in vitro* and *in vivo* studies.

```
                5                   10
Ser-Glu-Glu-Pro-Pro-Ile-Ser-Leu-Asp-Leu-Thr-Phe-His-Leu-
 15                  20                  25
Leu-Arg-Glu-Val-Leu-Glu-Met-Ala-Arg-Ala-Glu-Gln-Leu-Ala-
    30                  35                  40
Gln-Gln-Ala-His-Ser-Asn-Arg-Lys-Leu-Met-Glu-Ile-Ile
```

Fig. 6 Amino acid sequence of human CRH.

d. GRF Malacara *et al.*(1972) demonstrated the existence of a hypothalamic growth hormone-releasing factor (GRF). Peptides with the biological activity of hypothalamic GRF have been ectopically produced by pancreatic islet cell tumors and variously located carcinoids.

From a tumor of the pancreas that had caused acromegaly, Guillemin *et al.* (1982) and Ling *et al.* (1984) isolated and characterized a 44-amino acid peptide with growth hormone-releasing activity. The primary structure of the tumor-derived peptide is shown in Fig. 7. The synthetic replicate had full biological activity *in vitro* and *in vivo,* specifically to stimulate the secretion of immunoreactive growth hormone. The tumor-derived peptide is identical in biological activity and similar in physicochemical properties to the as yet uncharacterized GRF present in extracts of hypothalamic tissue, an amidated C terminus, and the other two peptides hpGRF-37 and hpGRF-40 being shown to correspond to the sequences 1–37 and 1–40 of hpGRF-44. The last two peptides possess a free C terminus. Because of the higher potency of hpGRF-44 in the *in vivo* assay and because it has an amidated C terminus, Ling *et al.* (1984) proposed that it was the mature form of the peptide and that hpGRF-37 and hpGRF-40 were postsecretory degradation products still endowed with biological activity.

Synthesis of GRF has been described by various investigators (Fujii *et al.*, 1984; Diaz *et al.*, 1985). Structure–activity studies (Coy *et al.*, 1985; Ohashi *et al.*, 1986, 1988) using GRF analogs have revealed that only the N-terminal 29-amino acid residues are required for full intrinsic GRF activity, the N-terminal Tyr being quite important. Clore *et al.* (1986) performed conformational analysis of GRF (1–29) using two-dimensional nuclear magnetic resonance (NMR) and revealed two regions of α-helical character between residues 6–13 and 16–29. Felix *et al.* (1988) synthesized analogs with extended α-helical region and with maximized amphiphilical α-helical structure; these analogs were found to exhibit increased biological potencies. They also synthesized a cyclic analog in an attempt to enhance the short half-life (6.8 min) reported for GRF (1–44)-NH_2.

e. Somatostatin Krulich *et al.* (1968) described the presence of a substance in hypothalamic extracts demonstrating inhibition of growth hormone secretion. They called it somatostatin; the name is derived from the Latin for "to halt growth." It has also been localized in extra-CNS sites and has been shown to

```
                5                   10                  15
Tyr-Ala-Asp-Ala-Ile-Phe-Thr-Asn-Ser-Tyr-Arg-Lys-Val-Leu-Gly-

                20                  25                  30
Gln-Leu-Ser-Ala-Arg-Lys-Leu-Leu-Gln-Asp-Ile-Met-Ser-Arg-Gln-

                35                  40                  44
Gln-Gly-Glu-Ser-Asn-Gln-Glu-Arg-Gly-Ala-Arg-Ala-Arg-Leu-NH2
```

Fig. 7 Amino acid sequence of human GRF.

```
Ala-Gly-Cys-Lys-Asn-Phe-Phe-Trp-Lys-Thr-Phe-Thr-Ser-Cys
        |_______________________________________________|
```

Fig. 8 Primary structure of somatostatin.

inhibit the secretion of many hormones other than growth hormone, including insulin, glucagon, and gastrin. Somatostatin is a cyclic tetradecapeptide (Fig. 8).

It is not yet known whether the diversity of somatostatin's multitudinous actions results from a common membrane effect (i.e., with regard to calcium transport), with organ specificity being dependent on local somatostatin generation, or whether specific segments of peptide have different effects on different target hormones. To date, based on these observations, attempts have been made to develop, for therapeutic purposes, analogs with longer duration of activity or with activity on oral administration as well as with selective inhibitory properties on the pancreas, the pituitary, or the GI tract (Folkers *et al.*, 1977: Yanaihara *et al.*, 1977). There have been reports of development of compounds having biological selectivity with regard to insulin release, glucagon release, or growth hormone release (Veber and Saperstein, 1979). Rivier (1974) has reported that Asp^5-deleted analogs preferentially inhibit insulin rather than glucagon or growth hormone secretion. Substitution of D- for L-cysteine^{14} yields an analog that is more potent in inhibiting glucagon and growth hormone secretion than insulin secretion (Brown *et al.*, 1977). Analogs in which the cysteine bridge is replaced by nonsulfur linkages are reported to retain growth hormone suppressive activity at doses that do not alter insulin or glucose release (Grant *et al.*, 1976).

Another approach to analog design has been based on a model for the biologically active conformation. Attempts to alter the duration of action have been through structural modifications such as acylation, reduction of the rate of metabolism by amino peptidases through the addition of glycine residues, replacement of various amino acids by the D-enantiomer, deletion of various amino acids, or replacement of reducible disulfide dimethylene groups. A new and promising approach to increasing metabolic stability is the introduction of conformational constraints in order to produce compounds with a conformation that interacts with receptors but has altered metabolic susceptibility (Hruby *et al.*, 1988). It is even possible that receptors for different biological actions may interact differently with different conformations of the same molecule. Recently, a series of studies involving analog synthesis, biological evaluation of analogs, and physical measurement, which have suggested a postulated bioactive conformation, has led to the design of a conformationally restricted somatostatin analog with increased duration in inhibiting insulin, glucagon, and growth hormone release but not gastric secretion (Veber, 1979). Cai *et al.* (1985) synthesized fragments of somatostatin for conformational studies and evaluation of activities. A potent cyclic hexapeptide analog of somatostatin was reported by Veber *et al.* (1981).

They hypothesized that the essential residues for somatostatin activity are Phe-Trp-Lys-Thr and that the Phe-Pro moiety induces the conformational constraint of the β-turn. Based on Veber's hypothesis, Nagai *et al.* (1988) replaced the Phe-Pro sequence with a β-turn dipeptide (BTD) and observed that the BTD analog showed weak activity in inhibiting growth hormone release from the pituitary. Coy *et al.* (1988) reported a receptor-selective somatostatin analog.

f. Oxytocin and Vasopressin The nonapeptide hormones oxytocin and vasopressin (Table V) are extracted from the posterior pituitary (du Vigneaud *et al.*, 1953; du Vigneaud, 1956). They have similar structures except that in vasopressin there is Phe at position 3 instead of Ile and either Arg (AVP) or Lys (LVP) at position 8 instead of Leu. The localization of oxytocin and vasopressin in hypothalamus was determined by Lederis (1961), Van Dyke *et al.* (1957), and Adamsons *et al.* (1956). The neurohypophyseal hormones exert their effect in the CNS; in addition, studies, mainly performed with peripheral nervous system in rats in aversively motivated tasks, suggest that vasopressin and related peptides affect learning and memory processes (De Wied, 1980). Besides, they act both in the circulatory system, causing vasoconstriction, and in the kidney, causing the increased uptake of water from the collecting duct (Rosas *et al.*, 1962). Oxytocin elicits smooth-muscle contraction, causing milk ejection and uterine contraction in mammals. More recent studies uncovered a multitude of effects of the neurohypophyseal hormones on CNS functions, ranging from brain development to maternal behavior, from temperature to cardiovascular regulation, and from sexual behavior to drug-seeking behavior. The other naturally occurring neurohypophyseal hormones include vasotocin and mesotocin.

Oxytocin was the first peptide hormone whose structure was determined and then proved by total synthesis. In addition, it was the first peptide hormone for

Table V

Amino Acid Sequences of Neurohypophyseal Hormones and Related Peptides

Hormone	Sequence
Oxytocin	H-Cys-Tyr-Ile-Gln-Asn-Cys-Pro-Leu-Gly-NH_2 (disulfide bridge Cys¹–Cys⁶)
Vasopressin	H-Cys-Tyr-Phe-Gln-Asn-Cys-Pro-Arg-(Lys)-Gly-NH_2
Vasotocin	H-Cys-Tyr-Ile-Gln-Asn-Cys-Pro-Arg-Gly-NH_2
Mesotocin	H-Cys-Tyr-Ile-Gln-Asn-Cys-Pro-Ile-Gly-NH_2

which a three-dimensional structure in solution was proposed (Urry and Walter, 1978); the first for which a complete assignment of the ^{1}H-NMR spectrum in aqueous solution was made (Brewster *et al.*, 1973; Brewster and Hruby, 1973); the first for which extensive dynamic properties in solution were determined (Deslauriers *et al.*, 1974; Glasel *et al.*, 1973) using NMR relaxation methods; and the first for which attempts were made to correlate conformation and dynamic properties of the hormone with biological activity (Walter *et al.*, 1971; Meraldi *et al.*, 1977).

Both oxytocin and vasopressin have a very short half-time of biological effect. If applied exogenously, a small amount is excreted intact in urine and a larger part is cleaved enzymatically. Although this is a physiologically important mechanism in that it prevents autointoxication of organisms with these hormones, in many cases it would be desirable to increase the half-time of their biological effect. First attempts in this direction concerned the higher resistance to enzymatic cleavage in the N-terminal part of the molecule. Many authors report this inactivation by cleavage of the hemiscystine–tyrosine bond (Tuppy, 1960). Enzymes responsible for this cleavage (oxytocinases) are, in principle, aminopeptidases and therefore it could be assumed that a suitable substitution of the α-amino group in cysteine in position 1 might prevent, or at least retard, the cleavage. The first analog of this type, *N*-glycyloxytocin, described by du Vigneaud and co-workers (1960), showed a prolonged action in avian depressor and rat pressor assays and inhibitory properties in the former test. Since then, a large number of analogs of both oxytocin and vasopressin have been synthesized and tested for various biological effects, e.g., memory effects, cardiovascular regulation, temperature regulation, antidiuretic effect, and uterotonic effect (Chan, 1965; Chan and Sawyer, 1961; Machova, 1971; Jost *et al.*, 1987). Extensive studies have been done on conformation–activity relationship (Melin *et al.*, 1981; Hruby, 1981, 1984; Hruby *et al.*, 1980; Struthers *et al.*, 1984).

2. Opioid Peptides

The potent effects of opium derivatives on the nervous system and gut, known for centuries, have led to their clinical use to produce calming, analgesic, euphoric, and antidiarrheal effects; however, the mechanisms underlying their widespread pharmacological actions were not understood until recently, and the consequences of opiate addiction have been profound in humans. The discovery and identification of the endogenous opioid peptides Met- and Leu-enkephalin (Met-Enk and Leu-Enk) by Hughes *et al.* (1975), followed by β-endorphin and the related peptides by Li and Chung (1976), presented an opportunity to understand the mechanisms of opiate actions and opened up a new era in neurobiological research. The search for opioid peptide analogs that have analgesic efficacy but are not addictive has been one of the most extensive pharmacological undertakings. Hundreds of analogs of enkephalins, endorphins, and dynorphins have been synthesized for SAR studies. The amino acid sequences of endogenous opioid peptides are shown in Table VI.

Given the morphine-like action of naturally occurring peptides, the enkephalins have undergone numerous physicochemical studies in attempts to find the possible structural similarity between morphine and enkephalins. The enkephalins compete with morphine for binding to analgesic receptors, and these bindings are inhibited by morphine antagonists such as naloxone, suggesting that the enkephalins may bind to the same receptor site as does morphine or other opiates. A synthetic analog of β-endorphin (β-endorphin 6–31) was shown to be a mixed agonist–antagonist (Li and Chung, 1976). This analog does not contain the Met-enkephalin segment and appears to possess measurable analgesic activity; also, the response was not blocked by naloxone. The naturally occurring

Table VI

Amino Acid Sequences of Endogenous Opioid Peptides

Peptide	Sequence
Met-Enkephalin	1 5 H-Tyr-Gly-Gly-Phe-Met-OH
Leu-Enkephalin	1 5 H-Tyr-Gly-Gly-Phe-Leu-OH
Dynorphin A (1–9)	1 5 9 H-Tyr-Gly-Gly-Phe-Leu-Arg-Arg-Ile-Arg-OH
Dynorphin (1–17)	1 5 10 15 17 H-Tyr-Gly-Gly-Phe-Leu-Arg-Arg-Ile-Arg-Pro-Lys-Leu-Lys-Trp-Asp-Asn-Gln-OH
Dynorphin B (rimorphin)	1 5 10 13 H-Tyr-Gly-Gly-Phe-Leu-Arg-Arg-Gln-Phe-Lys-Val-Val-Thr-OH
Dynorphin B (29) [Leu-morphin, rimorphin (29)]	1 5 10 15 H-Tyr-Gly-Gly-Phe-Leu-Arg-Arg-Gln-Phe-Lys-Val-Val-Thr-Arg-Ser-Gln-Glu-Asp- 20 25 29 Pro-Asn-Ala-Tyr-Tyr-Glu-Glu-Leu-Phe-Asp-Val-OH
β_h-Endorphin	1 5 10 15 H-Tyr-Gly-Gly-Phe-Met-Thr-Ser-Glu-Lys-Ser-Gln-Thr-Pro-Leu-Val-Thr-Leu-Phe- 20 25 30 31 Lys-Asn-Ala-Ile-Ile-Lys-Asn-Ala-Tyr-Lys-Lys-Gly-Glu-OH
α-Endorphin	1 5 10 15 16 H-Tyr-Gly-Gly-Phe-Met-Thr-Ser-Glu-Lys-Ser-Gln-Thr-Pro-Leu-Val-Thr-OH
γ-Endorphin	1 5 10 15 17 H-Tyr-Gly-Gly-Phe-Met-Thr-Ser-Glu-Lys-Ser-Gln-Thr-Pro-Leu-Val-Thr-Leu-OH
δ-Endorphin	1 5 10 15 H-Tyr-Gly-Gly-Phe-Met-Thr-Ser-Glu-Lys-Ser-Gln-Thr-Pro-Leu-Val-Thr-Leu-Phe- 20 25 27 Lys-Asn-Ala-Ile-Ile-Lys-Asn-Ala-Tyr-OH

antagonist β-endorphin 1–27 is four times more potent than naloxone in antagonizing analgesia. What kind of structure is involved in these properties? Dynorphin is an extension of Leu-Enk, yet it is 700 times more potent than Leu-Enk in the guinea pig ileum assay and about three times more potent in mouse vas deferens. What are the structural features of dynorphin that account for the increased potency? The complexity is reduced somewhat by the findings that (1) all the known endogenous mammalian opioids belong to one of three families: the enkephalin family, the endorphin family, or the dynorphin family; and (2) it is well established that there are at least three different types of opioid receptor, known as μ, δ, and κ (Martin *et al.*, 1976; Lord *et al.*, 1977), with the μ-opioid receptor being the classical morphine receptor, enkephalins being somewhat selective for the δ receptor, dynorphin for the κ receptor, and β endorphin being equipotent for both μ and δ receptors.

The concept of multiple opiate receptors offers a new strategy for the development of targeted therapy if specific *in vivo* effects can be associated with the occupation of specific receptor classes or combinations of receptor subtypes. μ Receptors appear to be involved in analgesia and, in particular, in heat-mediated nociception (Kosterlitz *et al.*, 1980; Romer, 1981; Ronai, *et al.*, 1981; Gacel *et al.*, 1981; Burkhardt *et al.*, 1982; Upton *et al.*, 1982) and chemical nociception (Schmauss *et al.*, 1983). They appear also to mediate the respiratory depressant effects of opiates. μ Receptors are involved in inhibition of intestinal motility (Ward and Takemori, 1983) and of small-intestinal fluid secretion (Coupar, 1983), and in the development of physical dependence (Romer, 1981).

δ Receptors appear to mediate respiratory depression (Florez and Pazos, 1982) and circulatory shock (Holaday *et al.*, 1982; Holaday and D'Amato, 1983). Spinal δ receptors are involved in intestinal transit (Porreca *et al.*, 1983).

κ receptors mediate analgesia, particularly pressure nociception (Upton *et al.*, 1982). They are also involved in diuresis (Leander, 1983a,b; Slizgi and Ludens, 1982) and feeding behavior (Morley *et al.*, 1982, 1983).

The presence of opiate receptors has been demonstrated in all vertebrates, including man (Hiller and Simon, 1976), and also, more recently in certain invertebrates (Stefeno and Captane, 1979; Stefano *et al.*, 1980). The opiate receptors are confined to neural tissue; their existence has been shown in the CNS of mammals and also in opiate-sensitive, isolated organs like the guinea pig ileum (Creese and Snyder, 1975; Zukin and Gintzler, 1980) and mouse vas deferens (Leslie *et al.*, 1979).

We describe here the SAR of the three classes of opioid peptides.

a. Enkephalins Met-Enk and the closely related Leu-Enk were the first endogenous opiates to be identified structurally (Hughes *et al.*, 1975). This discovery resulted in the synthesis of related peptides on an unprecedented scale. Over 1000 tetra- or pentapeptide analogs have been described in the general or patent literature, and many have been subjected to detailed pharmacological analysis. One of the most gratifying outcomes of these endeavors has been the emergence of analogs of high potency (equal to or greater than that of morphine) in almost every *in vivo* test of opiate-like activity following intravenous, subcutaneous, or oral administration of the compounds. Under such conditions, Met-Enk and Leu-Enk are generally inactive. Thus, by suitable molecular manipulation, problems inherent in the metabolism and transplant of peptides and in the penetration of peptides throughout absorptive barriers have been overcome, thus considerably increasing our knowledge of the associated molecular processes.

On examination of the SARs of enkephalin published by late 1980, one particularly striking observation was that highly potent enkephalin analogs could be prepared by substituting Gly^2 with a large variety of D-amino acids and replacing Met^5 (or Leu^5) with a large variety of L- or D-amino acids, leading to a potent analog, D-Ala^2, Leu^5-enkephalin amide (DADLE), a potent analgesic (Lee *et al.*, 1980). Sarantakis (1979) prepared and patented [D-Cys^2, L-Cys^5]-enkephalin. Shortly thereafter, Schiller and co-workers (1981) also prepared a series of cyclic amides and extensively examined their biological activities. This type of cyclization led to μ-selectivity. Mosberg *et al.* (1982, 1983) prepared a number of D-Pen^2, D(L)-Cys^5 cyclic enkephalinamide and enkephalin analogs. These compounds turned out to have considerable δ-receptor selectivity, as measured by comparison of inhibitory potencies in the guinea pig ileum (μ receptor) versus mouse vas deferens (δ receptor). These results led to the preparation of highly conformationally restricted bispenicillamide cyclic analogs, D-Pen^2, L-Pen^5-enkephalin and D-Pen^2, D-Pen^5-enkephalin. These analogs were found to be extraordinarily δ-receptor specific (Mosberg *et al.*, 1983). Roques and collaborators published a series of papers (Fournie-Zaluski *et al.*, 1981; Gacel *et al.*, 1980, 1981) reporting studies on a series of 2- and 6-substituted Leu-Enks that culminated in the selective δ-agonist "DSLET", Tyr-D-Ser-Gly-Phe-Leu-Thr, which is 22 times as potent as Met-Enk. A report from the same group (Zajac *et al.*, 1983) cites "DTLET" or deltakephin, Tyr-D-Thr-Gly-Phe-Leu-Thr, as the most potent and selective δ agonist in the series. Loew and collaborators (Judd *et al.*, 1987) reported four μ-selective peptides with *in vivo* antagonism to morphine analgesia. These peptides were modified by incorporating four modified tyrosine residues (*m*-Tyr, β-CH_3-*m*-Tyr, *N*-phenethyl-*m*-Tyr, and α,β-dimethyl-*m*-Tyr) into D-Ala^2, Met-enkephalinamide. The rationale for the modification of tyrosine residues was based on postulated similarities of peptide opioids with a particular class of μ-selective nonpeptide opioids, 3-phenylpiperidines, and the known requirement for antagonism in that class (Kugita *et al.*, 1965; Loew *et al.*, 1981; Cheng *et al.*, 1986; Jacoby *et al.*, 1981).

Data pertaining to the development of tolerance or dependence liability of Met- and Leu-Enk are contradictory (Bhargava, 1977; Wei and Loh, 1976; Tseng *et al.*, 1976). If tolerance does occur, it is weak, probably because of the very weak analgesic activity. However, abuse liability of potent enkephalin analogs has been well documented. The potent analogs FK 33-824 [Tyr-D-Ala-Gly-NMePhe-Met(o)ol] (Romer *et al.*, 1977), D-Ala^2-Met-enkephalinamide (Tortella and Moreton, 1980), and D-Met^2, Pro^5-enkephalinamide (Miglecz *et al.*, 1979) all produce acute dependence and tolerance in a variety of *in vivo* and *in vitro* systems. Furthermore, they were cross-tolerant with morphine. Thus, it appears that the stronger the opiate agonist activity of the known enkephalin analogs, the higher the abuse potential. In the case of opiate alkaloids, it has been known for some time that both agonist and antagonist properties seem to have a lower addiction liability than do pure agonists such as morphine (Archer *et al.*, 1964, 1973). Furthermore, small chemical modifications in morphine, particularly in the N-substituent, lead to antagonism. If agonism is not completely eliminated, a less-addicting analgesic results. By analogy to fused-ring opiates, it is reasonable to assume that if antagonism could be introduced into the enkephalins, addiction liability would be decreased.

The results on the SAR of enkephalins support the hypothesis that enkephalin, when bound to the receptor, assumes a morphine-like conformation (Fig. 9), with the tyrosine moiety corresponding to the tyramine portion of the morphine molecule and the side chains of residue 5, and perhaps 4 as well, interacting, by hydrophobic forces, with portions of the receptor that also interact with the C and D rings of opiate.

b. Endorphins β-endorphins, 31-amino acid fragments of a larger prohor-

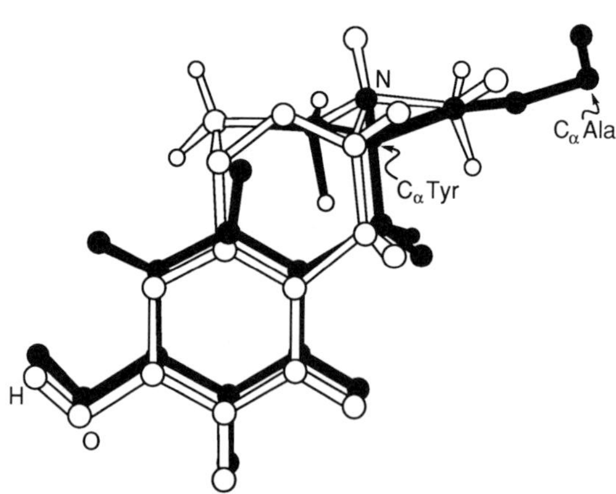

Fig. 9 Conformation of D-Ala^2-Met^5-enkephalinamide (black) overlapping benzomorphan fragment of morphine (white).

mone β-lipotropin, are potent endogenous opioid peptides with high receptor affinity and antinociceptive activity (Weiner *et al.*, 1984). β-Endorphin is the most potent species in all tests of analgesia. Met-Enk forms the N-terminal pentapeptide sequence of endorphins. The sequence of β-endorphin is remarkably conserved across a variety of species, which indicates that more than just the N-terminal Met-Enk-like portion of the peptides is important for activity. Several models of a β-endorphin–receptor complex have been proposed (Li *et al.*, 1980; Lee and Smith, 1980; Vaught *et al.*, 1982). A common feature of these models is the interaction of the N-terminal of β-endorphin with a presumptive enkephalin (δ) site and the C-terminal region with a presumptive morphine (μ) site (Yamashiro and Li, 1984).

β-Endorphins belong to a class of intermediate size bioactive peptides for which characterization of conformation profiles is most difficult. Such peptides pose discouraging difficulties for each of the three new disciplines: X-ray crystal structure determination, NMR studies, and theoretical energy-conformational studies. The latter, in principle, could be most useful for such studies. Such peptides are, in general, difficult to crystallize, have conformational flexibilities at room temperature, and have many possible stable structures, i.e., many local conformational minima of varying relative energies.

Recently, in an NMR study of β-endorphin, Jardetzky and collaborators (Lichtarge *et al.*, 1987) reported that, whereas conformational flexibility in water did not allow analysis of the spectra, dilution with methanol did. The extensive analysis of the NMR results, in water–methanol solution, including NOE spectra, indicated that the structure was consistent with a predominantly α-helical structure with the inclusion of a possible turn near residues 10–15. Loew *et al.* (1988) identified plausible initial structures of the full peptide by calculating and comparing the conformational preference of all possible extended tetrapeptide fragments of β-endorphin, starting from each of the first 28 residues. Comparisons of fragment energies suggested that two types of compact, folded β-endorphin conformers were plausible: a helix–turn–helix and an antiparallel β-sheet conformer. These structures were assembled, and total geometry optimization was performed using the empirical energy-based program AMBER. The results yielded an α-helical structure as the lowest energy form consistent with NMR studies of β-endorphin.

Since the discovery of β-endorphin, about 100 different analogs have been synthesized in an attempt to determine the importance of individual residues and regions to the affinity and activity of the peptide (Li, 1981; Nicholas *et al.*, 1982, 1984). These extensive SAR studies include replacement, omission, and addition of residues and incorporation of disulfide bridges. In another approach, variations in residues in the 13–31 regions were made based on the hypothesis that all that is required for opioid activity in β-endorphins is that this region form an amphiphilic helical structure.

The N-terminal pentapeptide sequence plays a crucial role in the activity of all endorphins, but there are interesting similarities and differences in SARs within this sequence compared with the enkephalins. The similarities are seen at the 1- and 4-positions. Thus, as in the case of enkephalins, an N-terminal tyrosine residue of L-configuration seems essential for activity, and there are also exact requirements at the Phe^4 position. The differences are more marked at the 2-position. Thus, whereas D-Ala^2 substitution in the enkephalins causes a marked increase in potency in guinea pig ileum (GPI) as well as in the mouse vas deferens (MVD) assay, similar substitution in β-endorphin increases potency only in the MVD assay (Coy *et al.*, 1977; Lemaire *et al.*, 1978) and causes a small fall in potency in the GPI assay (Lemaire *et al.*, 1978; Yamashiro *et al.*, 1977). Furthermore, it is inferred that the configuration requirements are different. L-Ala^2-β_c-endorphin has appreciable potency in the GPI assay (Li, 1979; Yamashiro *et al.*, 1978), whereas L-Ala^2-Met-Enk is almost inactive. Composite changes [e.g., D-Ala^2,Me-Phe^4,Met$(O)^5$] that provide enkephalin analogs of very high potency in the GPI assay and unchanged or weaker potency in the MVD assay have a reverse effect in the β-endorphin series; D-Ala^2,*N*-Me-Phe^4,Met$(O)^5$-β_s-endorphin, for example, has one-tenth the potency of β_s-endorphin in the GPI assay, but is 2–3 times more potent in a rat vas deferens assay (Lemaire *et al.*, 1978). The effect of structural change at positions other than the 1- to 5-position, as studied by C. H. Li (1979), are as follows. C-terminal changes in β_h-endorphin may cause an increase in potency. Thus, replacement of the C-terminal Glu with Gly or Gly-NH_2 provides analogs that are, respectively, 1.68 and 2.0 times more potent than β_h-endorphin (Li, 1979). In the Gly^{31} analog, further replacement of the Tyr^{27} by Phe causes only a small decrease in potency (Blake *et al.*, 1978b). In one study (Blake *et al.*, 1978a), the hydroxyl groups of the Thr and Ser at positions 6 and 7 were shown not to be of significance, since the $Ala^{6,7}$,Phe^{27},Gly^{31} analog, in which the sixth and seventh residues are replaced by Ala, was most equipotent. In another study (Blake *et al.*, 1979), the effect of reducing the conformational flexibility of the peptide chain by internal cystine bridges was examined. For this purpose the Ala^{26} and, in turn, Ser^7, Gln^{11}, and Leu^{17} were replaced by cysteine; oxidation of the resulting three dicysteine analogs provided analogs with internal disulfide bridging. The 11–26 and 17–26 bridged analogs were, respectively, more potent and equipotent compared with the parent analog. However, the 7–26 bridged analog was of very low potency. It was concluded that the 7–26 bridging brings the C-terminal region of β_h-endorphin close to the 1–5 region, thereby impending interaction of the latter with the opiate receptor.

The enkephalin moiety in β-endorphin is critical for the opiate activities since its deletion virtually abolishes these activities (Li, 1981). Truncation starting at the N terminus leads to an immediate and drastic loss of binding affinity as soon as Tyr[1] is deleted, followed by a progressive decline as residues 1–11, 1–15, and 1–19 are removed (Hammonds *et al.*, 1982).

c. Dynorphins Five dynorphin-related peptides—dynorphin A, dynorphin(1–8), dynorphin B, also called remorphin (Kilpatrick *et al.*, 1982a,b), α-neoendorphin, and β-neoendorphin—have been mapped in the rat brain. The 29-residue extended form of dynorphin B is called dynorphin B-29 or leumorphin (Suda *et al.*, 1983). All dynorphins are products of the same gene.

The first dynorphin peptide, dynorphin A, was discovered during the deliberate search for an endogenous opioid, in which several groups of investigators participated in the early 1970s. The biological activity of the pure natural peptide was quite astonishing. In the GPI assay it was by far the most potent of any opioid peptide yet examined—about 50 times more potent than β-endorphin, about 700 times more potent than Leu-Enk, and about 200 times more potent than normorphine. This remarkable potency dictated the choice of the name dynorphin, from the Greek *dyn-*, signifying strength or power. Synthetic 13-residue peptide dynorphin (1–13) was found to be just as potent as the natural dynorphin.

Dynorphin A is highly potent in both the GPI assay (δ receptor) and the MVD assay (μ receptor) (Goldstein *et al.*, 1979), not because the C-terminal extension of Leu-Enk enhances potency at the Leu-Enk receptor, but because the extension serves as an "address" to direct the peptide to a different receptor (κ instead of μ), which is highly specific for dynorphin A (Schwyzer, 1977). Evidence for κ-binding sites in guinea pig brain membranes has been adduced by Kosterlitz *et al.* (1981). Of the total opioid-binding sites in guinea pig brain, about 30% seemed to be of the κ type. κ-Opioid receptor has been identified both as a binding site and as a functional unit in tissues. Dynorphin A, dynorphin B, and α-neoendorphin are highly selective for it; dynorphin A (1–8) and β-neoendorphin are also κ-selective, but less so. Antibodies to dynorphin (1–13)–thyroglobulin conjugate do not cross-react with the enkephalin pentapeptides or β-endorphin.

Structure–activity studies of dynorphin A (1–13) can be summarized as follows. Each shortening of the chain leads to a modest decrease of potency, but decreases are larger when Lys[11] and Arg[7] are removed (Chavkin and Goldstein, 1981).

IV. Peptide Antibiotics

The peptide antibiotics form a large group, very few of which have found any therapeutic application. They are composed of peptide-linked amino acids, commonly including both D- and L-forms and some unusual compounds. Perlman and Bodanszky (1966) list the amino acid composition of 18 families of antibiotic peptides and 37 others. Characteristic non-amino acid moieties, such as fatty acids, also occur. Ring formation is common.

It is interesting that almost all peptide antibiotics have been isolated from the genus *Bacillus* and that no other type of antibiotic has emerged from this genus. Those that have been found useful in clinical medicine are gramicidin, bacitracin (isolated in the United States in 1945), and the polymyxins, discovered independently in Britain and America in 1947. We describe here the chemistry and biology of a few peptide antibiotics.

A. Alamethicin

Alamethicin (ALA) is a peptide antibiotic produced by the fungus *Trichoderma viride* (Reusser, 1967; Meyer and Reusser, 1967). Because of its amphiphilic character, ALA shows pronounced surface activity and adsorbs strongly to biological and artificial membranes. As a consequence, it causes lysis of human erythrocytes and damages the outer membrane of Ehrlich ascites tumor cells (Jung *et al.*, 1975).

Moreover, ALA induces aggregation and fusion of lecithin vesicles (Lau and Chan, 1974). The main interest in ALA, however, stems from the unique and specific way in which it affects the electrical properties of artificial lipid bilayer membranes (Mueller and Rudin, 1968). At very low concentrations ALA induces voltage-dependent conductances similar to those observed in nerve membranes (Mueller and Rudin, 1968; Eisenberg *et al.*, 1973; Boheim, 1974; Boheim and Hall, 1975). These effects can be understood by assuming that membrane-spanning ALA aggregates form ion-conducting channels (Hall, 1975; Baumann and Mueller, 1974; Gordon and Haydon, 1975).

Natural ALA is a mixture of closely related compounds (Payne *et al.*, 1970; Jung *et al.*, 1975; Rinehart *et al.*, 1977; Gisin *et al.*, 1977; Marshall and Balasubramanian, 1979). This explains, in part, why its structure has undergone several revisions. The first proposal, a cyclic structure (Fig. 10A) (Payne *et al.*, 1970), was found to be incorrect, and an open-chain sequence with an N-terminal Ac-Aib group and the C terminus R-Glu(Phol)-Gln was proposed (Jung *et al.*, 1975; Martin and Williams, 1975). Gisin *et al.* (1981) isolated the major component, ALA I, in pure form and compared it with the synthetic peptide (ALA I; Fig. 10B). The synthetic product corresponded within experimental error to the main component of natural ALA in several assays.

B. Polymyxins and Colistins

The polymyxins are a group of antibiotics that are bactericidal against most Gram-negative organisms. The original five polymyxins, A, B, C, D, and E, are derived from *Bacillus polymyxa* (Hoeprich, 1970). (The British investigators called the antibiotic "aerosporin" since they identified the bacillus as *Bacillus*

A

```
 ┌──────────────────────────────────────────────────────────────────────┐
  12          5                    10                  15                    19
c-Aib-Pro-Aib-Ala-Aib-Ala-Gln-Aib-Val-Aib-Gly-Leu-Aib-Pro-Val-Aib-Aib-Glu-Gln-OH
```

B

```
  1           5                    10                  15                    19
c-Aib-Pro-Aib-Ala-Aib-Ala-Gln-Aib-Val-Aib-Gly-Leu-Aib-Pro-Val-Aib-Aib-Glu-Gln-Phol
```

Fig. 10 Proposed sequences for alamethicin. See text for details. Aib, α-Aminoisobutyric acid; Phol, L-phenylalaninol.

aerosporus.) Colistin, obtained from a variant of Japanese origin (Koyama *et al.*, 1950) and polymyxin M, from a Russian strain (Il'inskaya and Rossovskaya, 1960; Khokhlov and Ch'ang-Ch'ing, 1961), are now recognized as being identical with polymyxins E and A, respectively (Wilkinson, 1967; Wilkinson and Lowe, 1964, 1966). Circulin A, isolated from a strain of *Bacillus circulans,* is related structurally to the polymyxins (Fujikawa *et al.*, 1965).

The polymyxins are basic cyclic decapeptides having a common type of structure (Fig. 11) with no free α-amino or free carboxyl groups. Their basicities are related to the presence of the uncommon amino acid αγ-diaminobutyric acid (Dab), and all contain Thr and a fatty acid, (+)-6-methyloctanoic acid (MOA) or isooctanoic acid (IOA), with MOA being present as an amide attached to one of the Dab residues. They differ in the nature of the three amino acids X, Y, and Z (Table VII). Those components yielding MOA on hydrolysis are referred to as

Table VII

Structures of the Polymyxin Group of Antibiotics[a]

Polymyxin	R	X	Y	Z
Polymyxin A1 or M1	MOA	D-Dab	D-Leu	Thr
Polymyxin A2 or M2	IOA	D-Dab	D-Leu	Thr
Polymixin B1	MOA	Dab	D-Phe	Leu
Polymyxin B2	IOA	Dab	D-Phe	Leu
Polymyxin D1	MOA	D-Ser	D-Leu	Thr
Polymyxin D2	IOA	D-Ser	D-Leu	Thr
Polymyxin E1 or colistin A	MOA	Dab	D-Leu	Leu
Polymixin E2 or colistin B	IOA	Dab	D-Leu	Leu
Polymixin	MOA	Dab	D-Leu	Ile

[a] R is the fatty acid contained in the common structure of the polymyxin group, either (+)-6-methyloctanoic acid (MOA) or isooctanoic acid (IOA). X, Y, and Z are amino acids. Dab, αγ-Diaminobutyric acid. See also Fig. 11.

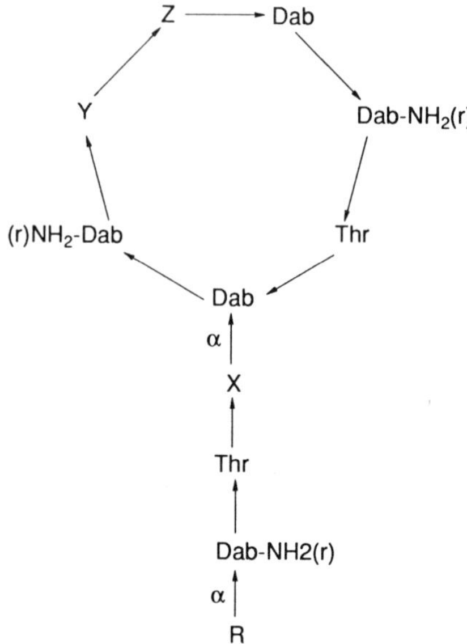

Fig. 11 Common structure of the polymyxin group of antibiotics. See text and Table VII for details.

polymyxins A1, B1, etc. and those yielding IOA are named polymyxins A2, B2, etc.

All of the polymyxins have a similar antibacterial spectrum. Nearly all species of Gram-negative bacilli are highly sensitive to polymyxin and, on a weight-for-weight basis, are usually more sensitive to polymyxin than to any other antibiotic. However, Gram-positive bacteria are resistant to polymyxins. The main therapeutic importance of the polymyxins lies in their activity against *Pseudomonas*.

Polymyxins bind to both bacterial and mammalian cell membranes. Because of this binding, the agents persist in the liver, kidneys, brain, heart, muscle, and lungs for as long as 72 hours (Kunin and Bugg, 1971). The major side effects of the polymyxins are renal dysfunction, neurotoxicity, and neuromuscular blockade. Possible hazards of their use must therefore be considered. Sulfomethyl derivatives were found to be considerably less toxic (Goodwin, 1970). The SAR of polymyxins has been explored very little; more research needs to be done in this respect.

C. Gramicidins

Gramicidins A (GA) and S (GS) are peptide antibiotics produced by *Bacillus brevis*. GA is a pentadecapetide (Fig. 12) and contains D--amino acids in a

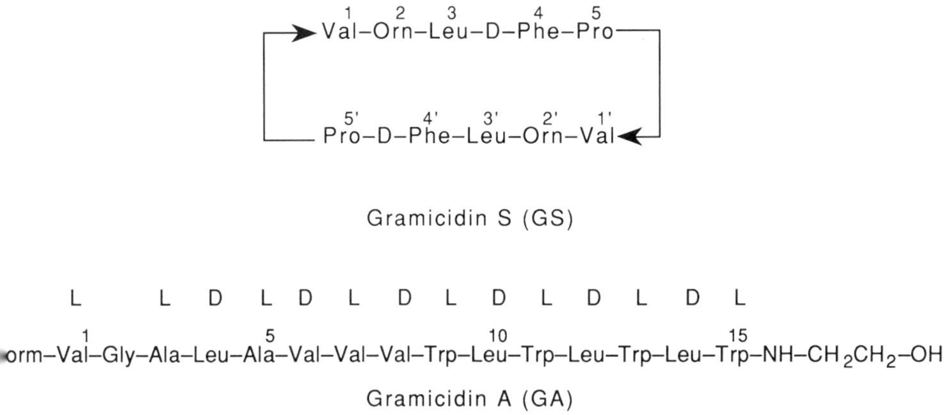

```
           1   2   3     4    5
    ──►Val–Orn–Leu–D–Phe–Pro──┐
   │                          │
   │   5'   4'    3'   2'  1' │
   └── Pro–D–Phe–Leu–Orn–Val◄─┘
```

Gramicidin S (GS)

```
  L     L   D   L   D   L   D   L   D   L   D   L   D   L
      1             5                  10                  15
Form–Val–Gly–Ala–Leu–Ala–Val–Val–Val–Trp–Leu–Trp–Leu–Trp–Leu–Trp–NH–CH2CH2–OH
```

Gramicidin A (GA)

Fig. 12 Structures of gramicidins S and A.

unique pattern that strictly observes alternation with residues of L-configuration (Sarges and Witkop, 1965). This gives rise to a hydrogen bond-stabilized conformation manifest in the β-helix (Urry, 1972). Peptides with β-helical structure are capable of embedding in lipid bilayers and transporting univalent cations via a channel mechanism; as such, GA can act as an antibacterial agent by affecting the cation permeability of membranes. On the other hand, Paulus and Sarkar (1976) and Sarkar *et al.* (1977) observed that GA can specifically inhibit transcription with purified bacterial RNA polymerase. Analogs of the linear gramicidins with amino acid exchanges and modifications in the N- and C-terminal regions have been synthesized and their ion transport-mediating properties determined (Bamberg *et al.*, 1978, 1979). Much work has been done on the structure–activity and conformational studies of gramicidins. Kato *et al.* (1970) studied the optical rotatory dispersion (ORD) of GS and reported a correlation between conformation and biological activity. Comparison of the ORD curves of biologically active GS analogs indicates that these compounds possess similar conformations irrespective of their primary structures. On the other hand, the biologically inactive decapeptide and cyclopentapeptide have a conformation distinctly different from that of their closely structurally related active analogs. Thus, there seems to be a definite relationship between the conformational states of the GS analog decapeptides and their antibacterial activity. Ivanov and Sychev (1983) studied the circular dichroism (CD) fluorescence and infrared (IR) spectra of covalently cross-linked GA dimers and observed that both GA and its bis derivatives form in membrane a variety of helical structures that are in equilibrium with each other.

Gramicidins are active against most species of aerobic and anaerobic Gram-positive bacteria, including mycobacteria. Gram-negative bacilli are completely insensitive, probably due to the presence of surface phospholipids, which inhibit the action of gramicidins. The latter are highly toxic to erythrocytes in liver and kidney.

D. Magainins

Magainins, a family of peptides with broad-spectrum antimicrobial activity, have been isolated from the skin of the African clawed frog *Xenopus leavis*. Magainin consists of two closely related peptides that each contain 23 amino acids (Zasloff, 1987) and differ by two subsititutions (Fig. 13). These peptides are water-soluble, nonhemolytic at their effective antimicrobial concentrations, and potentially amphiphilic.

Magainins are the first chemical defense system, apart from the immune system, that has been discovered in vertebrates. They probably are an animal's first line of defense against microbes, operating before the immune system springs into action. Magainins are found to be effective against bacteria such as *Escherichia coli,* staphylococci, streptococci, enterobacteria, and pseudomonades. Several other bacterial strains appear to be resistent, however. The peptides also kill *Candida albicans,* a common yeast that produces intractable infections in patients with acquired immune deficiency syndrome (AIDS) and other immune disorders. Especially dramatic is the effect of the peptides on protozoa such as amoebae and paramecia. Within minutes of being exposed to magainin at a concentration of 10 mg per milliliter, paramecia swell and then burst like "overstuffed water balloons," as described by Zasloff.

Chen *et al.* (1988) synthesized analogs of magainin 2 to enhance the α-helical structure. These analogs displayed an increase in antimicrobial activity of up to two orders of magnitude. Urrutia *et al.* (1989) recently described the ability of the magainin 2 peptide to assemble spontaneously into characteristic 13-nm-diameter filaments having a 30-nm periodic helical substructure. They suggest

Magainin 1: Gly[1]-Ile-Gly-Lys-Phe[5]-Leu-His-Ser-Ala-Gly[10]-Lys-Phe-Gly-Lys-Ala[15]-Phe-Val-Gly-Glu-Ile[20]-Met-Lys-Ser[23]

Magainin 2: Gly[1]-Ile-Gly-Lys-Phe[5]-Leu-His-Ser-Ala-Lys[10]-Lys-Phe-Gly-Lys-Ala[15]-Phe-Val-Gly-Glu-Ile[20]-Met-Asn-Ser[23]

Fig. 13 Amino acid sequence of magainins. Residues that differ between the two peptides are underlined.

that polymerization of magainin 2 may be involved in membrane-disrupting and antibiotic activities.

V. Peptide Vaccines

In recent years there has been considerable interest in the possibility of using synthetic peptides as viral, bacterial, and protozoan vaccines. Attached to appropriate carriers and mixed with an adjuvant, synthetic peptides may elicit antibodies capable of cross-reacting with proteins containing the same amino acid sequence as the immunizing peptide. Thus, peptide vaccines have been said to elicit antibodies of predetermined specificity (Lerner, 1982; Lerner *et al.*, 1981a,b).

The objective of any such vaccine is a protective immune response. This in turn requires the induction of neutralizing antibodies that bind proteinaceous virulence determinants of the microbe *in vivo;* in addition, immunity against viral pathogens may need to be associated with the development of a cytotoxic T cell response. Neutralizing antibodies of this kind satisfy two requirements. First, they bind to the surface-exposed regions of the native protein; these regions, which are accessible to the antigen combining site of the immunoglobulin molecule, are termed "epitopes" or, alternatively, "antigenic determinants." Second, neutralizing antibodies bind to these sites with an affinity that is high enough to perturb the pathogenic function of the microbial protein. In addition, neutralizing antibodies often have other functional attributes; for example, they may be opsonic, agglutinate the microbe, or fix complement.

When a native, folded protein is used as an immunogen, antibodies are normally elicited to only a part of the surface of the protein; these constitute the immunodominant antigenic determinants of the protein (Atassi, 1972, 1975; Atassi and Lee, 1978). As indicated in the studies of Atassi and colleagues with myoglobin and lysozyme, some of these determinants are linear, i.e., their antigenicity can be accounted for entirely by the primary structure of the region. An antigenic determinant can be said to be linear if antibody elicited to the determinant as a part of the immune response to the native protein has the same affinity for a peptide corresponding to the determinant as for the protein itself. However, as indicated in the studies of Berzofsky and colleagues (Berkower *et al.*, 1982) with myoglobin, other naturally occurring antigenic determinants consist of separate regions of primary structure, brought together as a discrete antigenic determinant by protein folding. These determinants are conformational and cannot be simulated by a small peptide lacking this kind of higher order structure. Thus, according to these studies, the use of synthetic peptides as immunogens would be restricted to surface-exposed regions of a protein that are immunodominant linear antigenic determinants. These studies were followed by experiments conducted by Lerner and colleagues (Lerner *et al.*, 1981a,b; Lerner, 1982) showing that peptides corresponding to surface-exposed regions that do not constitute immunodominant antigenic determinants of the native protein can nonetheless elicit antibodies that cross-react with the native protein. These studies suggested that a larger area of the protein's surface might be of more immunological interest than those regions comprising naturally occurring antigenic determinants. The results of the studies by Atassi *et al.* and by Lerner *et al.* cited above are not necessarily contradictory when it is recognized that immunogenicity (i.e., the capacity to stimulate an immune response) and antigenicity (i.e., the capacity to be bound by antibody) are properties that arise as a result of quite different biological events. As a result, surface-exposed regions of a protein that are not normally immunogenic can in principle be bound by antibody, elicited in this case by a peptide immunogen corresponding in primary structure to the region. The identification of regions with this kind of immunological potential is discussed below.

For microbial proteins of known crystal structure, surface-accessible regions can be identified directly by reference to the three-dimensional structure of the protein. However, when only the primary structure of the protein is known, the locations of surface-accessible regions can be predicted using algorithms that, in general, recognize the tendency of polar and charged amino acids to be solvent-exposed, in contrast to the tendency of hydrophobic amino acids to be buried in the interior of the molecule. One such algorithm, derived by Hopp and Woods (1981), predicts the location of antigenic determinants by analyzing the primary structure of a protein in order to deduce the site of greatest local hydrophilicity; this in turn was found to be within, or close to, an empirically determined antigenic determinant of several proteins, including the hepatitis B surface antigen. Kyte and Doolittle (1982) proposed an algorithm for the identification of hydropathic regions of a protein; although not derived for the purpose of predicting the location of antigenic determinants per se, this program has been employed by immunologists to identify solvent-exposed regions of proteins. When predictions of this kind are combined with algorithms for the prediction of secondary structure, particularly for the identification of regions likely to contain reverse turns, the probability of correctly finding a region of immunological interest seems to be enhanced. In other words, a predicted reverse turn within a hydrophilic segment of primary structure may have a reasonable probability of containing an antigenic determinant. Algorithms for the prediction of reverse or β-turns and for other elements of secondary structure have been proposed by Chou and Fasman (1978) and by Levin and Garnier (1988). The Chou and Fasman rules, which are derived from the statistical analysis of 29 globular proteins with known X-ray crystal structures, give the frequency of each amino acid within tetra-, penta-, and hexapeptide sequences that occur in one of three specific conformations: β-turn, β-sheet, or α-helix. From these frequencies, the probability that an individual amino acid or a given sequence will exist within one of these conformations can be derived. The frequency assigned to an amino acid is used to determine whether the amino acid will nucleate (form), break, or remain indifferent to a specific conformation, whether it be the α-helix, β-sheet, or β-turn. More recently, Levin and Garnier (1988) described an optimized version of a secondary structure–prediction method based on local homologies, using a new data base.

Even when these predictive algorithms are used to select a sequence for synthesis, many investigators have observed that the affinity of the resulting peptide antisera for the native protein is often too low to be useful. Thus, surface exposure by itself is an inadequate basis for the identification of a peptide that will reliably yield high-affinity antibodies for the native protein; in contrast, the affinity of the same antisera for the immunizing peptide is often high, usually 100 to 1000 times greater than the affinity of the antisera for the protein containing the same sequence. This disparity stems from structural differences between the immunizing peptide and the corresponding sequence of the folded protein.

Structural differences between a region of a protein and the corresponding peptide occur at several levels. First, unless the immunizing sequence is derived from the N- or C-terminal region of the protein, the immunizing peptide will have a nonnatural primary amine or carboxyl group (unless these have been modified during synthesis), and this in turn will result in the presence of nonnatural positive and negative charges at the respective terminus of the peptide. Second, the ends of the peptide will not be surrounded by all the flanking residues that normally encompass each amino acid (other than the N and C termini) within a protein. The role of these flanking residues for conformation and immune function is currently under study, but it seems certain that they alter the local mobility of the peptide backbone. Third, the immunogenicity of peptides is usually increased by conjugation of the peptide to a large carrier protein. The orientation of the coupled peptide with respect to the carrier protein has been shown to modify the immunogenicity of the peptide locally, the region of the peptide closest to the carrier protein being rendered less immunogenic (see Schwimmbeck *et al.*, 1987), perhaps through steric effects. Fourth, the conformation of the peptide and of the corresponding region of the folded protein may be different, for example, because the sequence within the protein adopts a particular secondary structure whereas the same sequence within a short peptide exists in a conformation that is less defined and more mobile. The significance of this effect for proteins containing disulfide bridges was first noted in studies with lysozyme and its loop peptide consisting of amino acid residues 63–83 and containing a disulfide bridge between residues 64 and 80. Antisera against native lysozyme reacted with the isolated loop peptide and, vice versa, antisera against the loop peptide reacted with intact lysozyme. However, antibodies against the loop peptide did not react with the open-chain peptide (Arnon and Sela, 1969;

Arnon *et al.*, 1971). Dreesman *et al.*, (1982) investigated the possibility of a synthetic peptide vaccine for hepatitis B virus (HBV). They chose the region between amino acids 117 and 137 because a cyclic disulfide could be formed between Cys-124 and Cys-137 (Fig. 14). After a single injection, the peptide elicited an antibody response in mice without linkage to a protein carrier. The peptide elicited the production of antibodies of a specificity similar to that produced by immunization with the sodium dodecylsulfate-denatured virus P25 polypeptide.

Brown *et al.* (1984) used synthetic peptides to study the affinity and level of antibody response to hepatitis B surface antigen (anti-HBs) in recipients of a plasma-derived hepatitis B vaccine. They observed that their cyclic peptide, comprising amino acid residues 139 to 147, bound to the antibodies with higher affinity than did the corresponding linear peptide.

The conformation effect has also been observed for proteins lacking disulfide bridges. Gariepy *et al.* (1986) examined the antigenic specificity of antibodies elicited to peptides corresponding to several regions of the calcium-binding protein calmodulin; in the calcium-saturated form of the molecule, these regions are known by X-ray crystallography to be α-helical, whereas in the calcium-free form, the helical content of the molecule decreases substantially. Antibodies to the calmodulin peptides bound only to calcium-free calmodulin, indicating that the regions of calmodulin corresponding to the peptide sequences were more antigenic in the absence of calcium, presumably because in this state they exhibited less helicity; as a result, they may have more closely resembled the conformation of the immunizing peptide. Tainer *et al.* (1984) showed that the atomic mobility of selected regions of myohemerythrin was correlated with the antigenicity of the same regions for antibodies elicited to peptides corresponding to the sequences of these regions. Taken together, these studies indicate that, in addition to surface exposure, the affinity of peptide antibodies for native proteins

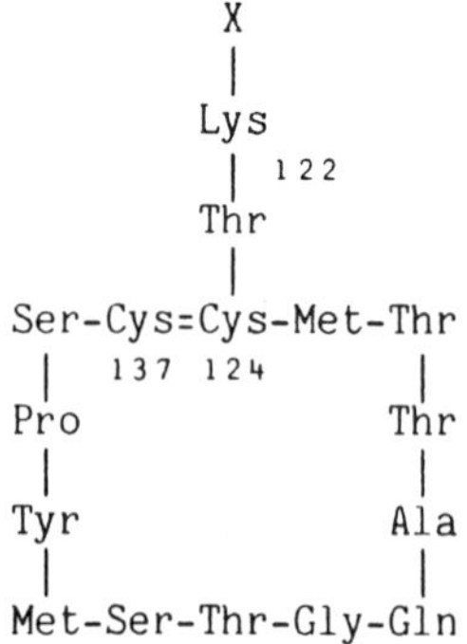

Fig. 14 Dreesman's hepatitis B virus peptide vaccine.

is positively correlated with the conformational relatedness between the peptide and corresponding region of the protein. In most instances, peptide antibodies will have the highest affinity for regions of proteins that are "peptide-like," i.e., highly flexible and lacking in defined secondary structure.

The concepts discussed above have evolved as a result of a growing number of studies using synthetic peptide vaccines. Among the earliest reports was a study by Anderer and Schlumberger (1965), who used a synthetic peptide corresponding to the C terminus of tobacco mosaic virus (TMV) coat protein for raising antibodies which reacted with the native protein and inactivated the infectivity of the virus. Subsequently, Fearney *et al.* (1971) and Langbeheim *et al.* (1976) prepared antibodies against the coat protein of TMV and coliphage MS2, respectively, using the same method. After the three-dimensional structure of TMV was established by X-ray crystallography in 1978, it became possible to interpret the immunochemical data in structural terms.

With the availability of computer programs for predicting regions of immunological interest in the amino acid sequence of a protein, attempts to develop peptide vaccines accelerated. Lerner and colleagues (1981a) used this approach in synthesizing 13 peptides from hepatitis B surface antigen; 7 of the 13 elicited an antipeptide response. Antisera against four of the remaining six peptides were reactive with hepatitis B surface antigen. Schoolnik and his associates (Rothbard *et al.*, 1985) synthesized peptides from the sequence of gonococcal pilin and tested them for their ability to be bound by polycloncal sera against pili isolated from homologous and heterologous gonococcal strains. They were able to define an antigenic determinant common to all strains of pili and two separate strain-specific epitopes. Itoh *et al.* (1986) described a 19-residue synthetic peptide vaccine involving the product of the pre-S(2) region of hepatitis B virus (HBV) DNA. When given to chimpanzees, the peptide raised antibodies that bound to viral particles and protected the animals from challenge with infectious doses of HBV. Neurath *et al.* (1988) designed synthetic peptides that mimicked the immunological and biological functions of the pre-S1 sequence of the HBV envelope protein. DiMarchi *et al.* (1986) designed a synthetic double-antigen peptide vaccine against foot-and-mouth disease (FMD) virus by combining two peptide antigens (141–158 and 200–213) and introducing a diproline spacer. The peptide was able to protect the cattle against FMD after a single immunization; this was the first example of protection using a synthetic peptide vaccine under conditions typical of those under which the potency of conventional vaccines is tested. More recently, a synthetic peptide vaccine against malaria was prepared by Etlinger *et al.* (1988), who injected into human volunteers an antimalaria (*Plasmodium falciperum*) sporozoite preparation consisting of a synthetic peptide Ac-Cys-$(NANP)_3$ coupled to tetanus toxoid and adsorbed to aluminum hydroxide. Antipeptide, anticircumsporozoite antibodies were detected in these volunteers.

Antigenically active peptides have also been synthesized for influenza (Green *et al.*, 1982; Shapira *et al.*, 1984), polio (Emini *et al.*, 1983), rabies (MacFarlan *et al.*, 1984), herpes simplex type I and type II (Weijer *et al.*, 1988; Watari *et al.*, 1987), and human immunodeficiency virus (Kennedy *et al.*, 1986; Chanh *et al.*, 1986; Ho *et al.*, 1987; Palker *et al.*, 1988). Jolivet *et al.* (1987) constructed a polyvalent synthetic vaccine consisting of two bacterial antigens (*Streptococcus pyogenes* M protein and diphtheria toxin), one viral antigen (hepatitis B surface antigen), and one parasitic antigen (circumsporozoite protein of *Plasmodium knowlesi*) covalently bound within the same construct. They demonstrated that the association of several peptides enhanced their respective immunogenicities compared with those of their homopolymers.

The selection of peptides for synthesis has been discussed in terms of the identification of surface-exposed regions of the target protein that, because of the "peptide-like" nature of the site, may be expected to give rise to high-affinity, cross-reacting antibodies as noted above. To enhance their immunogenicity, peptides with these properties are usually coupled as haptens to a large carrier protein and emulsified with an adjuvant before being presented to the immune system as a vaccine. Recent studies have explored the cellular basis for the immunogenicity of peptides in greater detail. Borras-Cuesta *et al.* (1987) demonstrated that two haptenic peptides could be rendered immunogenic if a well-characterized determinant recognized by T helper cells was synthesized as a colinear extension of these haptens. It has also been shown (Good *et al.*, 1987; Leclerc *et al.*, 1987) that immunogens could be constructed by coupling, via bifunctional reagents, two peptides representing a T cell determinant and a determinant recognized by B cells. These studies suggest that an essential requirement for the immunogenicity of a peptide is the simultaneous presence of T cell and B cell determinants. This idea was extended in a second study by Borras-Cuesta *et al.* (1988) showing that two synthetic peptides corresponding to residues 103–115 and 113–147 of the bovine rotavirus protein VP6, which do not themselves induce anti-rotavirus antibodies unless conjugated to bovine serum albumin, nonetheless could be rendered immunogenic if their sequences were extended by colinear synthesis of a well-characterized determinant that was recognized by T cells and represented a region of the influenza A virus hemagglutinin. Earlier in this section, the structural properties of B cell epitopes were discussed in terms of the presence of a hydrophilic domain that was associated with a predicted reverse turn. The newly recognized significance of T cell epitopes for the immunogenicity of peptides led to studies of their structural characteristics. DeLisi and Berzofsky (1985) proposed that T cell epitopes are likely to involve those sequences of a protein that can adopt stable amphipathic conformations. They suggested that amphipathicity, the presence of opposing hydrophilic and hydrophobic surfaces in some organized and stable secondary structure of the polypeptide, is required for a peptide's presentation to the T cell receptor (TcR). The hydrophobic surface could bind relatively nonspecifically to the antigen-binding site of class II major histocompatibility complex (MHC) antigens; the hydrophilic surface might then be recognized by a complementary TcR. Margalit *et al.* (1987) reported a computer algorithm designed to search for amphipathic structures in protein sequences. Rather than considering secondary structure, Rothbard and Taylor (1988) analyzed the primary structure of both helper and cytotoxic determinants and observed that a large percentage of them contain a linear pattern composed of a charged residue or a glycine followed by two hydrophobic residues. Reyes *et al.* (1989) reported on an algorithm to predict class II MHC-restricted peptides on the basis of their structural similarity to an amphipathic α-helix in class I. Their algorithm also predicted peptides that were presented to cytotoxic T cells by class I MHC molecules. Further studies using synthetically prepared immunogens containing both B cell and T cell determinants can be expected in the future.

According to Melnick (1986), if synthetic peptides could be made more effective as immunogens, the problem of liability associated with current vaccine development would be overcome. The vaccine would be a chemical rather than a biological product. Hence, vaccine preparation would no longer require the burdensome containment needed at present for producing large amounts of infectious agents—the source of all present vaccines, both live and inactivated. The vaccine would be a pure chemical of precisely known composition, every preparation being the same, with no possibility of contamination by extraneous microorganisms or other cellular products. Moreover, the storage and delivery of the vaccine would be facilitated because of the thermal stability of most peptide preparations.

References

Adamsons, K., Jr., Engel, S. L., Van Dyke, H. B., Schmidt-Nielson, B., and Schmidt-Nielsen, K. (1956). The distribution of oxytocin vasopressin (antidiuretic hormone) in the neurohypophysis of the camel. *Endocrinology (Baltimore)* **58,** 272–278.

Ahren, B., and Lundquist, I. (1988). Effects of petide PHI on basal and stimulated insulin and glucagon secretion in mouse. *Neuropeptides (Edinburgh)* **11,** 159–162.

Anagnostides, A. A., Mandas, K., Christofides, N. D., Yiangou, Y., Welbourn, R. B., Bloom, S. R., and Chadwick, V. S. (1983a). Peptide histidine isoleucine (PHI). A secretagogue in porcine intestine. *Dig. Dis. Sci.* **28,** 893–896.

Anagnostides, A. A., Christofides, N. D., Bloom, S. R., and Chadwick, V. S. (1983b). Peptide histidine isoleucine: A secretagogue in human intestine. *Gut* **24,** A 472.

Anastasi, A., Erspamer, V., and Bucci, M. (1973). Isolation and amino acid sequences of alytesin and bombesin, two analogous active tetradecapeptides form the skin of European discoglossid frogs. *Arch. Biochem. Biophys.* **148,** 443–446.

Anderer, F. A., and Schlumberger, H. D. (1965). Properties of different artificial antigens immunologically related to tobacco mosaic virus. *Biochim. Biophys. Acta* **97,** 503–509.

Andry, D. K., and Horita, A. (1977). Thyrotropin-releasing hormone: Physiological concomitant of behavioral excitation. *Pharmacol., Biochem. Behav.* **6,** 55–59.

Archer, S., Albertson, N., Harris, L., Pierson, A., and Bird, J. (1964). Pentazocine. Strong analgesics and analgesic antagonists in the benzomorphan series. *J. Med. Chem.* **7,** 123–127.

Archer, S., Albertson, N., and Pierson, A. (1973). Structure–activity relationships in the opioid antagonists. *In* "Agonist and Antagonist Actions of Narcotic Analgesic Drugs" (H. W. Kosterlitz *et al.,* eds.), pp. 25–29. Macmillan, London.

Arnon, R., and Sela, M. (1969). Antibodies to a unique region in lysozyme provoked by a synthetic antigen conjugate. *Proc. Natl. Acad. Sci. U.S.A.* **62,** 163–170.

Arnon, R., Maron, E., Sela, M., and Anfinson, C. B. (1971). Antibodies reactive with native lysozyme elicited by a completely synthetic antigen. *Proc. Natl. Acad. Sci. U.S.A.* **68,** 1450–1455.

Arshady, R., Atherton, E., Clive, D. L. J., and Sheppard, R. C. (1981). Peptide synthesis. I. Preparation and use of polar supports based on poly(dimethylacrylamide). *J. Chem. Soc., Perkin Trans. 1,* pp. 529–537.

Atassi, M. Z. (1972). Antigenic structure of proteins inferred from myoglobin as the first protein whose antigenic structure has reached completion. *In* "Specific Receptors of Antibodies, Antigens and Cells" (D. Pressman *et al.,* eds.), pp. 118–136. Karger, Basel.

Atassi, M. Z. (1975). Antigenic structure of myoglobin: The complete immunochemical anatomy of a protein and conclusions relating to antigenic structures of proteins. *Immunochemistry* **12,** 423–438.

Atassi, M. Z., and Lee, C. L. (1978). The precise and entire antigenic structure of native lysozyme. *Biochem. J.* **171,** 429–434.

Atherton, E., Logan, C. J., and Sheppard, R. C. (1981). Peptide synthesis II. Procedures for solid-phase synthesis using N^{α}-fluroenylmethoxycarbonylamino acids on polyamide supports. Synthesis of substance P and of acyl carrier protein 65–74 decapeptide. *J. Chem. Soc., Perkin Trans. 1,* pp. 538–559.

Baizman, E. R., Gordon, T. D., Hansen, P. E., Kiefer, D., Lopresti, D. M., McKay, F. C., Morgan, B. A., and Perrone, M. H. (1983). Structure and antagonist activity in a series of hexapeptide substance P analogs. *In* "Peptides" (Y. J. Hruby and D. H. Rich, eds.), pp. 437–440. Pierce Chemical Co., Rockford, Illinois.

Balasubramaniam, A., Grupp, I., Srivastava, L., Tatemoto, K., Murphy, R. F., Joffe, S. N., and Fischer, J. E. (1987). Synthesis of neuropeptide Y. *Int. J. Pept. Protein Res.* **29,** 78–83.

Bamberg, E., Apell, H.-J., Alpes, H., Gross, E., Morell, J. L., Harbaugh, J. F., Janko, K., and Läuger, P. (1978). Ion channels formed by chemical analogs of gramicidine A. *Fed. Proc., Fed. Am. Soc. Exp. Biol.* **37,** 2633–2638.

Bamberg, E., Apell, H.-J., Alpes, H., Läuger, P., Morell, J. L., and Gross, E. (1979). Formation of ion-transporting channels by analogs of gramicidin A. *In* "Peptides" (E. Gross and J. Meienhofer, eds.), pp. 629–634. Pierce Chemical Co., Rockford, Illinois.

Barnes, P. J., and Dixon, C. M. S. (1984). The effect of inhaled vasoactive intestinal peptide on bronchial reactivity to histamine in humans. *Am. Rev. Respir. Dis.* **130,** 162–166.

Baumann, G., and Mueller, P. (1974). A molecular model of membrane excitability. *J. Supramol. Struct.* **2,** 538–557.

Beale, J. S., White, R. P., and Huang, S. (1977). EEG and blood pressure effects of TRH in rabbits. *Neuropharmacology* **16,** 499–506.

Bentley, P. H., Kenner, G. W., and Sheppard, R. C. (1966). Structure of human gastrins I and II. *Nature (London)* **209,** 583–585.

Berkower, I., Buckenmeyer, G. K., Gurd, F. R. N., and Berzofsky, J. A. (1982). A possible immunodominant epitope recognized by murine T lymphocytes immune to different myoglobins. *Proc. Natl. Acad. Sci. U.S.A.* **79,** 4723–4727.

Beyerman, H. C., Izeboud, E., Kranenburg, P., and Voskamp, D. (1979). Synthesis of methionine-containing peptides via their sulfoxides. *In* "Peptides" (E. Gross and J. Meienhofer, eds.), pp. 333–336. Pierce Chemical Co., Rockford, Illinois.

Bhargava, H. N. (1977). Opiate-like action of methionine-enkephalin in inhibiting morphine abstinence syndrome. *Eur. J. Pharmacol.* **41,** 81–84.

Bienert, M., Klauschenz, E., Ehrlich, A., Katzwinkel, S., Niedrich, H., Toth, G., and Tephlan, J. (1979a). Tritium labelling in two phenylalanine residues of norleucine^{11}-substance P. *J. Labelled Compd. Radiopharm.* **16,** 673–679.

Bienert, M., Köller, G., Wohlfeil, R., Mehlis, B., Niedrich, H., and Kraft, R. (1979b). Synthese von Substanz P und Acylierten Teilsequenzen. *J. Prakt. Chem.* **321,** 721–740.

Blake, J., Tseng, L.-F., Chang, W.-C., and Li, C. H. (1978a). The synthesis and opiate activity of human β-endorphin analogs. *Int. J. Pept. Protein Res.* **11,** 323–328.

Blake, J., Chang, W.-C., and Li, C. H. (1978b). The synthesis and biological activity of human β-endorphin analogs with disulfide bridges. *Int. J. Pept. Protein Res.* **14,** 275–280.

Blake, J., Chang, W.-C., and Li, C. H. (1979). Synthesis and biological activity of human β-endorphin analogs with disulfide bridges. *Int. J. Pept. Protein Res.* **14,** 275–280.

Bloom, S. R., Christofides, N. D., Delamarter, J., Buell, G., Kavashima, E., and Polak, J. M. (1983). Diarrhoea in vipoma patients associated with cosecretion of a second active peptide (peptide histidine isoleucine) explained by single coding gene. *Lancet* **2,** 1163–1165.

Bodanszky, M., and Bodanszky, A. (1984). "The Practice of Peptide Synthesis." Springer-Verlag, Berlin.

Boheim, G. (1974). Statistical analysis of alamethicin channels in black lipid membranes. *J. Membr. Biol.* **19,** 227–303.

Boheim, G., and Hall, J. E. (1975). Oscillation phenomena in black lipid membranes induced by a single alamethicin pore. *Biochim. Biophys. Acta* **389,** 436–443.

Bolin, D. R., Sytwu, I.-I., Cottrell, J. M., Garippa, R. J., Brooks, C. C., and O'Donnell, M. (1988). Synthesis and airway smooth muscle relaxant activity of linear and cyclic vasoactive intestinal peptide analogs. *In* "Peptides" (G. R. Marshall, ed.), pp. 441–443. ESCOM, Leiden.

Borras-Cuesta, F., Petit-Camurdan, A., and Fedon, Y. (1987). Engineering of immunogenic peptides by co-linear synthesis of determinants recognized by B and T cells. *Eur. J. Immunol.* **17,** 1213–1215.

Borras-Cuesta, F., Fedon, Y., and Petit-Camurdan, A. (1988). Enhancement of peptide immunogenicity by linear polymerization. *Eur. J. Immunol.* **18,** 199–202.

Brandenburg, D. (1981). Modern aspects of insulin synthesis and semi synthesis. *In* "Perspectives in Peptide Chemistry" (A. Eberle, R. Geiger, and T. Weiland, eds), pp. 88–100. Karger, Basel.

Bregman, M. D., and Hruby, V. J. (1979). Synthesis and isolation of a glucagon antagonist. *FEBS Lett.* **101,** 191–194.

Bregman, M. D., Trivedi, D., and Hruby, V. J. (1980). Glucagon amino groups. Evaluation of modifications leading to antagonism and agonism. *J. Biol. Chem.* **255,** 11725–11731.

Brennan, L. J., McLoughlin, T. A., Mutt, V., Tatemoto, K., and Wood, J. R. (1982). Effects of PHI, a newly isolated peptide, on gall bladder function in the guinea pig. *J. Physiol. (London)* **329,** 71P–72P.

Brewster, A. I. R., and Hruby, V. J. (1973). 300 MHz nuclear magnetic resonance study of oxytocin in aqueous solution: Conformational implications. *Proc. Natl. Acad. Sci. U.S.A.* **70,** 3806–3809.

Brewster, A. I. R., Hruby, V. J., Glasel, J. A., and Tonelli, A. E. (1973). Proposed conformations of oxytocin and selected analogs in dimethyl sulfoxide as deduced from proton magnetic resonance studies. *Biochemistry* **12,** 5294–5304.

Brown, J. C., Cook, M. A., and Dryburgh, J. R. (1970). Motilin, a gastric motor activity stimulating polypeptide: The complete amino acid sequence. *Can. J. Biochem.* **51,** 533–537.

Brown, M. R., and Fischer, L. A. (1983). Central nervous system effects of corticotropin-releasing factor in the dog. *Brain Res.* **280,** 75–79.

Brown, M. R., and Fischer, L. A. (1985). Corticotropin-releasing factor: Effects on the autonomic nervous system and visceral system. *Fed. Proc., Fed. Am. Soc. Exp. Biol.* **44,** 243–248.

Brown, M. R., Rivier, J., and Vale, W. (1977). Somatostatin: Analogs with selected biological activities. *Science* **196,** 1467–1479.

Brown, S. E., Howard, C. R., Zuckerman, A. J., and Steward, M. W. (1984). Affinity of antibody responses in man to hepatitis B vaccine determined with synthetic peptides. *Lancet* **2,** 184–187.

Burkhardt, C., Frederickson, R. C. A., and Pasternak, G. W. (1982). Metkephamid (Tyr-D-Ala-Gly-Phe-N(Me)Met-NH_2), a potent opioid peptide: Receptor binding and analgesic properties. *Peptides (N.Y.)* **3,** 869–871.

Cai, R.-Z., Szoke, B., Fu, D., Redding, T. W., Colaluca, J., Torres-Aleman, I., and Schally, A. W. (1985). Synthesis and evaluation of activities of octapeptide analogs of somatostatin. *In* "Peptides" (C. M. Deber, V. J. Hruby, and K. D. Kopple, eds.), pp. 627–630. Pierce Chemical Co., Rockford, Illinois.

Carlquist, M., Kaiser, R., Tatemoto, K., Jornvall, H., and Mutt, V. (1984). A novel form of the polypeptide PHI isolated in high yield from bovine upper intestine. Relationship to other peptides of the glucagon–secretin family. *Eur. J. Biochem.* **144,** 243–247.

Chan, W. Y. (1965). Effects of neurohypophyseal hormones and their deamino analogs on renal excretion of sodium, potassium and water in rats. *Endocrinology (Baltimore)* **77,** 1097–1104.

Chan, W. Y., and Sawyer, W. H. (1961). Saluretic activity of neurohypophysial peptides in conscious dog. *Am. J. Physiol.* **210,** 799–803.

Chang, M. M., Leeman, S. E., and Niall, H. D. (1971). Amino acid sequence of substance P. *Nature (London), New Biol.* **232,** 86–87.

Chang, R. S., Lotti, V. J., Monoghan, R. L., Birnbaum, J., Stapley, E. O., Goetz, M. A., Albers-Schonberg, G., Patchett, A. A., Liesch, J. M., Hensens, O. D., and Springer, J. P. (1985). A potent nonpeptide cholecystokinin antagonist selective for peripheral tissues isolated from *Aspergillus alliaceus*. *Science* **230,** 177–179.

Chanh, T. C., Dreesman, G. R., Kanda, P., Linette, G. P., Sparrow, J. T., Ho, D. D., and Kennedy, R. C. (1986). Induction of anti-HIV neutralizing antibodies by synthetic peptides. *EMBO J.* **5,** 3065–3071.

Chavkin, C., and Goldstein, A. (1981). Specific receptor for the opioid peptide dynorphin: Structure–activity relationships. *Proc. Natl. Acad. Sci. U.S.A.* **78,** 6543–6547.

Chen, H.-C., Brown, J. H., Morell, J. L., and Huang, C. M. (1988). Synthetic magnesium analogues with improved antimicrobial activity. *FEBS Lett.* **236,** 462–466.

Cheng, A., Uyeno, E., Polgar, W., Toll, L., Lawson, J. A., DeGraw, J. I., Loew, G., Camerman, A., and Camerman, N. (1986). N-Substituent modulation of opiate agonist/antagonist activity in resolved 3-methyl-3-(*m*-hydroxyphenyl)piperidines. *J. Med. Chem.* **29,** 531–537.

Chou, P. Y., and Fasman, G. D. (1978). Empirical predictions of protein conformation. *Annu. Rev. Biochem.* **47,** 251–276.

Clore, G. M., Martin, S. R., and Gronenborn, A. M. (1986). Solution structure of human growth hormone-releasing factor. Combined use of circular dichroism and nuclear magnetic resonance spectroscopy. *J. Mol. Biol.* **191,** 553–561.

Corvera, S., Huerta-Bahena, J., Pelton, J. T., Hruby, V. J., Trivedi, D., and Garcia-Sainz, J. A. (1984). Metabolic effects and cyclic AMP levels produced by glucagon and forskolin in isolated rat hepatocytes. *Biochim. Biophys. Acta* **804,** 434–441.

Cote, T. E., and Epand, R. M. (1979). N^{α}-Trinitrophenyl glucagon. An inhibitor of glucagon-stimulated cyclic AMP production and its effects on glycogenolysis. *Biochim. Biophys. Acta* **582,** 295–306.

Coupar, I. M. (1983). Characterization of the opiate receptor population mediating inhibition of VIP-induced secretion from the small intestine of the rat. *Br. J. Pharmacol.* **80,** 371–376.

Coy, D. H., Gill, P., Kastin, A. J., Dupont, A., Cusan, L., Labric, F., Britton, D., and Fertel, R. (1977). Synthetic and biological studies on unmodified and modified fragments of human β-lipotropin with opioid activities. *In* "Peptides" (M. Goodman and J. Meienhofer, eds.), pp. 107–110. Wiley and Sons, New York.

Coy, D. H., Murphy, W. A., Sueiras-Diaz, J., Coy, E. J., and Lance, V. A. (1985). Structure–activity studies on the N-terminal region of growth hormone releasing factor. *J. Med. Chem.* **28,** 181–185.

Coy, D. H., Heiman, M. L., Rossowski, J., Murphy, W. A., Taylor, J. E., Moreau, S., and Moreau, J.-P. (1988). Receptor-selective somatostatin (SRIF) analogs. *In* "Peptides" (G. R. Marshall, ed.), pp. 462–464. ESCOM, Leiden.

Crawley, J. N., and Beinfeld, M. C. (1983). Rapid development of tolerance to the behavioral actions of cholecystokinin. *Nature (London)* **302,** 703–706.

Creese, I., and Snyder, S. H. (1975). Receptor binding and pharmacological activity in the guinea pig intestine. *J. Pharmacol. Exp. Ther.* **194,** 205–219.

Davies, J. G., Muir, A. V., and Offord, R. E. (1986). Identification of some cleavage sites of insulin by insulin proteinase. *Biochem. J.* **240,** 609–612.

DeLisi, C., and Berzofsky, J. A. (1985). T-Cell antigenic sites tend to be amphipathic structures. *Proc. Natl. Acad. Sci. U.S.A.* **82,** 7048–7052.

Deschenes, R. J., Lorenz, L. F., Haun, R. S., Roos, B. A., Collier, K. J., and Dixon, J. E. (1984). Cloning and sequence analysis of a cDNA encoding rat preprocholecystokinin. *Proc. Natl. Acad. Sci. U.S.A.* **81,** 726–730.

Deslauriers, R. Smith, I. C. P., and Walter, R. (1974). Conformational flexibility of the neurohypophyseal hormones oxytocin and lysine-vasopressin. A carbon-13 spin-lattice relaxation study of backbone and side chains. *J. Am. Chem. Soc.* **96,** 2289–2291.

De Wied, D. (1980). Behavioral actions of neurohypophyseal peptides. *Proc. R. Soc. London, Ser. B* **210,** 183–195.

Diaz, J., Geugan, R., Cabrera, P., Mellet, M., Muneaux, Y., Perreaut, P., Vedel, M., and Roncucci, R. (1985). Large scale synthesis of hGRF (1–44) NH2 (somatocrinin). *In* "Peptides" (C. M. Deber, V. J. Hruby, and K. D. Kopple, eds.), pp. 297–300. Pierce Chemical Co., Rockford, Illinois.

Dimaline, R., and Dockray, G. J. (1980). Actions of a new peptide from porcine intestine (PHI) on pancreatic secretion in the rat and turkey. *Life Sci.* **27,** 1947–1951.

DiMarchi, R., Brooke, G., Gale, C., Cracknell, V., Doel, T., and Mowat, N. (1986). Protection of cattle against foot-and-mouth disease by a synthetic peptide. *Science* **232,** 639–641.

Dockray, G. J. (1976). Immunochemical evidence of cholecystokininlike peptides in brain. *Nature (London)* **264,** 568–570.

Dockray, G. J., and Taylor, I. L. (1976). Heptadecapeptide gastrin: Measurement in blood by specific radioimmunoassay. *Gastroenterology* **71,** 971–977.

Dockray, G. J., Gregory, R. A., and Hutchinson, J. B. (1978). Isolation, structure and biological activity of two cholecystokinin octapeptides from sheep brain. *Nature (London)* **274,** 711–713.

Dodd, J., Kelly, J. S., and Said, S. I. (1979). Excitation of CA1 neurons of the rat hippocampus by the octacosapeptide (VIP). *Br. J. Pharmacol.* **66,** 125P.

Dreesman, G. R., Sanchez, Y., Ionescu-Matiu, I., Sparrow, J. T., Six, H. R., Peterson, D. L., Hollinger, F. B., and Melnick, J. L. (1982). Antibody to hepatitis B surface antigen after a single inoculation of uncoupled synthetic HBsAg peptides. *Nature (London)* **295,** 158–160.

du Vigneaud, V. (1956). Hormones of the posterior pituitary gland: Oxytocin and vasopressin. *Harvey Lect.* **50,** 1–26.

du Vigneaud, V., Lawler, H. C., and Popenoe, A. (1953). Enzymatic cleavage of glycinamide from vasopressin and a proposed structure for the pressor-antiduiretic hormone of the posterior pituitary. *J. Am. Chem. Soc.* **75,** 4880–4881.

du Vigneaud, V., Fitt, P. S., Bodanszky, M., and O'Connell, M. (1960). Synthesis and some pharmacological properties of a peptide derivative of oxytocin. *Proc. Soc. Exp. Biol. Med.* **104,** 653–656.

Eisenberg, M., Hall, J. E., and Mead, C. A. (1973). The nature of the voltage-dependent conductance induced by alamethicin in black lipid membranes. *J. Membr. Biol.* **14,** 143–176.

Emini, E. A., Jameson, B. A., and Wimmer, E. (1983). Priming for and induction of anti-polio virus neutralizing antibodies by synthetic peptides. *Nature (London)* **304,** 699–703.

Eng, J., Shiina, Y., Pan, Y.-C., Blacher, R., Chang, M., Stein, S., and Yalow, R. S. (1983). Pig brain contains cholecystokinin octapeptide and several cholecystokinin desoctapeptides. *Proc. Natl. Acad. Sci. U.S.A.* **80,** 6381–6385.

Eng, J., Du, B.-H., Pan, Y.-C. E., Chang, M., Hulmes, J. D., and Yalow, R. S. (1984). Purification and sequencing of a rat intestinal 22 amino acid C-terminal CCK fragment. *Peptides (N.Y.)* **5,** 1203–1206.

Erickson, B. W., and Merrifield, R. B. (1976). Solid-phase peptide synthesis. *In* "The Proteins" (H. Neurath and R. L. Hill, eds.), Vol. 2, pp. 255–527. Academic Press, New York.

Eriksson, L., and Gordon, A. (1981). Cardiovascular and behavioral changes after ICV infusion of TRH in the conscious goat. *Pharmacol. Biochem. Behav.* **14,** 901–905.

Etlinger, H. M., Felix, A. M., Gillessen, D., Heimer, E. P., Just, M., Pink, R. L., Sinigaglia, F., Sturchler, D., Takacs, B., Trzeciak, A., and Matile, H. (1988). Assessment in humans of a synthetic peptide-based vaccine against sporozoite stage of the human malaria parasite, *Plasmodium falciparum. J. Immunol.* **140,** 626–633.

Ewenson, A., Cohen, R., Levian-Teitelbaum, D., Chorev, M., Laufer, R., Selinger, Z., and Gilon, C. (1985). Synthesis, characterization and biological activity of ketomethylene pseudopeptide analogs related to the C-terminal hexapeptide of substance. *In* "Peptides" (C. M. Deber, V. J. Hruby, and K. D. Kopple, eds.), pp. 639–642. Pierce Chemical Co., Rockford, Illinois.

Eysselein, V. E., Reeve, J. R., Jr., Shively, J. E., Hawke, D., and Walsh, J. H. (1982). Partial structure of a large canine cholecystokinin (CCK58): Amino acid sequence. *Peptides (N.Y.)* **3,** 687–691.

Eysselein, V. E., Reeve, J. R., Jr., Shively, J. E., Miller, C., and Walsh, J. H. (1984). Isolation of a large precursor from canine brain. *Proc. Natl. Acad. Sci. U.S.A.* **81,** 6565–6568.

Faden, A. I., Jacobs, T. P., and Holaday, J. W. (1981). Thyrotropin-releasing hormone improves neurologic recovery after spinal trauma in cats. *N. Engl. J. Med.* **305,** 1063–1067.

Fearney, F. J., Leung, C. Y., Young, J. D., and Benjamini, E. (1971). The specificity of antibodies to a peptide determinant of the tobacco mosaic virus protein induced by immunization with the peptide conjugate. *Biochim. Biophy. Acta* **243,** 509–514.

Felix, A. M., Wang, C.-T., Heimer, E., Fournier, A., Bolin, D. R., Ahmad, M., Lambros, T., Mowles, T., and Miller, L. (1988). Synthesis and biological activity of novel linear and cyclic GRF analogs. *In* "Peptides" (G. R. Marshall, ed.), pp. 465–467. ESCOM, Leiden.

Fischer, L. A., Rivier, J., Rivier, C., Spiess, J., Vale, W., and Brown, M. R. (1982). Corticotropin-releasing factor: Central effects on mean arterial pressure and heart rate in rats. *Endocrinology (Baltimore)* **110,** 2222–2224.

Florez, J., and Pazos, A. (1982). Comparative effects of opioid peptides on respiration and analgesia in rats. *Life Sci.* **31,** 1275–1277.

Folkers, K., Chang, D., Yamaguchi, I., Wan, Y.-P., Rackur, G., and Fisher, G. (1977). Studies on structure and conformation of substance P towards affecting changes in biological activities. *In* "Substance P" (U. S. von Euler and B. Pernow, eds.), pp. 19–26. Raven Press, New York.

Fournie-Zaluski, M.-C., Gacel, G., Maigret, B., Premilat, S., and Roques, B. P. (1981). Structural requirements for specific recognition of μ or δ opiate receptors. *Mol. Pharmacol.* **20,** 484–491.

Franco, R., Costa, M., and Furness, J. B. (1979). Evidence that axons containing substance P in guinea pig ileum are of intrinsic origin. *Naunyn-Schmiedeberg's Arch. Pharmacol.* **307,** 5763.

Franzen, H., Ragnarsson, U., Arnasson, T., and Terenius, L. (1981). Synthesis and biological activity of substance P analogs. *In* "Peptides" (D. H. Rich and E. Gross, eds.), pp. 577–602. Pierce Chemical Co., Rockford, Illinois.

Freidinger, R. M., Anderson, P. S., Bock, M. G., Chang, R. S. L., DiPardo, R. M., Evans, B. E., Garsky, V. M., Lotti, V. J., Rittle, K. E., Veber, D. F., and Whitter, W. L. (1988). Design and comparison of nonpeptide and peptide CCK antagonists. *In* "Peptides" G. R. Marshall, ed.), pp. 97–100. ESCOM, Leiden.

Fujii, N., Shimokura, M., Akaji, K., Kiyama, S., and Yajima, H. (1984). Studies on peptides. CXVI. Synthesis of the protected decosapeptide corresponding to the C-terminal portion of human growth hormone releasing factor (GRF, somatocrinin). *Chem. Pharm. Bull.* **32,** 510–519.

Fukjikawa, K. Y., Suketa, Y, Hayashi, K., and Suzuki, T. (1965). Chemical structure of circulin A. *Experientia* **21,** 307, 308.

Gacel, G., Fournie-Zaluski, M. C., and Roques, B. P. (1980). D-Tyr-Ser-Gly-Phe-Leu-Thr, a highly preferential ligand for δ-opiate receptors. *FEBS Lett.* **118,** 245–247.

Gacel, G., Fournie-Zaluski, M.-C., Fellion, E., and Roques, B. P. (1981). Evidence of the preferential involvement of μ receptors in analgesia using enkephalins highly selective for periferal μ or δ receptors. *J. Med. Chem.* **24,** 1119–1124.

Gariepy, J., Mietzner, T. A., and Schoolnik, G. K. (1986). Peptide antisera as sequence-specific probes of protein conformational transitions: Calmodulin exhibits calcium-dependent changes in antigenicity. *Proc. Natl. Acad. Sci. U.S.A.* **83,** 8888–8892.]

Gaudreau, P., St.-Pierre, S., Pert, C. B., and Quirion, R. (1987). Structure–activity studies of C- and N-terminal fragments of cholecystokinin 26-33 in guinea pig isolated tissues. *Neuropeptides* **10,** 9–18.

Ghatei, M. A., Bloom, S. R., Laugevin, H., McGregor, G. P., Lee, Y. C., Adrian, T. E., O'Shaughnessy, D. J., Black, M. A., and Uttenthal, L. O. (1984). Regional distribution of bombesin and seven other regulatory peptides in the human brain. *Brain Res.* **293,** 101–109.

Ghiglione, M., Christofides, N. D., Yiangon, Y., Uttenthal, L. O., and Bloom, S. R. (1982). PHI stimulates intestinal fluid secretion. *Neuropeptides* **3,** 79–82.

Gisin, B. F., Koyabashi, S., and Hall, J. E. (1977). Synthesis of a 19-residue peptide with alamethicin-like activity. *Proc. Natl. Acad. Sci. U.S.A.* **74,** 115–119.

Gisin, B. F., Davis, D.G., Borowoska, Z. K., Hall, J. E., and Kobayashi, S. (1981). Synthesis of the major component of alamethicin. *J. Am. Chem. Soc.* **103,** 6373–6377.

Glasel, J. A., Hruby, V. J., McKelvy, J. F., and Spatola, A. F. (1973). Deuteron magnetic resonance studies on the microdynamical behavior of partially deuterated oxytocin with neurophysin. *J. Mol. Biol.* **79,** 555–575.

Goldstein, A., Tachibana, S., Lowney, L. I., Hunkapillar, M., and Hood, L. (1979). Dynorphin-(1-13), an extraordinarily potent opioid peptide. *Proc. Natl. Acad. Sci. U.S.A.* **76,** 6666–6670.

Good, M. F., Maloy, W. L., Lunde, M. N., Margalit, H., Cornette, J. L., Smith, G. L., Moss, B., Miller, L. H., and Berzofsky, J. A. (1987). Construction of synthetic immunogen: Use of new T-helper epitope on malaria circumsporozoite protein. *Science* **235,** 1059–1062.

Goodwin, N. J. (1970). Colistin and sodium colistimethate. *Med. Clin. North Am.* **54,** 1267–1276.

Gordon, L. G. M., and Haydon, D. (1975). Potential-dependent conductances in lipid membranes containing alamethicin. *Philos. Trans. R. Soc. London, Ser. B* **270,** 433–447.

Grant, N., Clark, D., Garsky, V., Jaunakais, I., McGregor, W., and Sarantakis, D. (1976). Dissociation of somatostatin effects. Peptides inhibiting the release of growth hormone but not glucagon or insulin in rats. *Life Sci.* **19,** 629–632.

Green, N., Alexander, H., Olsen, A., Alexander, S., Shinnick, T. M., Sutcliffe, J. G., and Lerner, R. A. (1982). Immunogenic structure of the influenza virus hemagglutinin. *Cell (Cambridge, Mass.)* **28,** 477–487.

Gregory, R. A., and Tracy, H. J. (1964). The constitution and properties of two gastrins extracted from hog antral mucosa. *Gut* **5,** 103–114.

Gregory, R. A., and Tracy, H. J. (1972). Isolation of two "big gastrins" from Zollinger-Ellison tumour tissue. *Lancet* **2,** 797–799.

Gregory, R. A., and Tracy, H. J. (1975). The chemistry of gastrins: Some recent advances. *In* "Gastrointestinal Hormones" (J. C. Thomas, ed.), pp. 13–24. Univ. of Texas Press, Austin.

Gregory, R. A., Dockray, G. J., Reeve, J. R., Jr., Shevely, J. E., and Miller, C. (1983). Isolation from porcine antral mucosa of a hexapeptide corresponding to the C-terminal sequence of gastrin. *Peptides (N.Y.)* **4,** 319–323.

Gross, E., and Meienhofer, J., eds. (1978–1985). "The Peptides," Vols. 1–7. Academic Press, New York.

Guillemin, R., Brazeau, P., Böhlen, P., Esch, F., Ling, N., and Wehrenberg, W. B. (1982). Growth hormone-releasing factor from a human pancreatic tumor that caused acromegaly. *Science* **218,** 585–587.

Hall, J. E. (1975). Toward a molecular understanding of excitability. Alamethicin in black lipid films. *Biophys. J.* **15,** 934–939.

Hammonds, R. J., Jr., Hammonds, A. S., Ling, N., and Puett, D. (1982). β-Endorphin and deletion peptides. *J. Biol. Chem.* **257,** 2990–2995.

Harper, A., and Raper, H. S. (1943). Pancreozymin, a stimulant of the secretion of pancreatic enzymes in extracts of the small intestine. *J. Physiol. (London)* **102,** 115–125.

Hashmonai, M., Go, V. L. W., Yaksh, T., and Szurszewski, J. H. (1987). Effects of central administration of motilin on migrating complexes in the dog. *Am. J. Physiol.* **252,** G195–G199.

Hefford, M. A., Oda, G., and Kaplan, H. (1986). Structure–function relationships in the free insulin monomer. *Biochem. J.* **237,** 663–668.

Hiller, J. M., and Simon, E. J. (1976). Studies on opiate receptors in animal and human brain. *In* "Tissue Responses to Addictive Drugs" (D. H. Ford and D. H. Clouet, eds.), pp. 335–353. Spectrum Publications, New York.

Hirning, L. D., and Burks, T. F. (1986). Neurogenic mechanism of action of motilin in the canine isolated small intestine *ex vivo*. *Eur. J. Pharmacol.* **128,** 241–248.

Ho, D. D., Sarngadharan, M. G., Hirsch, M. S., Schooley, R. T., Rota, T. R., Kennedy, R. C., Chanh, T. C., and Sato, V. L. (1987). Human immunodeficiency virus neutralizing antibodies recognize several conserved domains on the envelope glycoproteins. *J. Virol.* **61,** 2024–2028.

Hocart, S. J., Nekola, M. V., and Coy, D. H. (1987). Effect of reductive alkylation of D-lysine in position 6 on the histamine-releasing activity of luteinizing hormone-releasing hormone antagonists. *J. Med. Chem.* **30,** 739–743.

Hocart, S. J., Jiang, N. Y., Nekola, M. V., and Coy, D. H. (1988). The activity of reductive alkylation in solid phase peptide synthesis. *In* "Peptides" (G. R. Marshall, eds.), pp. 223–225. ESCOM, Leiden.

Hoeprich, P. D. (1970). The polymyxins. *Med. Clin. North Am.* **54,** 1257–1265.

Holaday, J. W., and D'Amato, F. J. (1983). Multiple opioid receptors: Evidence for μ-δ binding site interactions in endotoxic shock. *Life Sci.* **33,** Suppl. 1, 703–706.

Holaday, J. W., D'Amato, F. J., and Foden, A. I. (1981). Thyrotropin-releasing hormone improves cardiovascular function in experimental endotoxin and hemorrhagic shock. *Science* **213,** 216–218.

Holaday, J. W., Ruvio, B. A., Robles, L. E., Johnson, C. E., and D'Amato, R. J. (1982). M 154, 129, a putative δ antagonist, reverses endotoxic shock without altering morphine analgesia. *Life Sci.* **31,** 2209–2212.

Hopp, T. P., and Woods, K. R. (1981). Prediction of protein antigenic determinants from amino acid sequence. *Proc. Natl. Acad. Sci. U.S.A.* **78,** 3824–3828.

Horita, A., Carino, M. A., and Chestnut, R. M. (1976a). Influence of thyrotropin-releasing hormone on drug-induced narcosis and hypothermia in rabbits. *Psychopharmacol. Bull.* **49,** 57–62.

Horita, A., Carino, M. A., and Weitzman, R. E. (1976b). Role of catecholamines and vasopressin release in the TRH-induced vasopressor responce. *In* "Catacholamines: Basic and Clinical Frontiers" (E. Usclin *et al.*, eds.), pp. 1140–1142. Pergamon, New York.

Hruby, V. J. (1981). Structure and conformation related to the activity of peptide hormones. *In* "Perspectives in Peptide Chemistry" (A. Eberle, R. Geiger, and T. Weiland, eds.), pp. 207–220. Karger, Basel.

Hruby, V. J. (1984). Design of peptide super agonists and antagonists: Conformational and dynamic considerations. *In* "Conformationally Directed Drug Design" (J. A. Vida and M. Gordon, eds.), pp. 9–27. Am. Chem. Soc., Washington, D.C.

Hruby, V. J., Mosberg, H. I., Hadley, M. E., Chan, W. Y., and Powell, A. M. (1980). Synthesis, pharmacological, conformational, and dynamic studies of the potent hormone antagonists [1-penicillamine, 4-threonine]-oxytocin. Conformational and dynamic considerations in the design of antagonists. *Int. J. Pept. Protein Res.* **16,** 372–381.

Hruby, V. J., Kazmierski, W., Pelton, J. T., Shook, J. E., Knapp, R. J., Burks, T. K., and Yamamura, H. I. (1988). Design and conformational analysis of somatostatin analogs with exceptional mu opioid receptor selectivity, opioid antagonist activities and greatly reduced somatostatin-like activity: A new approach to receptor specific peptides. *In* "Peptide Chemistry 1987": (T. Shiba and S. Sakakibara, eds.), pp. 601–606. Protein Res. Found., Osaka.

Hughes, J., Smith, T. W., Kosterlitz, H. W., Fothergill, L. A., Morgan, B. A., and Morris, H. R. (1975). Identification of two related pentapeptides from the brain with potent opiate against activity. *Nature (London)* **258,** 577–579.

Il'inskaya, S. A., and Rossovskaya, V. S. (1960). A new type of polymyxin—polymyxin M. *Antibiotiki* **5,** 3–9.

Ishiguro, T., Fujita, S., Okano, R., Kato, N., Eguchi, C., and Matsuo, H. (1988). Synthesis of peptide fragments of neuropeptide Y: Potent inhibitors of calmodulin-stimulated phosphodiesterase. *Chem. Pharm. Bull.* **36,** 2720–2723.

Itoh, M., Obata, K., Yanaihara, N., and Okamoto, M. (1983). Human preprovasoactive intestinal polypeptide contains a novel PHI-27-like peptide, PHM-27. *Nature (London)* **304,** 547–549.

Itoh, Y., Takai, E., Ohnuma, H., Kitajima, K., Tsuda, F., Machida, A., Mishiro, S., Nakamura, T., Miyakawa, Y., and Mayumi, M. (1986). A synthetic peptide vaccine involving the product of the pre-S(2) region of hepatitis B virus DNA: Protective efficacy in chimpanzees. *Proc. Natl. Acad. Sci. U.S.A.* **83,** 9174–9178.

Ivanov, V. T., and Sychev, S. V. (1983). Spectral studies of gramicidin A and its derivatives in membranes. Ensuing models of ion channelling. *In* "Peptides" (V. J. Hruby and D. H. Rich, eds.), pp. 451–462. Pierce Chemical Co., Rockford, Illinois.

Jacoby, R. L., Boon, D., Darling, L. E., and Willette, R. E. (1981). Structure–activity studies on narcotic antagonists. 2. N-Substituted ethyl 3-(m- or p-hydroxyphenyl)nipecotates. *J. Med. Chem.* **24,** 218–221.

Jensen, R. T., Tatemoto, K., Mutt, V., Lemp, G. F., and Gardner, J. D. (1981). Actions of a newly isolated intestinal peptide PHI on pancreatic acini. *Am. J. Physiol.* **4,** G498–G502.

Jensen, R. T., Jones, S. W., Lu, I. A., Yu, J. C., Folkers, K., and Gardner, J. D. (1984a). Interaction of substance P antagonists with substance P receptors on dispersed pancreatic acini. *Biochim. Biophys. Acta* **804,** 181–191.

Jensen, R. T., Jones, S. W., Folkers, K., and Gardner, J. D. (1948b). A synthetic peptide that is a bombesin receptor antagonist. *Nature (London)* **309,** 61–63.

Jessell, T., and Iversen, L. L. (1977). Opiate analgesics inhibit substance P release from rat trigeminal nucleus. *Nature (London)* **268,** 549–551.

Jolivet, M. E., Audibert, F. M., Gras-Masse, H., Tartar, A. L., Schlesinger, D. H., Wirtz, R., and Chédid, L. A. (1987). Induction of biologically active antibodies by a polyvalent synthetic vaccine constructed without carriers. *Infect. Immun.* **55,** 1498–1502.

Jost, K., Lebl, M., and Brtnik, F., eds. (1987). "Handbook of Neurohypophyseal Hormone Analogs," Vols. 1 and 2, Parts 1 and 2. CRC Press, Boca Raton, Florida.

Judd, A. K., Lawson, J. A., Olsen, C. M., Toll, L. R., Polgar, W. E., Uyeno, E. T., Keys, C. J., and Loew, G. H. (1987). Novel μ-selective Met-enkephalinamide analogs with antagonist activity. *Int. J. Pept. Protein Res.* **30,** 299–317.

Jung, G., Dubischar, N., and Leibfritz, D. (1975). Conformational changes of alamethicin induced by solvent and temperature. *Eur. J. Biochem.* **54,** 395–409.

Kato, T., Waki, M., Matsuura, S., and Izumiya, N. (1970). The correlation between conformation and biological activity of gramicidin S analogs. *J. Biochem. (Tokyo)* **68,** 751–753.

Kato, Y., Iwasaki, Y., Iwasaki, J. Abe, H., Yanaihara, N., and Imura, H. (1978). Prolactin release by vasoactive intestinal polypeptide in rats. *Endocrinology (Baltimore)* **103,** 554–558.

Kennedy, R. C., Henkel, R. D., Pauletti, D., Allan, J. S., Lee, T. H., Essex, M., and Dreesman, G. R. (1986). Antiserum to a synthetic peptide recognizes the HTLV-III envelope glycoprotein. *Science* **231,** 1556–1559.

Khokhlov, A. S., and Ch'ih Ch'ang-Ch'ing. (1961). A new type of polymyxin—polymyxin M. *Biokhimiya* **26,** 267–296.

Kilpatrick, D. L., Wahlström, A., Lahm, H. W., Blacher, R., Ezra, E., Fleminger, G., and Udenfriend, J. (1982a). Characterization of rimorphin, a new [Leu]enkephalin-containing peptide from bovine posterior pituitary gland. *Life Sci.* **31,** 1849–1852.

Kilpatrick, D. L., Wahlström, A., Lahm, H. W., Blacher, R., and Udenfriend, J. (1982b). Rimorphin, a unique, naturally occurring [Leu]enkephalin-containing peptide found in association with dynorphin and α-neo-endorphin. *Proc. Natl. Acad. Sci. U.S.A.* **79,** 6480–6483.

Kimball, C. P., and Murlin, J. R. (1923). Aqueous extracts of pancreas. III. Some precipitation reactions of insulin. *J. Biol. Chem.* **58,** 337–346.

Kimmel, J. R., Hayden, J., and Pollock, H. G. (1975). Isolation and characterization of a new pancreatic polypeptide hormone. *J. Biol. Chem.* **250,** 9369–9376.

Kiyama, S., Ooi, Y., Kitagawa, K., Nakamura, T., Akita, T., Kogire, M., Hosotani, R., Inoue, K., Tobe, T., and Yajima, H. (1987). Synthesis of porcine neuropeptide Y (NPY) in solution. *Int. J. Pept. Protein Res.* **29,** 533–544.

Koivusalo, F., Paakari, I., Leppaluoto, J., and Karppanen, H. (1979). The effect of centrally administered TRH on blood pressure, heart rate and ventilation in rat. *Acta Physiol. Scand.* **106,** 83–86.

Kosterlitz, H. W., Lord, J. A. H., Paterson, S. J., and Waterfield, A. A. (1980). Effects of changes in the structure of enkephaline and of narcotic analgesic drugs on their interactions with mu- and delta-receptors. *Br. J. Pharmacol.* **68,** 333–342.

Kosterlitz, H. W., Paterson, S. J., and Robsen, L. E. (1981). Characterization of the κ-subtype of the opiate receptor in the guinea-pig brain. *Br. J. Pharmacol.* **73,** 939–949.

Koyama, Y., Kurosawa, A., Tsuchiya, A., and Takakuda, K. (1950). A new antibiotic "colistin," produced by spore-forming soil bacteria. *J. Antibiot., Ser. B* **3,** 457–458.

Krulich, L., Dhariwal, A. P. S., and McCann, S. M. (1968). Stimulatory and inhibitory effects of purified hypothalamic extracts on growth hormone release from rat pituitary in vitro. *Endocrinology (Baltimore)* **83,** 783–790.

Kugita, H., Oine, T., Inoue, H., and Hayashi, G. (1965). 3-Alkyl-3-phenylpiperidine derivatives as analgesics. II. *J. Med. Chem.* **8,** 313–316.

Kunin, C. M., and Bugg, A. (1971). Binding of polymyxin antibiotics to tissues: The major determinant of distribution and persistence in the body. *J. Infect. Dis.* **124,** 394–400.

Kuno, S., Li, W., Fujii, N., Adachi, H., Bessho, K., Segawa, T., Nakata, Y., Inoue, A., and Yajima, H. (1986). Studies on peptides CXLVI. Synthesis of Gln15-motilin and examination of its immunological properties. *Chem. Pharm. Bull.* **34,** 4811–4816.

Kyte, J., and Doolittle, R. F. (1982). A simple method for displaying the hydropathic character of a protein. *J. Mol. Biol.* **157,** 105–132.

Labroo, V. M., Feurerstein, G., and Cohen, L. A. (1985). Synthesis and cardiovascular activity of imidazole-substituted analogs of TRH. *In* "Peptides" (C. M. Deber, V. J. Hruby, and K. D. Kopple, eds.), pp. 703–706. Pierce Chemical Co., Rockford, Illinois.

Lamers, C., Harrison, A., Ippoliti, A., and Walsh, J. H. (1979). Failure to demonstrate CCK-octapeptide in the circulation during fasting and after a meal. *Gastroenterology* **76,** 1179.

Langbeheim, H., Arnon, R., and Sela, M. (1976). Antiviral effect on MS-2 coliphage obtained with a synthetic antigen. *Proc. Natl. Acad. Sci. U.S.A.* **73,** 4636–4640.

Larsson, L. I., Farhenkrug, J., de Muckadell, O. S., Sundler, F., Hakanson, R., and Rehfield, J. F. (1976). Localization of vasoactive intestinal polypeptide (VIP) to central and peripheral neurons. *Proc. Natl. Acad. Sci. U.S.A.* **73,** 3197–3200.

Lau, A. Y., and Chan, S. (1974). Nuclear magnetic resonance studies of the interaction of alamethicin with lecithin bilayers. *Biochemistry* **13,** 4942–4948.

Leander, J. D. (1983a). Evidence that nalorphine, butorphine and oxilorphan are partial agonists at a κ-opioid receptor. *Eur. J. Pharmacol.* **86,** 467–470.

Leander, J. D. (1983b). A κ opioid effect: Increased urination in the rat. *J. Pharmacol. Exp. Ther.* **224,** 89–94.

Leban, J., Rackur, G., Yamaguchi, I., Folkers, K., Björkroth, U., Rosell, S., Yanaihara, N., and Yanaihara, C. (1979). Synthesis of substance P analogs and agonistic and antagonistic activities. *Acta Chem. Scand., Ser. B* **B33,** 664–668.

Leclerc, C., Przewlocki, G., Schutze, M. P., and Chédid, L. (1987). A synthetic vaccine constructed by copolymerization of B and T cell determinant. *Eur. J. Immunol.* **17,** 269–273.

Lederis, K. (1961). Vasopressin and oxytocin in the mammalian hypothalamus. *Gen. Comp. Endocrinol.* **1,** 80–89.

Lee, N. M., and Smith, A. P. (1980). A protein–lipid model of the opiate receptor. *Life Sci.* **26,** 1459–1464.

Lee, N. M., Leybin, L., Chang, J. K., and Loh, H. H. (1980). Opiate and peptide interaction: Effect of enkephalins on morphine analgesia. *Eur. J. Pharmacol.* **68,** 181–185.

Lemaire, S., Bérubé, A., Derome, G., Lemaire, I., Magnan, J., Regoli, D., and St.-Pierre, S. (1978). Synthesis and biological activity of β-endorphin and analogs. Additional evidence for multiple opiate receptors. *J. Med. Chem.* **21,** 1232–1235.

Lenz, H. J., Hester, S. E., and Brown, M. R. (1985). Corticotropin-releasing factor: Mechanisms to inhibit gastric acid secretion in conscious dogs. *J. Clin. Invest.* **75,** 889–895.

Lerner, R. A. (1982). Tapping immunological repertoire to produce antibodies of predeterminable specificity. *Nature (London)* **229,** 593–596.

Lerner, R. A., Green, N., Alexander, H., Liu, F. T. J., Sutcliffe, J. G., and Shinnick, T. M. (1981a). Chemically synthesized peptides predicted from the nucleotide sequence of the hepatitis B virus genome elicit antibodies reactive with the native envelope protein of Dane particles. *Proc. Natl. Acad. Sci. U.S.A.* **78,** 3404–3407.

Lerner, R. A., Sutcliffe, J. G., and Shinnick, T. M. (1981b). Antibodies to chemically synthesized peptides predicted from DNA sequences as probes of gene expression. *Cell (Cambridge, Mass.)* **23,** 309–310.

Leslie, F. M., Chavkin, C., and Cox, B. M. (1979). Ligand specificity of opioid binding sites in brain and peripheral tissues. *In* "Endogenous and Exogenous Opiate Agonists and Antagonists" (E. L. Way, ed.), pp. 109–112. Pergamon, New York.

Levin, J. M., and Garnier, J. (1988). Improvements in a secondary structure prediction method based on a search for local sequence homologies and its use as a model building tool. *Biochim. Biophys. Acta* **955,** 283–295.

Li, C. H. (1979). B-Endorphine: Aspects of structure–activity relationship. *In* "Endorphins 1978" (L. Graf, M. Palkovitis, and A. Z. Ronai, eds.), pp. 15–31. Akadémiai Kiadó, Budapest.

Li, C. H. (1981). β-Endorphin: Synthetic analogs and structure–activity relationships. *In* "Hormonal Proteins and Peptides" (C. H. Li, ed.), Vol. 10, pp. 1–34. Academic Press, New York.

Li, C. H., and Chung, D. (1976). Isolation and structure of an untriakonta peptide with opiate activity from camel pituitary glands. *Proc. Natl. Acad. Sci. U.S.A.* **73,** 1145–1148.

Li, C. H., Yamashiro, D., Tseng, L.-F., Chang, W.-C., and Ferrara, P. (1980). β-Endorphin omission analogs: Dissociation of immunoreactivity from other biological activity. *Proc. Natl. Acad. Sci. U.S.A.* **77,** 3211–3214.

Lichtarge, O., Jardetzky, O., and Li, C. H. (1987). Secondary structure determination of human β-endorphin by ^{1}H NMR spectroscopy. *Biochemistry* **26,** 5916–5925.

Ling, N., Esch, F., Böhlen, P., Brazeau, P., Wehrenberg, W., and Guillemin, R. (1984). Isolation, primary structure and synthesis of human hypothalamic somatocrinin: Growth hormone-releasing factor. *Proc. Natl. Acad. Sci. U.S.A.* **81,** 4302–4306.

Loew, G., Burt, S. K., and Hashimoto, G. M. (1981). Quantum chemical studies of the origin of agonist and antagonist activity in 3- and 4-phenylpiperidines. *NIDA Res. Monogr.* **34,** 399–405.

Loew, G., Collins, J., Payne, P., Judd, A. K., and Wacknow, K. H. (1988). Energy conformational studies of β-endorphins: Identification of plausible folded conformers. *Int. J. Quantum Chem., Quantum Biol. Symp.* **15,** 055–066.

Lord, J. A., Waterfield, A. A., Hughes, J., and Kosterlitz, H. W. (1977). Endogenous opioid peptides: Multiple agonists and receptors. *Nature (London)* **267,** 495–499.

Lundberg, J. M., and Tatemoto, K. (1982). Vascular effects of the peptides PYY and PHI: Comparison with APP and VIP. *Eur. J. Pharmacol.* **83,** 143–146.

Lux, W. E., Jr., Feuerstein, G., and Faden, A. I. (1983). Altercation of leukotriene D4 hypotension by thyrotropin-releasing hormone. *Nature (London)* **302,** 822–824.

MacCannell, K. L., and Lederis, K. (1983). Mammalian pharmacology of the fish neuropeptide urotensin I. *Fed. Proc., Fed. Am. Soc. Exp. Biol.* **42,** 91–95.

MacFarlan, R. I., Dietzschold, B., Wiktor, T. J., Kiel, M., Houghton, R., Lerner, R. A., Sutcliffe, J. G., and Koprowski, H. (1984). T-Cell responses to cleaved rabies virus glycoprotein and to synthetic peptides. *J. Immunol.* **133,** 2748–2752.

Machova, A. (1971). Effect of methyloxytocin on renal excretion of water and electrolytes in the rat. *Physiol. Bohemoslov.* **20,** 515–522.

Malacara, J. M., Valverda, R. C., Reichlin, S., and Bollinger, J. (1972). Elevation of plasma radioimmunoassayable growth hormone in the rat induced by porcine hypothalamic extract. *Endocrinology (Baltimore)* **91,** 1189–1198.

Margalit, H., Spouge, J. L., Cornette, J. L., Cease, K. B., DeLisi, C., and Berzofsky, J. (1987). Prediction of immunodominant helper T cell antigenic sites from the primary sequence. *J. Immunol.* **138,** 2213–2229.

Markussen, J., Damagaard, U., Diers, I., Fiil, N., Hansen, M. T., Larsen, P., Norris, F., Norris, K., Schou, O., Snel, L., Thim, L., and Voigt, H. O. (1987). Biosynthesis of human insulin in yeast via single-chain precursors. *In* "Peptides" (D. Theodoropoulos, ed.), pp. 189–194. De Gruyter, Berlin and New York.

Markussen, J., Hansen, M. T., Norris, K., and Sorensen, E. (1988). Synthesis of insulin substituted in position A17, B13, B27 and in the terminals of the B-chain, combining genetic engineering and tryptic transpeptidation in organic-aqueous medium. *In* "Peptide Chemistry 1987" (T. Shiba and S. Sakakibara, eds.), pp. 417–422. Protein Res. Found., Osaka.

Marshall, G. R., and Balasubramanian, T. M. (1979). Alamethicin: Purification, characterization, conformational and synthetic studies. *N* "Peptides" (E. Gross and J. Meienhofer, eds.), pp. 639–646. Pierce Chemical Co., Rockford, Illinois.

Martin, D. R., and Williams, R. J. (1975). The nature and function of alamethicin *Biochem. Soc. Trans.* **3,** 166, 167.

Martin, W. R., Eades, C. G., Thompson, J. A., Huppler, R. E., and Gilbert, P. E. (1976). The effects of morphine and morphine-like drugs in the nondependent and morphine-dependent chronic spinal dog. *J. Pharmacol. Exp. Ther.* **197,** 517–532.

McKee, R. L., Trivedi, D., Zechel, C., Johnson, D., Brendel, K., and Hruby, V. J. (1988). Activities of glucagon antagonists on normal liver: Evidence for cAMP-independent events. *In* "Peptides" (G. R. Marshall, ed.), pp. 341–343. ESCOM, Leiden.

Melin, P., Vilhardt, H., Lidenberg, G., Larsson, L. E., and Akerland, M. (1981). Inhibitory effect of O-alkylated analogues of oxytocin and vasopressin in human and rat myometrial activity. *J. Endocrinol.* **88,** 173–180.

Melnick, J. L. (1986). Beginning of the development of synthetic peptides as viral vaccines. *Ann. Inst. Pasteur/Virol.* **137E,** 497–528.

Meraldi, J. P., Hruby, V. J., and Brewster, A. I. R. (1977). Relative conformational rigidity in oxytocin and [1-penicillamine]-oxytocin: A proposal for the relationship of conformational flexibility to peptide hormone agonism and antagonism. *Proc. Natl. Acad. Sci. U.S.A.* **74,** 1373–1377.

Merrifield, R. B. (1963). Solid phase peptide synthesis. The synthesis of a tetrapeptide. *J. Am. Chem. Soc.* **85,** 2149–2154.

Meyer, C. E., and Reusser, F. (1967). A polypeptide antibacterial agent isolated from *Trichoderma viride. Experientia* **23,** 85–86.

Miglecz, E., Szekely, J. F., and Dunai-Kovacs, Z. (1979). Comparison of tolerance development and dependence capacities of morphine, β-endorphin, and [D-Met^2,Pro^5]-enkephalinamide. *Psychopharmacology* **62,** 29–34.

Minemino, N., Kangawa, K., and Matsuo, H. (1983). Neuromedin B: A novel bombesin-like peptide identified in porcine spinal cord. *Biochem. Biophys. Res. Commun.* **114,** 541–548.

Minemino, N., Kangawa, K., and Matsuo, H. (1984). Neuromedin C: A bombesin-like peptide identified in porcine spinal cord. *Biochem. Biophys. Res. Commun.* **119,** 14–20.

Morgan, B. A., Bower, J. D., Dettmar, P. W., Metcalf, G., Schaffer, D. J., and Brown, R. (1979). Novel TRH analogs with increased neuropharmacological activity. *In* "Peptides" (E. Gross and J. Meienhofer, eds.), pp. 909–912. Pierce Chemical Co., Rockford, Illinois.

Morgan, B. A., Singh, J., Baizman, E., Bentley, H., Keifer, D., and Ward, S. (1988). Structure–function studies in a series of tachykinin antagonists containing a conformationally constrained tryptophan analog. *In* "Peptides" (G. R. Marshall, ed.), pp. 508, 509. ESCOM, Leiden.

Morice, A., Unwin, R. J., and Sever, P. S. (1983). Vasoactive intestinal peptide as a bronchodilator in asthmatic subjects. *Lancet* **2,** 1225–1227.

Morley, J. E., Levine, A. S., Grace, M., and Kneip, J. (1982). An investigation of the role of κ opiate receptor agonists in the initiation of feeding. *Life Sci.* **31,** 2617–2626.

Morley, J. E., Levine, A. S., Grace, M., Kneip, J., and Zeugner, H. (1983). The effect of opioid-benzodiazepine, trifluadom, on ingestive behaviors. *Eur. J. Pharmacol.* **93,** 265–269.

Morley, J. S. (1968a). Structure–function relationships in gastrin-like peptides. *Proc. Ry. Soc. London, Ser. B.* **170,** 97–111.

Morley, J. S. (1968b). Structure–activity relationships. *Fed. Proc., Fed. Am. Soc. Exp. Biol.* **27,** 1314–1317.

Moroder, L., Göhring, W., Jaeger, E., Thamm, P., Wünsch, E., Tatemoto, K., and Mutt, V. (1981). On the synthesis of PHI. *In* "Peptides" (D. H. Rich and E. Gross, eds.), pp. 49–52. Pierce Chemical Co., Rockford, Illinois.

Mosberg, H. I., Hurst, R., Hruby, V. J., Galligan, J. J., Burks, T. F., Gee, K., and Yamamura, H. I.

(1982). [D-Pen[2], L-Cys[5]]-enkephalinamide and [D-Pen[2], D-Cys[5]]-enkephalinamide, conformationally constrained cyclic enkaphalinamide analogs with delta receptor specificity. *Biochem. Biophys. Res. Commun.* **106,** 506–512.

Mosberg, H. I., Hurst, R., Hruby, V. J., Galligan, J. J., Burks, T. F., Gee, K., and Yamamura, H. I. (1983). Conformationally constrained cyclic enkaphalin analogs with pronounced delta opioid receptor agonist selectivity. *Life Sci.* **32,** 2565–2569.

Moss, R. L., and McCann, S. M. (1973). Induction of mating behavior in rats by luteinizing hormone-releasing factor. *Science* **181,** 177–179.

Mueller, P., and Rudin, D. O. (1968). Action potentials induced in biomolecular lipid membranes. *Nature (London)* **217,** 713–719.

Murphy, G. J., Hruby, V. J., Trivedi, D., Wakelam, M. J. O., and Houslay, M. D. (1987). The rapid desensitization of glucagon-stimulated adenylate cyclase is a cyclic AMP-independent process that can be mimicked by hormones which stimulate inositol phospholipid metabolism. *Biochem. J.* **243,** 39–46.

Mutt, V. (1976). Further investigations on intestinal hormonal polypeptides. *Clin. Endocrinol.* **5,** Suppl., 175s–183s.

Mutt, V. (1980). Cholecystokinin: Isolation, structure, and functions. *In* "Gastrointestinal Hormones" (G. B. Jerzy, ed.), pp. 169–221. Raven Press, New York.

Mutt, V., and Jorpes, J. E. (1967). Contemporary developments in the biochemistry of the gastrointestinal hormones. *Recent Prog. Horm. Res.* **23,** 483–503.

Mutt, V., and Jorpes, E. (1971). Hormonal polypeptides of the upper intestine. *Biochem. J.* **125,** 57P, 58P.

Mutt, V., Jorpes, J. E., and Magnusson, S. (1970). Structure of porcine secretin. The amino acid sequence. *Eur. J. Biochem.* **15,** 513–519.

Nagai, U., Kato, R., Sato, K., Ling, N., Matsuzaki, T., and Tomotake, Y. (1988). Synthesis and properties of some peptides related to the bicyclic β-turn diapeptide (BTD). *In* "Peptides" (G. R. Marshall, ed.), pp. 129–130. ESCOM, Leiden.

Nestor, J. J., Jr. (1984). Development of agonistic LHRH. *In* "LHRH and Its Analogs: Contraceptive and Therapeutic Applications" (B. J. Vickery, J. J. Nestor, Jr., and E. S. E. Hafez, eds.), pp. 3–10. MTP Press Ltd., Lancaster.

Nestor, J. J., Jr., Ho, T. L., Simpson, R. A., Horner, B. L., Jones, G. H., McRae, G. I., and Vickery, B. H. (1982). Synthesis and biological activity of some very hydrophobic superagonist analogues of luteinizing hormone-releasing hormone. *J. Med. Chem.* **25,** 795–801.

Nestor, J. J., Jr., Ho, T. L., Tahilramani, R., Horner, B. L., Simpson, R. A., Jones, G. H., McRae, G. I., and Vickery, B. H. (1984). LHRH agonists and antagonists containing very hydrophobic amino acids. *In* LHRH and Its Analogs: Contraceptive and Therapeutic Applications" (B. J. Vickery, J. J. Nestor, Jr., and E. S. E. Hafez, eds.), pp. 23–33. MTP Press Ltd., Lancaster.

Nestor, J. J., Jr., Tahilramani, R., Ho, T. L., McRae, G. I., and Vickery, B. H. (1985). Potent LHRH agonists containing N^G, N^G,-dialkyl-D-homoarginines. *In* "Peptides" (C. M. Deber, V. J. Hruby, and K. D. Kopple, eds.), pp. 557–560. Pierce Chemical Co., Rockford, Illinois.

Neubert, K., Mensfeld, H.-W., Hartrodt, B., Berger, E., Jakubke, H.-D., Bergmann, J., and Mehlis, B. (1979). Synthesis of cyclic peptides related to modified partial sequences of substance P. *In* "Peptides 1978" (I. Z. Siemion and G. Kupryszewski, eds.), pp. 455–459. Wroclaw Univ. Press, Wroclaw.

Neurath, A. R., Strick, N., Kent, S. B. J., Parker, K., Seto, B., and Girard, M. (1988). Design of synthetic peptides mimicking the immunologic functions of the pre-S1 sequence of the hepatitis-B virus envelope protein. *In* "Vaccines '88, New Chemical and Genetic Approaches to Vaccination" (H. Ginsberg, F. Brown, R. A. Lerner, and R. M. Chanock, eds.), pp. 229–234. Cold Spring Harbor Lab., Cold Spring Harbor, New York.

Nicholas, P., Hammonds, R. G., Jr., and Li, C. H. (1982). β-Endorphin: Opiate receptor binding activities of six naturally occurring β-endorphin homologs studied by using tritiated human hormone and naloxone as primary ligands—effects of sodium ion. *Proc. Natl. Acad. Sci. U.S.A.* **79,** 2191.

Nicholas, P., Hammonds, R. G., Jr., and Li, C. H. (1984). β-Endorphin-induced analgesia is inhibited by synthetic analogs of β-endorphin. *Proc. Natl. Acad. Sci. U.S.A.* **81,** 3074–3077.

Nutt, R. F., Hisschmann, R., and Veber, D. F. (1979). Synthesis of ⟨AAD-His-(4R,5R)-5-methyl-TZL-NH_2, a TRH analog with high CNS activity. *In* "Peptides" (E. Gross and J. Meienhofer, eds.), pp. 913–916. Pierce Chemical Co., Rockford, Illinois.

Oehme, P., Hilse, H., Morgenstern, E., and Göres, E. (1980). Does substance P produce analgesia or hyperalgesia. *Science* **208,** 305–307.

Ohashi, S., Shiraki, M., Sawano, S., Ozaki, S., Akimoto, K., Takaoka, T., Hirose, S., and Kurihara, T. (1986). Structure and activities of hGRF analogs. *In* "Peptide Chemistry 1985" (Y. Kiso, ed.), pp. 45–50. Protein Res. Found., Osaka.

Ohashi, S., Shiraki, M., Sawano, S., Seki, M., and Ozaki, S. (1988). Structure and activities of human growth hormone-releasing factor (hGRF) analogs(II). *In* "Peptide Chemistry 1987" (T. Shiba and S. Sakakibara, eds.), pp. 521–524. Protein Res. Found., Osaka.

Ono, N., Lumpkin, M. D., Samson, W. K., McDonald, J. K., and McCann, S. M. (1984). Intrahypothalamic action of corticotrophin-releasing factor to inhibit growth hormone and LH release in the rat. *Life Sci.* **35,** 1117–1123.

Otsuka, M., Konishi, S., and Takahashi, T. (1975). Hypothalamic substance P as a candidate for transmitter of primary afferent neurons. *Fed. Proc., Fed. Am. Soc. Exp. Biol.* **34,** 1922–1928.

Palker, T. J., Clark, M. E., Langlois, A. J., Matthews, T. J., Weinhold, K. J., Randall, R. R., Bolognesi, D. P., and Haynes, B. F. (1988). Type specific neutralization of the human immunodeficiency virus with antibodies to env-encoded synthetic peptides. *Proc. Natl. Acad. Sci. U.S.A.* **85,** 1932–1936.

Paulus, H., and Sarkar, N. (1976). Regulation of transcription by peptide antibiotics. *In* "Molecular Mechanisms in the Control of Gene Expression" (D. P. Nierlich, W. J. Rutter, and C. F. Fox., eds.), pp. 177–194. Academic Press, New York.

Payne, R., Jakes, R., and Hartley, B. S. (1970). The primary structure of alamethicin. *Biochem. J.* **117,** 757–766.

Perlman, D., and Bodanszky, M. (1966). Structural relationships among peptide antibiotics. *Antimicrob. Agents Chemother.*, pp. 122–131.

Pfaff, D. W. (1973). Luteinizing hormone-releasing factor potentiates lordosis behavior in hypophysectomized, ovariectomized female rats. *Science* **182,** 1148–1149.

Phillis, J. W., and Kirkpatrick, J. R. (1979). Actions of various gastrointestinal peptides on the isolated amphibious spinal cord. *Can. J. Physiol. Pharmacol.* **57,** 887–899.

Polak, J. M., Pearse, A. G. E., Garaud, J. C., and Bloom, S. R. (1974). Cellular localization of a vasoactive intestinal peptide in the mammalian and avian gastrointestinal tract. *Gut* **15,** 720–724.

Porreca, F., Mosberg, H. I., Hurst, R., Hruby, V. J., and Burks, T. F. (1983). A comparison of the analgesic and gastrointestinal transit effects of [D-Pen^2, L-Cys^5]enkephalin after intracerebroventricular and intrathecal administration to mice. *Life Sci.* **33,** Suppl. 1, 457–460.

Prange, A. J., Jr., Wilson, I. C., Lara, P. P., Alltop, L. B., and Breese, G. R. (1972). Effects of thyrotropin-releasing hormone in depression. *Lancet* **2,** 999–1002.

Prange, A. J., Jr., Breese, G. R., Cott, J. M., Martin, B. R., Cooper, B. R., Wilson, I. C., and Plotnikoff, N. P. (1974). Thyrotropin-releasing hormone: Antagonism of pentobarbital in rodents. *Life Sci.* **14,** 447–455.

Reeve, J. R., Jr., Eysselein, V. E., Walsh, J. H., Sankaran, H., Deveney, C. W., Tourtellotte, W. W., Miller, C., and Shively, J. E. (1984). Isolation and characterization of biologically active and inactive cholecystokinin-octapeptides from human brain. *Peptides (N.Y.)* **5,** 959–966.

Renfeld, R. F. (1981). Four basic characteristics of gastrin-cholecystokinin system. *Am. J. Physiol., Gastrointest. Liver Physiol.* **255.**

Reusser, F. (1967). Biosynthesis of antibiotic U-22,324, a cyclic polypeptide. *J. Biol. Chem.* **242,** 243–247.

Reyes, V. E., Chin, L. T., and Humphreys, R. E. (1989). Selection of class I MHC-restricted peptides with the strip-of-helix hydrophobicity algorithm. *Mol. Immunol.* **25,** 867–871.

Riggs, A. D., Itakura, K., Hirose, T., Kraszewski, A., Crea, R., Goeddel, D., Kleid, D., Yansura, D., Bolivar, F., and Heyneker, H. (1979). Chemical DNA synthesis as an approach to peptide synthesis: The human insulin project. *In* "Peptides" (E. Gross and J. Meienhofer, eds.), pp. 985–992. Pierce Chemical Co., Rockford, Illinois.

Rinehart, K. L., Jr., Cook, J. C., Jr., Meng, H., Olsen, K. L., and Pandey, R. C. (1977). Mass spectrometic determination of molecular formulas for membrane-modifying antibiotics. *Nature (London)* **269,** 832–833.

Rivier, C., and Vale, W. (1984a). Influence of corticotropin-releasing factor on reproductive functions in the rat. *Endocrinology (Baltimore)* **114,** 914–921.

Rivier, C., and Vale, W. (1984b). Corticotropin-releasing factor (CRF) acts centrally to inhibit growth hormone secretion in the rat. *Endocrinology (Baltimore)* **114,** 2409–2411.

Rivier, C., and Vale, W. (1985). Effects of corticotropin-releasing factor, neurohypophyseal peptide and catecholamines on pituitary function. *Fed. Proc., Fed. Am. Soc. Exp. Biol.* **44,** 189–195.

Rivier, C., Rivier, J., and Vale, W. (1982). Inhibition of adrenocorticotropin hormone secretion in the rat by immunoneutralization of corticotropin-releasing factor. *Science* **218,** 377–379.

Rivier, C., Rivier, J., and Vale, W. (1984). Synthetic competitive antagonists of corticotropin-releasing factor: Effects on ACTH secretion in the rat. *Science* **224,** 889–891.

Rivier, J. (1974). Somatostatin. Total solid phase synthesis. *J. Am. Chem. Soc.* **96,** 2986–2992.

Rivier, J., and Brown, M. (1978). Bombesin, bombesin analogues and related peptides: Effects on thermoregulation. *Biochemistry* **17,** 1766–1771.

Rivier, J., Rivier, C., Galycan, R., Yamamoto, G., and Vale, W. (1988). Corticotropin-releasing factor: Characterization of new analogs. *In* "Peptide Chemistry 1987" (T. Shiba and S. Sakakibara, eds.), pp. 597–600. Protein Res. Found., Osaka.

Robberecht, P., Tatemoto, K., Chatelain, P., Waelbroeck, M., Delhaye, M., Taton, G., De Neef, P., Camus, J. C., Heuse, D., and Christophe, J. (1982). Effect of PHI on vasoactive intestinal peptide receptors and adenylate cyclase activity in lung membranes. A comparison in man, rat, mouse, and guinea pig. *Regul. Pept.* **4,** 241–250.

Robberecht, P., Coy, D. H., De Neef, P., Camus, J. C., Cauvin, A., Waelbroeck, M., and Christophe, J. (1987). [D-Phe4] peptide histidine-isoleucineamide ([D-Phe4]PHI), a highly selective vasoactive-intestinal-peptide (VIP) agonist, discriminates VIP-preferring from secretin-preferring receptors in rat pancreatic membranes. *Eur. J. Biochem.* **165,** 243–249.

Rodriguez, M., Fulcrand, P., Lignon, M.-F., Galas, M.-C., Bali, J.-P., Magous, R., Dubreuil, P., Laur, J., and Martinez, J. (1988). On the importance of the peptide bonds in the C-terminal tetrapeptide of gastrin and in the C-terminal heptapeptide of cholecystokinin. *In* "Peptides" (G. R. Marshall, ed.), pp. 101–104. ESCOM, Leiden.

Romer, D. (1981). Opioid analgesics. *Pain, Suppl.* **1,** S235.

Romer, D., Buescher, H. H., Hill, R. C., Pless, J., Bauer, W., Cardinaux, F., Closse, A., Hauser, D., and Huguenin, R. (1977). A synthetic enkephalin analogue with prolonged parenteral and analgesic activity. *Nature (London)* **268,** 547–549.

Ronai, A. Z., Berzetei, I. P., Szekely, J. I., Miglecz, E., Kurgyis, J., and Bajuscz, S. (1981). Enkephalin-like character and analgesia. *Eur. J. Pharmacol.* **69,** 263–271.

Rosamond, J. D., Comstock, J. M., Thomas, N. J., Clark, A. M., Blosser, J. C., Simmons, R. D., Gawlak, D. L., Loss, M. E., Augello-Vaisey, S. J., Spatola, A. F., and Benovitz, D. E. (1988).

Structural requirements for the satiety effect of CCK-8. *In* "Peptides" (G. R. Marshall, ed.), pp. 610–612. ESCOM, Leiden.

Rosas, R., Barnafi, L., Pereda, T., and Croxatto, H. (1962). Effect of oxytocin structural changes on rat renal excretion of Na, K and water. *Am. J. Physiol.* **202,** 901–904.

Rothbard, J. B., and Taylor, W. R. (1988). A sequence pattern common to T cell epitopes. *EMBO J.* **7,** 93–100.

Rothbard, J. B., Fernandez, R., Wang, L., Teng, N. N. H., and Schoolnik, G. K. (1985). Antibodies to peptides corresponding to a conserved sequence of gonococcal pilins block bacterial adhesion. *Proc. Natl. Acad. Sci. U.S.A.* **82,** 915–919.

Rubini, E., Chorev, M., Gilon, C., Friedman, Z. Y., Wormser, U., and Selinger, Z. (1981). Enzymatically stable, partially modified retro-inverso analogs of substance P. Synthesis and biological activity. *In* "Peptides" (D. H. Rich and E. Gross, eds.), pp. 593–597. Pierce Chemical Co., Rockford, Illinois.

Said, S. I. (1967). Vasoactive substances in the lung. *U. S., Public Health Serv. Publ.* **1787.**

Said, S. I., and Mutt, V. (1970). Polypeptide with broad biological activity: Isolation from small intestine. *Science* **169,** 1217, 1218.

Said, S. I., and Porter, J. C. (1979). Vasoactive intestinal polypeptide: Release into hypophyseal portal blood. *Life Sci.* **24,** 227–230.

Said, S. I., Kitamura, S., Yoshida, T., Preskitt, J., and Holden, L. D. (1974). Humoral control of airways. *Ann. N.Y. Acad. Sci.* **221,** 103–114.

Sarantakis, D. (1979). Analgesic polypeptide U.S. Patent 4, 148, 786.

Sarges, R., and Witkop, B. (1965). Gramicidin 8. The structure of valine- and isoleucine-gramicidine C. *Biochemistry* **4,** 2491–2494.

Sarkar, N., Langley, D., and Paulus, H. (1977). Biological function of gramicidin: Selective inhibition of RNA polymerase. *Proc. Natl. Acad. Sci. U.S.A.* **74,** 1478–1482.

Sasaki, K., Dockerill, S., Adamaiak, D. A., Tickle, I. J., and Blundell, T. (1975). X-Ray analysis of glucagon and its relationship to receptor binding. *Nature (London)* **257,** 751–757.

Schiller, P. W., Eggimann, B., Di Malo, J., Lemieux, C., and Nguyen, T. M.-D. (1981). Cyclic enkaphalin analogs containing a cystine bridge. *Biochem. Biophys. Res. Commun.* **101,** 337–343.

Schmauss, C., Yaksh, T. L., Shimohigashi, Y., Harty, G., Jensen, T., and Rodbard, D. (1983). Differential association of spinal μ, δ, and κ opioid receptors with cutaneous, thermal and visceral chemical nociceptive stimuli in the rat. *Life Sci.* **33,** Suppl. 1, 653–656.

Schwimmbeck, P. L., Yu, D. T. Y., and Oldstone, M. B. A. (1987). Autoantibodies to HLA B27 in the sera of HLA B27 patients with ankylosing spondylitis and Reiter's syndrome. *J. Exp. Med.* **166,** 173–181.

Schwyzer, R. (1977). ACTH: A short introductory review. *Ann. N.Y. Acad. Sci.* **297,** 3–26.

Shapira, M., Jibson, M., Muller, G., and Arnon, R. (1984). Immunity and protection against influenza virus by synthetic peptide corresponding to antigenic sites of hemagglutinin. *Proc. Natl. Acad. Sci. U.S.A.* **81,** 2461–2465.

Skrabanek, P., and Powell, D. (1977). Substance P. *In* "Annual Research Reviews: Endocrinology," Vol. 1. Churchill-Livingstone, Edinburgh and London.

Slizgi, G. R., and Ludens, J. H. (1982). Studies on the nature and mechanism of the diuretic activity of the opioid analgesic ethyl-ketocyclazocine. *J. Pharmacol. Exp. Ther.* **220,** 585–591.

Smith, J. R., Carino, M. A., and Horita, A. (1976). Interaction of various anesthetic agents with TRH: Effects on temperature and arousal in rabbits. *Proc. West. Pharmacol. Soc.* **19,** 214, 215.

Stefano, G. B., and Captane, E. J. (1979). Enkephalins increase dopamine levels in the CNS of a marine mollusc. *Life Sci.* **24,** 1617–1622.

Stefano, G. B., Kream, R. M., and Zukin, S. (1980). Demonstration of stereospecific opiate binding in nervous tissue of marine mollusc *Mytilus edulis*. *Brain Res.* **181,** 440–445.

Stewart, J. M., and Channabasavaiah, K. (1979). Evolutionary aspects of some neuropeptides. *Fed. Proc., Fed. Am. Soc. Exp. Biol.* **38,** 2302–2308.

Stewart, J. M., and Young, J. D. (1984). "Solid Phase Peptide Synthesis." Pierce Chemical Co., Rockford, Illinois.

Stewart, J. M., Getto, C. J., Nesdner, K., Reeve, E. B., Krivoy, W. A., and Zimmerman, E. (1976). Substance P and analgesia. *Nature (London)* **262,** 784, 785.

Stezowski, J. J., and Eekle, E. (1983). Structural properties of TRH analogs: Probing structure–CNS activity relationships at the molecular level. *In* "Peptides" (V. J. Hruby and D. H. Rich, eds.), pp. 809–812. Pierce Chemical Co., Rockford, Illinois.

Struthers, R. S., Hagler, A. T., and Rivier, J. (1984). Design of peptide analogs. *In* "Conformationally Directed Drug Design" (J. A. Vida and M. Gordon, eds.), pp. 239–261. Am. Chem. Soc., Washington, D.C.

Suda, M., Nakao, K., Yoshimasa, T., Ikeda, Y., Sakamoto, M., Yanaihara, N., Numa, S., and Imura, H. (1983). A novel opioid peptide, leumorphine, acts as an agonist at the κ-opiate receptor. *Life Sci.* **32,** 2769–2775.

Szecowka, J., Tatemoto, K., Mutt, V., and Effendic, S. (1980). Interaction of a newly isolated intestinal polypeptide (PHI) with glucose and arginine to effect the secretion of insulin and glucagon. *Life Sci.* **26,** 435–438.

Tache, Y., Goto, Y., Gunion, M. W., Vale, W., Rivier, J., and Brown, M. (1983). Inhibition of gastric acid secretion in rats by intracerebral injection of rat corticotropin-releasing factor. *Science* **222,** 935–937.

Tainer, J. A., Getzoff, E. D., Alexander, H., Houghten, R. A., Olson, A. J., Lerner, R. A., and Hendrickson, W. A. (1984). The reactivity of anti-peptide antibodies is a function of the atomic mobility of sites in a protein. *Nature (London)* **312,** 127–134.

Takahashi, Y., Kato, K., Hayaschizaki, Y., Wakabayashi, T., Ohtsuka, E., Matsuki, S., Ikehara, M., and Matsubara, K. (1985). Molecular cloning of the human cholecystokinin gene by use of a synthetic probe containing deoxyinosine. *Proc. Natl. Acad. Sci. U.S.A.* **82,** 1931–1935.

Tatemoto, K. (1982a). Isolation and characterization of peptide YY (PYY), a candidate gut hormone that inhibits pancreatic exocrine secretion. *Proc. Natl. Acad. Sci. U.S.A.* **79,** 2514–2518.

Tatemoto, K. (1982b). Neuropeptide Y: Complete amino acid sequence of the brain peptide. *Proc. Natl. Acad. Sci. U.S.A.* **79,** 5485–5489.

Tatemoto, K., and Mutt, V. (1980). Isolation of two novel candidate hormones using a chemical method for naturally occurring polypeptides. *Nature (London)* **285,** 417–418.

Tatemoto, K., and Mutt, V. (1981). Isolation and characterization of the intestinal peptide porcine PHI (PHI-27), a new member of the glucagon-secretin family. *Proc. Natl. Acad. Sci. U.S.A.* **78,** 6603–6607.

Tatemoto, K., Carlquist, M., and Mutt, V. (1982). Neuropeptide Y: A novel brain peptide with structural similarities to peptide YY and pancreatic polypeptide. *Nature (London)* **296,** 659–660.

Tatemoto, K., Carlquist, M., McDonald, T. J., and Mutt, V. (1983). Isolation of a brain peptide identical to the intestinal PHI (peptide A1). *FEBS Lett.* **164,** 124-128.

Theodoropoulos, D., Poulos, C., Pinas, N., Couture, R., Regoli, D., and Escher, E. (1981). Evaluation of the biological importance of the three primary amides in substance P hepatapeptides 5-11. *In* "Peptides" (D. H. Rich and E. Gross, eds.), pp. 603–606. Pierce Chemical Co., Rockford, Illionis.

Tortella, F. C., and Moreton, J. E. (1980). D-Ala^2-methionine enkaphalinamide self-administration in the morphine-dependent rat. *Psychopharmacology (Berlin)* **69,** 143–147.

Tracy, H. J., and Gregory, R. A. (1964). Physiological properties of a series of synthetic peptides structurally related to gastrin I. *Nature (London)* **204,** 935–938.

Traczyk, W. Z. (1977). Circulatory effects of substance P, SP_{6-11} and $[pGlu^6]SP_{6-11}$ hexapeptides. *In* "Substance P" (U. S. von Euler and B. Pernow, eds.), pp. 297–309. Raven Press, New York.

Tregear, G. W., Niall, H. D., Potts, J. T., Jr., Leeman, S. F., and Chang, M. M. (1971). Synthesis of substance P. *Nature (London) New Biol.* **232,** 87–88.

Tseng, L. F., Loh, H. H., and Li, C. H. (1976). Beta-Endorphin: Cross tolerance to and cross physical dependence on morphine. *Proc. Natl. Acad. Sci. U.S.A* **73,** 4187–4189.

Tuppy, H. (1960). Enzyme inactivation and degradation of oxytocin and vasopressin. *In* "Polpeptides which Affect Smooth Muscle and Blood Vessels" (M. Schachter, ed.), pp. 49–58. Pergamon, Oxford.

Unger, R. H. (1978). Role of glucagon in the pathogenesis of diabetes: The status of the controversy. *Metabol. Clin. Exp.* **27,** 1691–1709.

Upton, N., Sewell, R. D. E., and Spencer, P. S. J. (1982). Differentiation of potent μ and κ-opiate agonists using heat and pressure antinociceptive profiles and combined potency analysis. *Eur. J. Pharmacol.* **78,** 421–429.

Urrutia, R., Uruciani, R. A., Barker, J. L., and Kachar, B. (1989). Spontaneous polymerization of the antibiotic pepitide magainin 2. *FEBS Lett.* **247,** 17–21.

Urry, D. W. (1972). The gramicidin A transmembrane channel: A proposed π(L,D) helix. *Proc. Natl. Acad. Sci. U.S.A.* **68,** 762–676.

Urry, D. W., and Walter, R. (1978). Proposed conformation of oxytocin in solution. *Proc. Natl. Acad. Sci. U.S.A.* **68,** 956–958.

Vale, W., Spiess, J., Rivier, C., and Rivier, J. (1981). Characterization of a 41-residue ovine hypothalamic peptide that stimulates secretion of corticotropin and beta-endorphin. *Science* **213,** 1394–1397.

Vale, W., Rivier, C., Brown, M. R., Speiss, J., Koob, G., Swanson, L., Bilezikjian, L., Bloom, F., and Rivier, J. (1983). Chemical and biological characterization of corticotropin-releasing factor. *Recent Prog. Horm. Res.* **39,** 245–270.

Vanderhaegen, J. J., Signeau, J. C., and Gepts, W. (1975). New peptide in the vertebrate CNS reacting with antigastrin antibodies. *Nature (London)* **257,** 604, 605.

Van Dyke, H. B., Adamson, K., Jr., and Engel, S. L. (1957). The storage and liberation of neurohypophyseal hormones. *In* "The Neurohypophysis" (H. Heller, ed.), pp. 65–76. Academic Press, New York.

Vaught, J. L., Rothman, R. B., and Westfall, T. C. (1982). Mu and delta receptors: Their role in analgesia and in the differential effects of opioid peptides on analgesia. *Life Sci.* **30,** 1443–1455.

Veber, D. F. (1979). Conformational considerations in the design of somatostatin analogs showing increased metabolic stability. *In* "Peptides" (E. Gross and J. Meienhofer, eds.), pp. 409–419. Pierce Chemical Co., Rockford, Illinois.

Veber, D. F., and Saperstein, R. (1979). Somatostatin. *Annu. Rep. Med. Chem.* **14,** 209–218.

Veber, D. F., Freidinger, R. M., Perlow, D. S., Paleveda, W. J., Jr., Holly, F. W., Strachan, R. G., Nutt, R. F., Arison, B., Homnick, C., Randall, W. C., Giltzer, M. S., Saperstein, R., and Hirschmann, R. (1981). A potent cyclic hexapeptide analogue of somatostatin. *Nature (London)* **292,** 55–58.

Vijayan, E., and McCann, S. M. (1977). Suppression of feeding and drinking activity in rats following intraventricular injection of thyrotropin-releasing hormone (TRH). *Endocrinology (Baltimore)* **100,** 1727–1730.

Vijayan, E., Samson, W. K., Said, S., and McCann, S. M. (1979). Vasoactive intestinal peptide: Evidence for a hypothalamic site of action to release growth hormone, luteinizing hormone, and prolactin in conscious ovariectomized rats. *Endocrinology (Baltimore)* **104,** 53–57.

von Euler, V. S., and Gaddum, J. H. (1931). An unidentified depressor substance in certain tissue extracts. *J. Physiol. (London)* **72,** 74–87.

Walter, R., Schwartz, I. L., Darnell, J. H., and Urry, D. W. (1971). Relation of the conformation of oxytocin to the biology of neurohypophyseal hormones. *Proc. Natl. Acad. Sci. U.S.A.* **68,** 1355–1359.

Ward, S. J., and Takemori, A. E. (1983). Relative involvement of receptor subtypes in opiate-induced inhibition of gastrointestinal transit in mice. *J. Pharmacol. Exp. Ther.* **224,** 359–363.

Watari, E., Dietzschold, B., Szokan, G., and Herber-Katz, E. (1987). A synthetic peptide induces long-term protection from lethal infection with herpes simplex virus 2. *J. Exp. Med.* **165,** 459–470.

Wei, E., and Loh, H. H. (1976). Physical dependence of opiate-like peptides. *Science* **193,** 1262, 1263.

Weijer, W. J., Drijfhout, J. W., Geerigs, H. J., Bloemhoff, W., Feijlbrief, M., Bos, C. A., Hoogerhout, P., Kerling, K. E. T., Popken-Boer, T., Slopsema, K., Wilterdink, J. B., Welling, G. W., and Welling-Wester, S. (1988). Antibodies against synthetic peptides of the herpes simplex virus type 1 glycoprotein D and their capability to neutralize viral infectivity in vitro. *Virology* **62,** 501–510.

Weiner, S. J., Kollman, P. A., Case, D. A., Singh, U. C., Ghio, C., Alagona, G., Profeta, S., and Weiner, P. J. (1984). A new force field for molecular mechanical simulation of nucleic acids and proteins. *J. Am. Chem. Soc.* **106,** 765–784.

Wilkinson, S. (1967). Identification of the polymyxins. *Antimicrob. Agents Chemother.* pp. 651–654.

Wilkinson, S., and Lowe, L. A. (1964). Structure of polymyxin B2 and polymyxin E1. *Nature (London)* **204,** 185.

Wilkinson, S., and Lowe, L. A. (1966). Structure of polymyxin A and the question of identity with the polymyxin M. *Nature (London)* **212,** 311.

Wright, D. E., and Rodbell, M. (1979). Glucagon (1-6) binds to the glucagon receptor and activates adenylate cyclase. *J. Biol. Chem.* **254,** 268–269.

Wright, D. E., Hruby, V. J., and Rodbell, M. (1978). A reassessment of structure–function relationships in glucagon. Glucagon (1-21) is a full agonist. *J. Biol. Chem.* **253,** 6338–6340.

Yamashiro, D., and Li, C. H. (1984). B-Endorphin: Structure and activity. *Peptides (N.Y.)* **6,** 191–217.

Yamashiro, D., Tseng, L. F., Doneen, B. A., Loh, H. H., and Li, C. H. (1977). β-Endorphin: Synthesis and morphine like activity of analogs with D-amino acid residues in positions 1, 2, 4, and 5. *Int. J. Pept. Protein Res.* **10,** 159–166.

Yamashiro, D., Li, C. H., Tseng, L.-R. F., and Loth, H. H. (1978). B-Endorphins: Synthesis and analgesic activity of several analogs modified in positions 2 and 5. *Int. J. Pept. Protein Res.* **11,** 251–257.

Yanaihara, N., Yanaihara, C., Hirohashi, M., Sato, H., Iizuka, Y., Hashimoto, T., and Sakagami, M. (1977). Substance P analogs: Synthesis and biological and immunological properties. *In* "Substance P" (U. S. von Euler and B. Pernow, eds.), pp. 27–33. Raven Press, New York.

Yanaihara, N., Kadowaki, M., Yagi, N,. Inoue, T., Sakabe, M., Ishikawa, J., Hashimoto, Y., Mochizuki, T., and Yanaihara, C. (1988). Galanin: A unique feature in structure–function relationship. *In* "Peptide Chemistry 1987" (T. Shiba and S. Sakakibara, eds.), pp. 487–490. Protein Res. Found., Osaka.

Yang, S.-Z., Wang, S.-M., and Niu, C.-I. (1988). Solid phase synthesis of the A chain of insulin and partial synthesis of crystalline porcine insulin from the synthetic A chain and the natural B chain. *In* "Peptide Chemistry 1987" (T. Shiba and S. Sakakibara, eds.), pp. 405–408. Protein Res. Found., Osaka.

Yasui, A., Naruse, S., Yanaihara, C., Ozaki, T., Hoshino, M., Mochizuki, T., Daniel, E. E., and Yanaihara, N. (1987). Corelease of PHI and VIP by vagal stimulation in dog. *Am. J. Physiol.* **253,** G13–G19.

Yiangou, Y., Requejo, F., Polak, J. M., and Bloom, S. R. (1986). Characterization of a novel prepro VIP derived peptide. *Biochem. Biophys. Res. Commun.* **139,** 1142–1149.

Zajac, J.-M., Gacel, G., Petit, F., Dodey, P., Rossignol, P., and Roques, B. P. (1983). Deltakephaline, Tyr-D-Thr-Gly-Phe-Leu-Thr: A new highly potent and fully specific agonist for opiate δ-receptors. *Biochem. Biophys. Res. Commun.* **111,** 390–397.

Zasloff, M. (1987). Magainins, a class of antimicrobial peptides from *Xenopus* skin: Isolation, characterization of two active forms, and partial cDNA sequence of a precursor. *Proc. Natl. Acad. Sci. U.S.A.* **84,** 5449–5453.

Zhou, Z. Z., Eng, J., Pan, Y.-C. E., Chang, M., Hulmes, J.-D., Raufman, J. P., and Yalow, R. S. (1985). Unique cholecystokinin peptides isolated from guinea pig intestine. *Peptides (N.Y.)* **7,** 337–341.

Zukin, S. R., and Gintzler, A. R. (1980). Guanyl nucleotide interactions with opiate receptors in guinea pig brain and ileum. *Brain Res.* **186,** 486–491.

Subject Index